THE LIVING
BRAND NAME SHO...
Third Ed...

MW00963608

MICHAEL E. DeBAKEY, M.D.
ANTONIO M. GOTTO, JR., M.D., D.PHIL.
LYNNE W. SCOTT, M.A., R.D.
JOHN P. FOREYT, PH.D.
with
Mary C. McMann, M.P.H., R.D.
Suzanne Jaax, M.S., R.D.
Edited by
Suzanne Simpson, B.A.

THE LIVING HEART BRAND NAME SHOPPER'S GUIDE

Third Edition

MASTERMEDIA LIMITED
NEW YORK

Copyright © 1995 Michael E. DeBakey, Antonio M. Gotto, Jr., Lynne W. Scott, and John P. Foreyt

All rights reserved, including the right of reproduction in whole or in part in any form.

First edition, 1992. Second edition, 1993. Third edition, 1995.

Published by MasterMedia Limited.

MASTERMEDIA and colophon are registered trademarks of MasterMedia Limited.

Inclusion of a food in this guide does not imply an endorsement and is not meant to classify any food as "good" or "bad."

Library of Congress Cataloging-in-Publication Data

The Living Heart brand name shopper's guide / Michael E. DeBakey ... [et al.]
   p. cm.
  Includes index.
  ISBN 1-57-101-024-6 (paper)
  1. Food–Cholesterol content–Tables. 2. Low-cholesterol diet. 3. Low-fat diet.
  4. Coronary heart disease–Prevention.
1. DeBakey, Michael E. (Michael Ellis), 1908–
TX553.C43L58 1992
641.1'4–dc20   91-42946

                                                                        CIP

Production services by Cranston Communications, Inc., Dearborn, Michigan
Manufactured in the United States of America
10 9 8 7 6 5 4 3 2 1

TABLE OF CONTENTS

FOOD SECTIONS

FOOD SECTIONS

PREFACE

Public interest in diet and how its specific components affect health continues to grow. As the Food and Drug Administration (FDA) and U.S. Department of Agriculture (USDA) guidelines for more complete nutrient labeling of foods become established, people are becoming increasingly familiar with major health concerns about the American diet: too many calories and too much fat, saturated fat, cholesterol, and sodium, and intakes that are too low in fiber and some vitamins and minerals. *The Living Heart Brand Name Shopper's Guide* was originally written, and has been revised, to provide practical information about how to improve health by the wise selection of food.

The Guide is unique in several ways. It is the first book to identify for shoppers both brand name and generic foods that are good choices. Most of the cutoff points used to evaluate foods for inclusion in this book are consistent with the FDA and USDA definitions of "low fat," "low saturated fat," and "lean." The Guide describes how to plan and follow a diet to lower blood cholesterol and triglyceride, weight, and blood pressure. In addition, it includes information on managing diabetes and on reducing the risk for certain types of cancer by increasing fiber. Users of the first two editions of *The Living Heart Brand Name Shopper's Guide* tell us that the book succeeded in making it easier to select foods in the supermarket. We believe that people interested in improving their health through the wise selection of food will find the third edition of the Guide to be valuable as well.

ACKNOWLEDGMENTS

It was a pleasure to work on the third edition of *The Living Heart Brand Name Shopper's Guide* with the same individuals who played key roles in preparing the first two editions, which were released in 1992 and 1993. We are grateful to Myrthala Miranda-Guzman, who entered all the information from the food manufacturers into the computer. Her expertise in data management, coupled with her standard of excellence, buoyed us through our assessment of a tremendous amount of information. We are grateful as well to Laura Frey for managing the letters sent to food manufacturers and the return of nutrient information from them, and for typing the manuscript. We very much appreciate the assistance provided by Danièle Brauchi and Cathy Renteria throughout the revision of the book. We thank Marieta Carlson for her help with the chapter on diabetes, and for recommending that the Food Sections include a column for carbohydrate.

A special thank you goes to Susan Stautberg, president of MasterMedia, for creatively promoting the first two editions of *The Living Heart Brand Name Shopper's Guide.* Working with Susan, our enthusiastic and innovative publisher, continues to be an invigorating and rewarding experience.

We also wish to express our appreciation to the food manufacturers who responded to our inquiries and allowed us to include their products in the Guide. And finally, and very importantly, we thank the numerous readers of the first two editions of *The Living Heart Brand Name Shopper's Guide* who took the time to send us names of foods to evaluate for this book.

INTRODUCTION

The Living Heart series of books began with publication in 1977 of *The Living Heart,* a book explaining the nature of heart disease. *The Living Heart Diet* followed in 1984. It combined information on diet and heart disease and hundreds of heart-healthy recipes, and became a *New York Times* Best Seller; more than 1 million copies are in print. A revised edition, *The New Living Heart Diet,* is scheduled for publication in early 1996.

The first edition of *The Living Heart Brand Name Shopper's Guide,* released in the spring of 1992, provided information on health topics of general interest and listed nutrient information on more than 5,000 foods. The book was extremely popular — more than 441,000 copies were printed and distributed through bookstores across the country and by a large pharmaceutical company. The second edition, which was released in the summer of 1993, extended the health-related information and contained nutrient information on about 6,100 foods.

The present edition of *The Living Heart Brand Name Shopper's Guide* continues to add the new low-fat foods that have become available (and to delete foods that are no longer being manufactured); its food listings now represent about 5,500 foods. Moreover, it has been redesigned specifically to assist you in selecting a diet to help:

- Lower blood cholesterol and triglyceride levels
- Lose weight
- Lower high blood pressure
- Manage diabetes
- Reduce cancer risk by increasing fiber

The Guide now includes values for carbohydrate and for fiber, in addition to the calories, fat, saturated fat, and sodium included in earlier editions. Another change is that values for dietary cholesterol are no longer included. Cholesterol is found only in animal foods (see page 21); the small amounts of cholesterol shown in the Nutrition Facts portion of the labels of other foods are present because an animal food (such as egg yolk, milk, or meat) has been used as an ingredient in that food.

The style for printing the Food Sections in this edition of the Guide has been updated. When several products have the same brand name, the brand name is listed only once (with all the flavors or varieties printed under it) rather than repeated. In addition, different flavors of some products are combined into one entry to save space. These changes should make the lists easier to use.

THE LIVING HEART
BRAND NAME SHOPPER'S GUIDE
Third Edition

Chapter 1

Using *The Living Heart Brand Name Shopper's Guide* to Make Dietary Changes

The Living Heart Brand Name Shopper's Guide emphasizes choosing supermarket foods that are low in fat and saturated fat. It is designed to help you make wise food choices in order to:

- Lower blood cholesterol and triglyceride levels (see page 16)
- Lose weight (see page 26)
- Lower high blood pressure (see page 39)
- Manage diabetes (see page 45)
- Reduce cancer risk by increasing fiber (see page 48)

Whether you are making dietary changes because your physician recommends you do so or simply because you feel it is the right thing to do, the Guide will help you identify which foods to eat to help you accomplish your health goals. *The New Living Heart Diet* (another book by the same authors) includes extensive information on each of the topics mentioned above.

The Guide is unique in that it lists only those brand name foods that are fat free or low in fat or saturated fat. If a food is low in fat, it is also low in saturated fat, but not all foods that are low in saturated fat are low in total fat (for example, canola oil). Because fat is not the whole picture in healthier eating, the Guide also provides values for calories, carbohydrate, fiber, and sodium for each food listed. This additional information will further help you make good food choices. Some of the fat-free and low-fat foods are low in calories, but others are moderately high in calories. The only test a brand name food had to pass for inclusion in the Guide was that it is fat free or low in fat or saturated fat (see page 52).

To make the Guide easy to use, it is divided into sections similar to the way foods are grouped in most supermarkets. For example, fresh meat, poultry, and fish are grouped together, frozen dinners are grouped together, and all types of crackers are grouped together. A quick and easy reference for finding any Food Section in the book appears on page xi.

If you are seeing a registered dietitian or other health professional for help in lowering blood cholesterol or triglyceride, losing weight, reducing blood pressure, or controlling diabetes, this book can be used along with the other materials that person gives you. For example, the Guide provides specific brand names to accompany lists of foods to choose or decrease. It can also be used with heart-healthy cookbooks to identify ingredients that are low in fat, such as low-fat brands of cheese and sour cream.

Although the focus of the Guide is brand name foods that are low in fat and saturated fat, foods that are higher in these components are listed at the beginning of some food sections (for example, Dairy Products, Desserts, Meats) under the headings "Higher-Fat Foods" or "Higher-Saturated-Fat Foods." The foods that are higher in fat or saturated fat are *not* recommended for regular use; they are included for comparison purposes only. These higher-fat foods, such as regular cheese, bacon, ice cream, and chocolate candy, are not listed by brand name. These short lists of foods will help you see how high the fat content is in some common foods — for example, regular ice cream and cheddar cheese compared with ice milk, low-fat frozen yogurt, and low-fat cheese.

The important lists of foods in each food section are "Lower-Fat Foods" and "Lower-Saturated-Fat Foods." For a food to be included in these lists, one serving of the food may not exceed a specified level — called a cutoff point — of fat or saturated fat. Cutoff points are described on page 52.

STARTING TO MAKE DIETARY CHANGES

Making dietary changes can be a difficult task. One of the reasons changing our eating habits is so hard is that we learned to like certain foods when we were children and have been enjoying them ever since. Food preferences are very individual. And food can mean different things to different people. Some people eat when they are happy, others when they are sad, and still others eat because of either emotional state. People may eat as a response to boredom, anxiety, or loneliness. Food acts as a companion for some people; it can always be counted on and never lets you down, even when people and events around you change. For some people, food may be the only consistent thing in their lives; it always tastes the same: good.

It is important for you to assess honestly your present eating habits before starting to make dietary changes. Begin by asking yourself some questions, such as:

- How often do I eat foods high in calories and fat?
- What are my favorite high-fat foods?
- Am I more likely to choose foods higher in fat when I'm eating at home or away from home?
- How often do I eat away from home?
- How many meals do I eat each day? Do I snack between meals? How often?
- How much alcohol do I consume?
- Why do I want to begin making changes *now?*

It is also a good idea to take a look at your exercise habits. Regular moderate exercise plays an important role in weight control in addition to having many other beneficial health effects.

Next, you will need to set reasonable goals on the basis of your assessment, and begin to make gradual changes to meet the goals. If your favorite high-fat food is ice cream, for example, you might try finding a satisfactory substitute, such as ice milk or low-fat frozen yogurt, that is lower in fat and calories. If you snack an average of three times each day, you might try cutting back to twice, then once each day. Don't expect to change everything at once, or to make extreme changes overnight in long time habits. Give yourself a reasonable amount of time to adopt one aspect of a new, healthier lifestyle before making the next change.

Chapters 2 through 6 provide guidelines for using *The Living Heart Brand Name Shopper's Guide* to accomplish your personal health goals, such as losing weight, reducing blood cholesterol or triglyceride, lowering blood pressure, managing diabetes, or increasing fiber. The Food Sections, which start on page 59, provide values for about 5,500 foods to help you choose those products whose use can help you reach your health goals.

COOKING TIPS TO HELP YOU MAKE DIETARY CHANGES

Incorporating desirable changes into your eating habits may require that you learn some new ways to cook your favorite foods. Two important modifications for healthier cooking are reducing fat and reducing sodium (salt). Eating less fat is the mainstay of an eating pattern to lower blood cholesterol and triglyceride levels and to lose weight, and losing weight helps lower high blood pressure and manage diabetes. Decreasing use of foods high in sodium can also help lower high blood pressure.

TIPS FOR LOWER-FAT COOKING

Here are some tips for cutting the fat in your cooking:

- Start with lower-fat ingredients, such as those listed in this guide. Also, see page 263 in the Appendix for recipe substitutions to lower fat and/or dietary cholesterol.
- Broil, bake, roast, or stew lean cuts of meat, skinless poultry, or fish. If you love fried foods, try "fat-free frying" in a nonstick pan; you can use a cooking spray (page 142) to prevent sticking and to add flavor. Season pasta, rice, potatoes, and cooked vegetables with herbs, spices, spray margarine, flavored cooking spray, or a fat substitute (page 142).
- Choose mixes, such as cake and muffin mixes, that provide instructions for preparing a reduced-fat product. Or reduce the fat in foods prepared from mixes by adding less fat than is called for in the directions, replacing whole eggs with egg whites or egg substitute, and replacing whole milk with skim, 1/2%, or 1% low-fat milk. Try substituting applesauce, puréed fruit, or plain, nonfat yogurt for some or all of the fat in baked products, such as brownies and some types of cakes.
- Lower-fat cooking has become more popular in recent years, and several appliances and cooking utensils on the market make low-fat cooking easier. Countertop convection ovens, which cook by circulating hot air around food on a rack, cook foods quickly while retaining moisture. Specialized steamers for rice or for vegetables are also popular. The slowcooker (for example, the Crock Pot) is regaining popularity because it provides an easy way to cook very lean cuts of meat until they are quite tender. The pressure cooker can be used to cook meat and vegetables in a short time. Hot-air poppers and microwave

poppers continue to be favorites of popcorn lovers; try flavoring the popcorn with a butter-flavored cooking spray (page 142) or a spray margarine. Simple utensils such as the pitcher designed to separate fat from meat drippings are a good and inexpensive investment.

When a small amount of fat is needed for cooking or as an ingredient in a recipe, use fats that are low in saturated fat (listed on pages 142 to 145).

The following recipe illustrates how to substitute lower-fat ingredients for those higher in fat. Fettuccine Alfredo is a delicious and popular but notoriously high-fat dish. Making just three substitutions in dairy products and not adding fat to the fettuccine during cooking as indicated in the original recipe cuts the total fat by 70%, the saturated fat by 75%, and the dietary cholesterol by almost half. Pages listing brand names of foods used are shown in parentheses.

CHICKEN FETTUCCINE ALFREDO*

Lower-Fat Recipe	Higher-Fat Recipe Identical Except Uses
2 tablespoons tub margarine (page 142)	2 tablespoons butter
1 pound chicken meat, no skin, cut into bite-size pieces	
1 tablespoon all-purpose flour	
3 large cloves garlic, minced	
1 can (12 ounces) canned evaporated skimmed milk (page 119)	1½ cups whipping cream
½ pound fresh mushrooms, sliced	
¾ cup grated reduced-fat Parmesan cheese (page 113)	¾ cup grated Parmesan cheese
¼ cup white wine	
1 teaspoon fresh sweet basil, chopped, OR ½ teaspoon dried sweet basil	
1 teaspoon chopped fresh parsley	
1 package (9 ounces) fettuccine, prepared according to package directions, omitting salt and fat	1 package (9 ounces) fettuccine prepared according to package directions, adding salt and fat

Instructions for the **lower-fat** version are:

1. In a nonstick skillet, melt margarine; add chicken and cook until tender. Remove chicken from skillet and set aside.
2. Add flour to remaining liquid in skillet and cook over low heat, stirring constantly, until the mixture stops bubbling and becomes a golden paste.
3. Add garlic and continue stirring until the garlic softens.
4. Add evaporated milk and simmer over medium heat, stirring constantly, until milk thickens.
5. Add mushrooms and continue cooking over low heat until mushrooms soften.
6. Add Parmesan cheese and stir well. Simmer, stirring often, until cheese melts and is blended thoroughly. Remove skillet from heat.
7. Stir in wine, basil, parsley, and chicken; stir until all ingredients are hot. Serve immediately over fettuccine.

Yield: 8 cups

One cup of the lower-fat recipe contains:

Calories	Fat g	Saturated Fat g	Cholesterol mg	Carbohydrate g	Fiber g	Sodium mg
278	7	3	66	29	2	317

If the recipe is made with the higher-fat ingredients, 1 cup contains:

Calories	Fat g	Saturated Fat g	Cholesterol mg	Carbohydrate g	Fiber g	Sodium mg
419	25	12	117	25	1	388

*From *The New Living Heart Diet*, by DeBakey, M.E., Gotto, A.M., Scott, L.W., et al., Simon & Schuster, New York, 1996.

g = grams; mg = milligrams.

Often, the primary change to lower fat in your recipe will be to use leaner meat in place of higher-fat cuts. In the following recipe for Breakfast Casserole, you can decrease both fat and sodium by using easy-to-make homemade sausage without the salt.

BREAKFAST CASSEROLE

Lower-Fat Recipe	*Higher-Fat Recipe* *Identical Except Uses*
nonstick cooking spray (page 142)	2 teaspoons oil
1 recipe Homemade Sausage made without salt (see next page)	1 pound ground pork sausage
3 slices day-old bread	
1½ cups egg substitute (page 140)	
1 large can (12 ounces) plus 1 small can (5 ounces) canned evaporated skimmed milk (page 119)	6 eggs 17 ounces evaporated milk
1½ teaspoons dry mustard	
½ cup shredded part-skim mozzarella cheese (page 113)	½ cup shredded cheddar cheese
Mexican salsa (optional) (page 97)	

Instructions for the **lower-fat** version are:

1. Spray 9- x 13-inch baking dish with nonstick spray.
2. In mixing bowl, combine ingredients for sausage listed below. Cook sausage in skillet and stir to break meat into small pieces. Cook until well done.
3. Drain meat in colander, then spread on paper towels until cool.
4. Cut bread into cubes and arrange in bottom of casserole dish. Spread sausage on top of bread.
5. In separate dish, combine egg substitute, milk, and mustard. Pour over sausage and bread.
6. Cover and refrigerate overnight. (May be frozen. To defrost, set in refrigerator overnight.)
7. Set oven at 350°F and place uncovered casserole dish in oven while it is heating. Cook 45 minutes or until light brown around edges and knife inserted in center comes out clean.
8. Top with cheese and return to oven until cheese melts. Serve hot with salsa.

Yield: 6 servings

Homemade Sausage

1   pound very lean ground beef
½   teaspoon ground sage
¼   teaspoon dried thyme
1   teaspoon pepper
1   teaspoon liquid smoke
1   teaspoon salt (optional)

One serving of the lower-fat version of the casserole contains:

Calories	Fat g	Saturated Fat g	Cholesterol mg	Carbohydrate g	Fiber g	Sodium mg
243	8	3	50	13	1	322

If optional salt is added to the Homemade Sausage recipe, the sodium in the Breakfast Casserole will be 677 mg.

If the Breakfast Casserole is made with the higher-fat ingredients, 1 serving contains:

Calories	Fat g	Saturated Fat g	Cholesterol mg	Carbohydrate g	Fiber g	Sodium mg
401	27	12	253	16	0	735

---

*From The New Living Heart Diet, by DeBakey, M.E., Gotto, A.M., Scott, L.W., et al., Simon & Schuster, New York, 1996.

g = grams; mg = milligrams.

TIPS FOR LOWER-FAT HOLIDAY COOKING

Holiday meals often present a problem for people trying to avoid high-fat eating, whether it is to lower an elevated blood cholesterol level, to lose weight, or simply to follow a heart-healthy lifestyle. Traditional holiday fare can be quite high in calories, fat, saturated fat, and cholesterol, as shown on the next page.

```
+--------------------------------------------------+
|          Traditional Holiday Menu                |
|         Roasted Turkey with Dressing             |
|                Turkey Gravy                      |
| Candied Yams                Cranberry Sauce      |
| Broccoli with Cheese Sauce  Mashed Potatoes      |
|         Fruit Salad with Whipped Cream           |
| Crescent Roll                        Butter      |
|         Pumpkin Pie with Whipped Cream           |
| Coffee                               Tea         |
+--------------------------------------------------+
```

One serving of this traditional holiday meal provides:

    2,205 calories

    111 grams of fat

    55 grams of saturated fat

    475 milligrams of cholesterol

    218 grams of carbohydrate

    15 grams of fiber

    3,392 milligrams of sodium

This one meal provides as many calories as many people need in an entire day. Someone eating *only* this meal for the day would get 45% of calories from fat and 22% of calories from saturated fat, as well as the 475 milligrams (mg) of cholesterol. On a heart-healthy diet (see page 18), total fat should not exceed 30% of calories, saturated fat should not exceed 10% of calories, and dietary cholesterol should not exceed 300 mg per day. The traditional holiday meal obviously cannot be considered heart healthy.

One reason that is often given for not using lower-fat cooking methods is that they are harder to use and are more time consuming. This is just not true. Supermarkets have an abundance of foods that make it possible, with some careful planning, to prepare a delicious holiday meal while spending much less time in the kitchen. The information in this guide will help you identify low-fat foods and ingredients to make your holiday meal festive, healthy, and easy to prepare. In addition to being quick and easy, the following Thanksgiving meal contains about 700 fewer calories, only 28% of the fat, and 18% of the saturated fat provided by the traditional menu.

```
┌─────────────────────────────────────────────────────┐
│         Quick-and-Easy "Lite" Thanksgiving Menu      │
│              Roasted Turkey with Dressing            │
│                     Turkey Gravy                     │
│  Candied Yams                       Cranberry Sauce  │
│  Broccoli with Cheese-Flavored Sauce   Mashed Potatoes │
│            Fruit Salad with Whipped Topping          │
│  Dinner Roll                             Margarine   │
│            Pumpkin Pie with Whipped Topping          │
│  Coffee                                        Tea   │
└─────────────────────────────────────────────────────┘
```

One serving of this quick-and-easy "lite" holiday meal prepared using the tips below provides:

     1,489 calories

     31 grams of fat

     10 grams of saturated fat

     135 milligrams of cholesterol

     225 grams of carbohydrate

     13 grams of fiber

     3,288 milligrams of sodium

Here are some tips for choosing foods for the quick-and-easy holiday meal.

- Select a turkey that is non-basted, if you are roasting a whole bird; white meat is lower in calories and fat than dark meat.
- Reduce the fat typically present in stuffing made with a mix by preparing the mix without added fat or by using diet margarine* and adding about half the amount listed in package directions.
- Select a commercial turkey gravy* with no more than 2 grams of fat per serving.
- Choose canned sweet potatoes with no more than 1 gram of fat per serving.
- Select frozen broccoli in cheese-flavored sauce* with no more than 3 grams of fat per serving.
- Prepare mashed potatoes with diet margarine* and skim or evaporated skim milk.*
- Use lite whipped topping* as dressing for fruit salad.

- Serve diet margarine* with plain dinner rolls,* which are lower in calories and fat than crescent or other "buttery" rolls.
- Prepare pumpkin pie filling* using evaporated skim milk* and egg substitute.* Choose a pie shell with less than 5 grams of fat per serving; fat-free commercial pie crusts are now available. (Even if you use a pie shell with more than 3 grams of fat per serving, preparing a fat-free filling will still result in a dessert that is lower in fat.) Top with lite whipped topping* with no more than 2 grams of fat per serving.

TIPS FOR LOWER-SODIUM COOKING

To add flavor when cooking without salt or other sources of sodium, such as MSG (monosodium glutamate), use more herbs, spices, and low-sodium seasoning mixtures; fruit juices, such as lemon, lime, and orange juice; flavored vinegars; and table wine (remember that "cooking wine" has added salt). There is a list of recipe substitutions to lower sodium on page 264 of the Appendix.

If you are not sure if a food is high in sodium, read the label. The sodium content for a serving is listed in milligrams. A percent Daily Value is also listed on the label; this number indicates the percent of 2,400 mg of sodium (the daily intake recommended as the upper limit by the Food and Drug Administration) provided in one serving of the food. A little more than 1 teaspoon of salt contains 2,400 mg of sodium. Next, compare the sodium content listed on the label of several products and select one that is low. For example, 1/4 cup of regular tomato sauce contains about 300 mg of sodium; the same amount of a "no-salt-added" tomato sauce contains 20 mg of sodium. The sodium value is shown for each food in this book; some foods are high in sodium and others are low. Compare the sodium listed on the label for regular and lower-sodium ingredients to see how much sodium you can save.

---

*Specific brand names of products low in calories, fat, saturated fat, and cholesterol appear in this guide. Check the table of contents, the thumb guide (page xi), or the index to locate the food you are interested in finding.

A recipe for Italian Meat Sauce with regular and lower-sodium ingredients is shown below. A change as simple as using no-salt-added instead of regular canned tomatoes and tomato juice reduced the sodium in this recipe from 257 mg to 43 mg of sodium, a decrease of 214 mg of sodium.

ITALIAN MEAT SAUCE*

Lower-Sodium Recipe	Higher-Sodium Recipe Identical Except Uses
1 pound very lean ground beef	
1 large onion, chopped	
2 cloves garlic, minced	
1 can (14½ ounces) no-salt-added canned tomatoes, undrained (page 255)	1 can (14½ ounces) stewed tomatoes, undrained
11 ounces no-salt-added tomato juice (page 168)	11 ounces tomato juice
1 teaspoon fennel seeds	
½ cup chopped fresh parsley	
¼ teaspoon coarsely ground pepper	
½ tablespoon dried oregano	
½ teaspoon dried sweet basil	
½ teaspoon dried thyme	
¼ teaspoon marjoram	
⅓ cup dry red wine, such as Chianti	

1. In a large pan, bring about 1 quart of water to a boil. Crumble the ground beef into the water and stir constantly. When water starts to boil again, pour water and the meat into a large strainer sitting in sink.
2. Place meat in a large saucepan or Dutch oven; add onion and garlic and cook until onion is tender.
3. Add remaining ingredients except wine. Bring to a boil; reduce heat, cover loosely, and simmer 1½ hours, stirring occasionally.
4. Add wine and simmer 30 minutes, stirring occasionally.
5. Serve meat sauce over pasta cooked in unsalted water.

Yield: 8 servings

One serving (²/₃ cup) of the lower-sodium meat sauce contains:

Calories	Fat g	Saturated Fat g	Cholesterol mg	Carbohydrate g	Fiber g	Sodium mg
119	5	2	32	7	2	43

The higher-sodium version provides 257 mg of sodium per ²/₃-cup serving.

---

*From *The New Living Heart Diet,* by DeBakey, M.E., Gotto, A.M., Scott, L.W., et al., Simon & Schuster, New York, 1996.

g = grams; mg = milligrams.

Chapter 2

Using *The Living Heart Brand Name Shopper's Guide* to Prevent or Treat High Cholesterol and Triglyceride Levels

An elevated level of blood cholesterol, more particularly LDL-cholesterol ("bad cholesterol"), is a major risk factor for coronary heart disease (CHD). Restricting fat, saturated fat, and cholesterol in the diet (see below) and reaching a desirable weight (see page 26) are the primary dietary measures to lower elevated levels of total cholesterol and LDL-cholesterol.

A direct link between elevated blood triglyceride levels and the development of CHD has not been definitely established. However, many physicians recommend that their patients try to reduce elevated blood triglyceride levels using diet, weight control, and exercise, or, sometimes, these lifestyle measures combined with medication.

The following tables list the classifications of blood levels of total cholesterol, LDL-cholesterol, HDL-cholesterol ("good cholesterol"), and triglyceride for adults (20 years of age and older). The first table classifies total cholesterol and LDL-cholesterol levels in adults who show no evidence of CHD or other atherosclerotic disease. Atherosclerotic diseases are those characterized by the narrowing of arteries due to the formation of plaque in the artery wall.

CLASSIFICATIONS OF TOTAL CHOLESTEROL AND LDL-CHOLESTEROL LEVELS IN ADULTS WITHOUT EVIDENCE OF ATHEROSCLEROTIC DISEASE

Total cholesterol

Desirable	Less than 200 mg/dL
Borderline-high	200–239 mg/dL
High	240 mg/dL or greater

LDL-cholesterol
Desirable   Less than 130 mg/dL
Borderline-high   130–159 mg/dL
High   160 mg/dL or greater

mg/dL = milligrams per deciliter.

The next table classifies LDL-cholesterol levels for those adults who are known to have CHD or other atherosclerotic disease (for example, atherosclerosis in the legs or a history of stroke).

CLASSIFICATIONS OF LDL-CHOLESTEROL LEVELS IN ADULTS
KNOWN TO HAVE ATHEROSCLEROTIC DISEASE
Acceptable LDL-cholesterol   100 mg/dL or less
Higher-than-acceptable LDL-cholesterol More than 100 mg/dL

mg/dL = milligrams per deciliter.

The table below classifies levels of HDL-cholesterol and triglyceride in all adults. HDL-cholesterol is sometimes referred to as an "anti-risk," or protective, factor because a low level is associated with increased risk for CHD and a high level is associated with decreased risk. You want lower levels of total cholesterol, LDL-cholesterol, and triglyceride but higher levels of HDL-cholesterol.

CLASSIFICATIONS OF HDL-CHOLESTEROL AND
TRIGLYCERIDE LEVELS IN ALL ADULTS
HDL-cholesterol
Low (increased CHD risk)   Less than 35 mg/dL
Acceptable   35 mg/dL or greater
High (protective level of HDL) 60 mg/dL or greater

Triglyceride
Normal   Less than 200 mg/dL
Borderline-high   200–400 mg/dL
High   400–1,000 mg/dL
Very high   1,000 mg/dL or greater

mg/dL = milligrams per deciliter.

DIETARY CHANGES

A diet low in fat, saturated fat, and cholesterol and providing adequate calories to maintain a desirable weight is used to decrease levels of both blood cholesterol and triglyceride. Decreasing the amount of fat in your diet is the most efficient way to reduce your intake of saturated fat, and reducing saturated fat intake is the most important dietary step in lowering blood cholesterol levels. Limiting dietary cholesterol is also a factor in lowering blood cholesterol levels, but it is of less importance than limiting saturated fat. The dietary measures to decrease an elevated blood triglyceride level include 1) weight loss, when appropriate, 2) reduction of fat, saturated fat, and cholesterol intakes, 3) restriction of alcohol intake (in some people), and 4) reduction of simple carbohydrate (such as in candy, soda, and desserts) in people with a high intake.

Eating less fat also helps you decrease the calories you consume *if* you do not replace those calories by eating more carbohydrate or protein. Remember, just because a food is labeled "fat free" does *not* mean that it is "calorie free." Some fat-free foods have about the same number of calories as their regular-fat counterparts.

The two levels of fat discussed in the following sections are 1) a diet with no more than 30% of calories from fat, and 2) a very low fat diet (about 20% of calories from fat). Both levels of fat intake can help lower blood cholesterol and triglyceride and reduce body weight.

DIET PROVIDING NO MORE THAN
30% OF CALORIES FROM FAT

An eating pattern in which no more than 30% of calories come from fat is recommended for all healthy Americans age 2 years or older. It is also recommended that all Americans decrease their intake of saturated fat to 8% to 10% of calories and cholesterol to less than 300 milligrams per day, as well as control their calorie intake to reach their desirable body weight.

The Living Heart Brand Name Shopper's Guide can help you with each of the following three methods of controlling your fat and saturated fat intake.
• Count grams of fat and saturated fat
• Select foods lower in fat and saturated fat
• Count servings of food from each food group

COUNT GRAMS OF FAT AND SATURATED FAT

How many grams of fat equal 30% of calories, and how many grams of saturated fat equal 8% of calories? The answers depend on your calorie needs. The following tables provide estimates of how many calories it takes to maintain your present weight, and the maximum grams of fat and saturated fat allowed at each calorie level. These tables are based on a person with a medium frame who is doing light activity. If your frame is small or large or if you are less or more active, see pages 26 to 30 for more information on estimating your calorie needs.

MEN
MAXIMUM GRAMS OF FAT (30% OF CALORIES)
AND SATURATED FAT (8% OF CALORIES)

Height*	Desirable Weight† (pounds)	Calories‡	Grams of Fat Equal to 30% of Calories	Grams of Saturated Fat Equal to 8% of Calories
5'5"	130–143	2,050	68	18
5'6"	134–147	2,100	70	19
5'7"	138–152	2,200	73	20
5'8"	142–156	2,250	75	20
5'9"	146–160	2,300	77	20
5'10"	150–165	2,350	78	21
5'11"	154–170	2,450	82	22
6'0"	158–175	2,500	83	22
6'1"	162–180	2,550	85	23
6'2"	167–185	2,650	88	24
6'3"	172–190	2,700	90	24

Adapted from 1959 Metropolitan Life Insurance Company, New York City.
* Table adjusted for measurement of height without shoes.
† Medium frame size (see page 27).
‡ Light activity level (see page 30).

WOMEN
MAXIMUM GRAMS OF FAT (30% OF CALORIES)
AND SATURATED FAT (8% OF CALORIES)

Height*	Desirable Weight† (pounds)	Calories‡	Grams of Fat Equal to 30% of Calories	Grams of Saturated Fat Equal to 8% of Calories
5'0"	107–119	1,700	57	15
5'1"	110–122	1,750	58	16
5'2"	113–126	1,800	60	16
5'3"	116–130	1,850	62	16
5'4"	120–135	1,900	63	17
5'5"	124–139	1,950	65	17
5'6"	128–143	2,050	68	18
5'7"	132–147	2,100	70	19
5'8"	136–151	2,150	72	19
5'9"	140–155	2,200	73	20
5'10"	144–159	2,250	75	20

Adapted from 1959 Metropolitan Life Insurance Company, New York City.
* Table adjusted for measurement of height without shoes.
† Medium frame size (see page 27).
‡ Light activity level (see page 30).

This book is an excellent source of information on the grams of fat and saturated fat in generic and brand name foods; values for brand name products can also be found in the Nutrition Facts portion of the label on the foods you eat. If you eat away from home, use *The Living Heart Guide to Eating Out,* another book by the same authors (see back page for order form), to estimate the grams of fat and saturated fat in restaurant and fast foods. Remember, you can compensate for eating some foods that are high in fat or saturated fat by selecting other foods that are very low in these components. Compensating in this way will enable you to keep your total intake below the maximum grams of fat and saturated fat shown in the tables above.

SELECT FOODS LOWER IN FAT AND SATURATED FAT

You can choose from among the thousands of supermarket foods listed in this book, all of which are low in saturated fat and most of which are also low in fat. As you can see from looking at the fresh fruits and vegetables, these foods contain very little, if any, fat or saturated fat. The Guide includes foods such as avocado, oil, margarine, salad dressing, olives, nuts, and seeds that are high in fat but low in saturated fat; these foods may be eaten in limited amounts on a diet with no more than 30% of calories from fat. Recipe substitutions that you can use to lower fat and/or cholesterol in the foods you cook appear on page 263 in the Appendix. *The Living Heart Guide to Eating Out* lists 160 practical tips for choosing lower-fat foods when eating away from home, which can be used in addition to the general information below.

Now more than ever, it is possible to find delicious lower-fat foods in many restaurants. A few simple rules of thumb will make it easier for you to enjoy "eating low fat" when away from home.

- Choose foods that are cooked at the time they are ordered, that is, that are not prepared ahead of time. This allows you to ask that foods be prepared with little or no added fat. A good choice might be a chicken breast or fish that is grilled instead of fried.
- Select lean cuts of meat and trim all visible fat from the served portion. Remove and discard skin from servings of chicken or other poultry.
- Request that gravies, sauces, and dressings be served on the side so that you can control the amount you eat.
- Try baked potatoes with salsa, lemon, or ketchup instead of butter, sour cream, bacon, and cheese.
- Eat bread or rolls without butter.

- If you eat dessert, choose fruit, fruited gelatin, angel food cake without icing, sorbet, sherbet, or low-fat frozen yogurt.

COUNT SERVINGS OF FOOD FROM EACH FOOD GROUP

Counting servings of food is described on pages 31 to 38 of Chapter 3. This method is excellent for lowering your intake of fat and saturated fat.

LIMITING CHOLESTEROL INTAKE

Limiting dietary cholesterol is an important part of an eating plan to lower blood cholesterol. Since dietary cholesterol is found only in animal foods (meat, poultry, fish, dairy products, and egg yolk), cholesterol values have not been provided for all the foods in the Guide. At times you may find a small amount of cholesterol listed on the label of foods, such as cake, cookies, and crackers that are included in the Guide; this is because egg, milk, or another animal product was being used as an ingredient. The following table shows common sources of dietary cholesterol.

CHOLESTEROL CONTENT OF SELECTED FOODS

Food	Cholesterol mg
Meat, poultry, or fish (3 ounces cooked)	
Lean beef, pork, lamb, and poultry	75
Liver	330
Finfish	20–100
Shrimp	165
Dairy products	
Cheese, hard (1 ounce)	20–35
Cottage cheese, regular (1/2 cup)	15
Ricotta (1/2 cup)	65
Ice cream (1/2 cup)	
Regular	25
Rich	45
Milk (1 cup)	
Whole	35
2% fat	20
1% fat	10
Skim	5
Sour cream (2 tablespoons)	20
Yogurt (1 cup)	
Regular, plain	30
Fruited	25
Low-fat, fruited	10
Nonfat, plain	4
Egg yolk (1 medium)	215

Cholesterol values rounded to nearest 5; mg = milligrams.

As a rule, if you consume a maximum of 6 ounces total of lean meat, skinless poultry, and/or fish per day, limit your egg yolks to 3 per week, and use low-fat or fat-free dairy products, your average intake of cholesterol will not exceed 300 milligrams per day.

VERY LOW FAT DIET

Some people find it necessary to lower their fat intake to about 20% of calories in order to achieve a desirable blood cholesterol level. A diet in which 20% of calories come from fat also reduces saturated fat and usually reduces calories. The Women's Health Initiative is a long-term study that utilizes an eating plan with 20% of calories from fat and 7% of calories from saturated fat with an emphasis on the consumption of complex carbohydrate and high-fiber foods. Results of this study of about 63,000 postmenopausal women across the country will provide even more information about the effects of a low-fat diet on health.

A reduction in fat to about 20% of calories will usually decrease calorie intake, which can result in weight loss. If you do not need to lose weight, you will need to replace the calories from fat with calories from carbohydrate, primarily complex carbohydrate. To prevent weight loss, increase your consumption of foods that contain little or no fat, such as the starchy foods, vegetables, fruits, and fat-free dairy products.

There are two methods that are effective in helping you limit your fat intake to about 20% of calories.

- Count grams of fat
- Select foods that are very low in fat and saturated fat

COUNT GRAMS OF FAT
The following tables provide estimates of the maximum grams of fat on a diet with 20% of calories from fat.

MEN
MAXIMUM GRAMS OF FAT AT 20% OF CALORIES

Height*	Desirable Weight† (pounds)	Calories‡	Grams of Fat Equal to 20% of Calories
5'5"	130–143	2,050	46
5'6"	134–147	2,100	47
5'7"	138–152	2,200	49
5'8"	142–156	2,250	50
5'9"	146–160	2,300	51
5'10"	150–165	2,350	52
5'11"	154–170	2,450	54
6'0"	158–175	2,500	56
6'1"	162–180	2,550	57
6'2"	167–185	2,650	59
6'3"	172–190	2,700	60

Adapted from 1959 Metropolitan Life Insurance Company, New York City.
* Table adjusted for measurement of height without shoes.
† Medium frame size (see page 27).
‡ Light activity level (see page 30).

WOMEN
MAXIMUM GRAMS OF FAT AT 20% OF CALORIES

Height*	Desirable Weight† (pounds)	Calories‡	Grams of Fat Equal to 20% of Calories
5'0"	107–119	1,700	38
5'1"	110–122	1,750	39
5'2"	113–126	1,800	40
5'3"	116–130	1,850	41
5'4"	120–135	1,900	42
5'5"	124–139	1,950	43
5'6"	128–143	2,050	46
5'7"	132–147	2,100	47
5'8"	136–151	2,150	48
5'9"	140–155	2,200	49
5'10"	144–159	2,250	50

Adapted from 1959 Metropolitan Life Insurance Company, New York City.
* Table adjusted for measurement of height without shoes.
† Medium frame size (see page 27).
‡ Light activity level (see page 30).

It is not necessary to count grams of saturated fat at this fat level. When fat intake is 20% of calories or less, saturated fat intake is automatically low.

SELECT FOODS THAT ARE VERY LOW IN FAT AND SATURATED FAT

A 20% fat diet typically consists of eating the following each day:

- 6 or more servings of bread, cereals, pasta, and/or rice
- 3 or more servings of vegetables
- 2 or more servings of fruit
- A maximum of 5 ounces total of the leanest cuts of meat, white meat of poultry (without skin), and/or fish. These meats are often labeled "extra lean," which means they contain 5 grams of fat or less per 3.5 ounces of cooked meat. For canned fish (see page 183 of food table), select tuna packed in water (1 gram of fat in 3 oz) instead of tuna packed in oil (7 grams of fat in 3 oz) or sockeye salmon (6 grams of fat in 3 oz). For fresh or frozen fish (see page 184), choose cod or haddock (each 1 gram of fat in 3 oz) or snapper (2 grams of fat in 3 oz) instead of catfish or Atlantic salmon (each 7 grams of fat in 3 oz). In poultry, white meat (without skin) is lower in fat than dark meat. The amount of meat eaten will need to be limited to 3 ounces per day if higher-fat meats are consumed. Meat, poultry, and fish should be cooked without added fat. Try combining smaller portions of meat with other foods, including rice, pasta, and vegetables. Legumes (beans, peas, and lentils) are a good source of protein and can be substituted for meat.
- 2 to 4 servings of fat-free (skim) dairy products
- Fat-free spreads, salad dressings, and mayonnaise. Oils low in saturated fat (olive, canola, safflower, sunflower, corn, soybean) may be used in small amounts. Fortunately, a wide variety of lower-fat margarines and fat-free salad dressings are available. It will be necessary to learn to cook without added fat. Try "sautéing" in wine, flavored vinegars, or clear broths, or use cooking sprays.
- Sweets and desserts that contain little or no fat may be included in moderation.

In addition, you may eat a maximum of 1 egg yolk per *week*; there is no limit on egg whites.

SELECTING VERY LOW FAT FOODS WHEN EATING AWAY FROM HOME

When you are following an eating plan with about 20% of calories from fat, you will need to pay special attention to foods selected when eating away from home. It is more challenging to choose low-fat foods in a restaurant than at home. *The Living Heart Guide to Eating Out* can help you estimate the grams of fat in restaurant foods. If a higher-fat food is eaten, it is important to compensate for the extra fat by choosing other foods that are very low in fat. This will help keep your total fat intake within your goal. You may choose to eat the very low fat foods at the same meal, or at another meal the same day. There may even be times when compensating carries over to the next day.

Chapter 3

Using *The Living Heart Brand Name Shopper's Guide* to Control Weight

Calorie intake is of interest to most health-minded people. Overweight continues to be the number-one nutrition problem in the United States. It is estimated that 35% of women and 31% of men age 20 years and older are obese, that is, 20% or more above their desirable weight; even more are overweight to a lesser extent. Excess weight contributes to a number of disorders, including coronary heart disease, high blood pressure, and diabetes.

A good weight control program consists of two important parts:

- Decreasing calories
- Increasing physical activity

A gradual loss of 1 to 2 pounds per week is much better than a rapid weight loss. Weight that is lost rapidly is usually regained. A slower rate of weight loss that is accompanied by a permanent change in eating and exercise habits is more likely to help you keep weight off.

Remember:
- Losing just 1 pound per week for a year equals a loss of 52 pounds.
- It is not how much weight you lose that is important—it is how much weight you keep off for the rest of your life.

DETERMINING YOUR CALORIE NEEDS

Before beginning any weight control program, it is a good idea to determine the approximate number of calories you need each day to maintain your desirable weight. To do this, you need to know your height, frame size, and activity level so that you can use the calorie-level tables below.

1. *Height.* Measure your height without shoes.

2. *Frame size.* Use one of the following two simple tests to determine your frame size. For the first method, which requires no equipment, place the thumb and index finger of one hand around your other wrist. Be sure your thumb and index finger go around the radius and ulna bones at your wrist (the smallest part, closest to your hand).

- If thumb and index finger *overlap,* you have a *small* frame.
- If thumb and index finger *just touch,* you have a *medium* frame.
- If thumb and index finger *do not meet,* you have a *large* frame.

A second way to determine frame size is to use a flexible measuring tape to measure around your wrist at the smallest area, nearest your hand. Match your wrist measurement with your height in the table below to get your frame size.

| Height | Wrist Size | | |
	Small Frame	Medium Frame	Large Frame
Under 5'3"	Less than 5½"	5½" to 5¾"	Greater than 5¾"
5'3" to 5'4"	Less than 6"	6" to 6¼"	Greater than 6¼"
Over 5'4"	Less than 6¼"	6¼" to 6½"	Greater than 6½"

3. *Activity level.* (continued on page 30)

Height Without Shoes	Frame Size	Desirable Weight (Pounds)	Calories			
			Very Light Activity	Light Activity	Moderate Activity	Heavy Activity
5'5"	Small	129 (124–133)	1,700	1,950	2,200	2,600
	Medium	137 (130–143)	1,800	2,050	2,350	2,750
	Large	147 (138–156)	1,900	2,200	2,500	2,950
5'6"	Small	133 (128–137)	1,750	2,000	2,250	2,650
	Medium	141 (134–147)	1,850	2,100	2,400	2,800
	Large	152 (142–161)	2,000	2,300	2,600	3,050
5'7"	Small	137 (132–141)	1,800	2,050	2,350	2,750
	Medium	145 (138–152)	1,900	2,200	2,450	2,900
	Large	157 (147–166)	2,050	2,350	2,650	3,150
5'8"	Small	141 (136–145)	1,850	2,100	2,400	2,850
	Medium	149 (142–156)	1,950	2,250	2,550	3,000
	Large	161 (151–170)	2,100	2,400	2,750	3,200
5'9"	Small	145 (140–150)	1,900	2,200	2,450	2,900
	Medium	153 (146–160)	2,000	2,300	2,600	3,050
	Large	165 (155–174)	2,150	2,500	2,800	3,300
5'10"	Small	149 (144–154)	1,950	2,250	2,550	3,000
	Medium	158 (150–165)	2,050	2,350	2,700	3,150
	Large	169 (159–179)	2,200	2,550	2,850	3,400
5'11"	Small	153 (148–158)	2,000	2,300	2,600	3,050
	Medium	162 (154–170)	2,100	2,450	2,750	3,250
	Large	174 (164–184)	2,250	2,600	2,950	3,500
6'0"	Small	157 (152–162)	2,050	2,350	2,650	3,150
	Medium	167 (158–175)	2,150	2,500	2,850	3,350
	Large	179 (168–189)	2,350	2,700	3,050	3,600
6'1"	Small	162 (156–167)	2,100	2,450	2,750	3,250
	Medium	171 (162–180)	2,200	2,550	2,900	3,400
	Large	184 (173–194)	2,400	2,750	3,150	3,700
6'2"	Small	166 (160–171)	2,150	2,500	2,800	3,300
	Medium	176 (167–185)	2,300	2,650	3,000	3,500
	Large	189 (178–199)	2,450	2,850	3,200	3,800
6'3"	Small	170 (164–175)	2,200	2,550	2,900	3,400
	Medium	181 (172–190)	2,350	2,700	3,100	3,600
	Large	193 (182–204)	2,500	2,900	3,300	3,850

Adapted from 1959 Metropolitan Life Insurance Company, New York City. These tables are based on 1959 rather than 1983 Metropolitan Life Insurance Company height–weight tables because the earlier tables specify lower weights, which are more appropriate to health-related concerns.

WOMEN

Height Without Shoes	Frame Size	Desirable Weight (Pounds)	Calories			
			Very Light Activity	Light Activity	Moderate Activity	Heavy Activity
5'0"	Small	106 (102–110)	1,400	1,600	1,800	2,100
	Medium	113 (107–119)	1,450	1,700	1,900	2,250
	Large	123 (115–131)	1,600	1,850	2,100	2,450
5'1"	Small	109 (105–113)	1,400	1,650	1,850	2,200
	Medium	116 (110–122)	1,500	1,750	1,950	2,300
	Large	126 (118–134)	1,650	1,900	2,150	2,500
5'2"	Small	112 (108–116)	1,450	1,700	1,900	2,250
	Medium	119 (113–126)	1,550	1,800	2,000	2,400
	Large	129 (121–138)	1,700	1,950	2,200	2,600
5'3"	Small	115 (111–119)	1,500	1,750	1,950	2,300
	Medium	123 (116–130)	1,600	1,850	2,100	2,450
	Large	133 (125–142)	1,750	2,000	2,250	2,650
5'4"	Small	118 (114–123)	1,550	1,750	2,000	2,350
	Medium	127 (120–135)	1,650	1,900	2,150	2,550
	Large	137 (129–146)	1,800	2,050	2,350	2,750
5'5"	Small	122 (118–127)	1,600	1,850	2,050	2,450
	Medium	131 (124–139)	1,700	1,950	2,250	2,600
	Large	141 (133–150)	1,800	2,100	2,400	2,800
5'6"	Small	126 (122–131)	1,650	1,900	2,150	2,500
	Medium	135 (128–143)	1,750	2,050	2,300	2,700
	Large	145 (137–154)	1,900	2,200	2,450	2,900
5'7"	Small	130 (126–135)	1,700	1,950	2,200	2,600
	Medium	139 (132–147)	1,800	2,100	2,350	2,800
	Large	149 (141–158)	1,950	2,250	2,550	3,000
5'8"	Small	135 (130–140)	1,750	2,050	2,300	2,700
	Medium	143 (136–151)	1,850	2,150	2,450	2,850
	Large	154 (145–163)	2,000	2,300	2,600	3,100
5'9"	Small	139 (134–144)	1,800	2,100	2,350	2,800
	Medium	147 (140–155)	1,900	2,200	2,500	2,950
	Large	158 (149–168)	2,050	2,350	2,700	3,150
5'10"	Small	143 (138–148)	1,850	2,150	2,450	2,850
	Medium	151 (144–159)	1,950	2,250	2,550	3,000
	Large	163 (153–173)	2,100	2,450	2,750	3,250

Adapted from 1959 Metropolitan Life Insurance Company, New York City. These tables are based on 1959 rather than 1983 Metropolitan Life Insurance Company height–weight tables because the earlier tables specify lower weights, which are more appropriate to health-related concerns.

3. *Activity level.* Consider all your activities for a typical day. That includes the amount of time you spend resting, walking around your house, sitting at a desk, watching television, and exercising. Then, use the list below to determine your level of activity.

ACTIVITY LEVEL

- Very Light Activity
  Seated and standing activities, such as working in a laboratory, driving, typing, sewing, ironing, cooking, playing cards, playing a musical instrument
- Light Activity
  Walking on a level surface at 2.5 to 3 miles per hour, garage work, electrical work, restaurant work, carpentry, house cleaning, child care, sailing, playing golf or table tennis
- Moderate Activity
  Walking 3.5 to 4 miles per hour, weeding, carrying a load, cycling, skiing, playing tennis, dancing
- Heavy Activity
  Playing basketball, football, or soccer, walking uphill with a load, climbing, heavy manual labor such as digging

Adapted from National Research Council. *Recommended Dietary Allowance,* 10th edition. National Academy Press, Washington, D.C., 1989.

4. *Calorie level.* Use your height, frame size, and level of activity with the table for men (page 28) or the table for women (page 29) to determine the approximate number of calories needed to maintain the desirable weight listed in the third column of the table.

DIETARY CHANGES

Here are three ways in which you can use *The Living Heart Brand Name Shopper's Guide* to help you control your calorie intake:

- Select lower-fat foods (these are also usually lower in calories)
- Count calories
- Count servings of food from each food group

You may need to try each method to determine which one works best for you. If you do not like a structured approach, you may prefer the first method: selecting lower-fat foods. If you like structure, try counting servings of food (see page 31).

SELECT LOWER-FAT FOODS

Decreasing your intake of fat is a good way to limit calories. Fat provides more than twice the calories of carbohydrate or protein: fat provides 9 calories per gram and carbohydrate and protein each provide 4 calories per gram. A decrease in fat intake can result in weight loss if the calories are not replaced by eating more carbohydrate or protein. There are many foods on the market that contain little or no fat but still provide a lot of calories. When you are trying to lose weight, it is important for you to be aware of the calories in all the foods you eat.

Most people find it fairly easy to select lower-fat foods (see page 20 for additional discussion of this method). Emphasis is placed on eating more vegetables and fruits; moderate amounts of starchy foods (such as bread, cereal, pasta, and rice); low-fat or fat-free dairy products; and lean meat, poultry (without skin), and fish. The values given in this book will help you choose foods that are lower in fat and calories. *The Living Heart Guide to Eating Out,* another book by the same authors, can help you select lower-fat foods when you eat away from home. It contains values for fat for 750 restaurant foods and 880 fast foods.

COUNT CALORIES

Counting calories means keeping a written record of everything that you eat and drink and calculating the calories provided by these foods. You can find the calorie content for thousands of foods in the Guide; calorie count is also listed in the Nutrition Facts portion of food labels. *The Living Heart Guide to Eating Out* can be used to estimate calories in restaurant and fast foods.

The method of "compensating" can be used with calorie counting. For example, if you eat a high-calorie food, compensate for the extra calories by selecting other foods that are much lower in calories for the remainder of the day and possibly the next day. In this way you can keep your intake close to your desired calorie level. The tables on pages 28 and 29 provide estimates of calorie intake to maintain your present weight or to lose weight. In order to lose about 1 pound per week, you need to reduce the calories it takes to maintain your weight by about 500 per day; you can do this by eating 500 calories less each day, by increasing physical activity to burn 500 calories more each day, or by a combination of both calorie restriction and exercise.

COUNT SERVINGS OF FOOD FROM EACH FOOD GROUP

An eating plan in which you count servings of food is a good way to eat approximately the same number of calories and about the same amount of carbohydrate, protein, and fat every day. First, you will need to estimate the calories you need each day (see pages 26 to 30). Next, find the nearest calorie level in the table below to determine the number of servings from each food group that will provide your desired calorie intake. Beginning below, there is a brief description of each food group, including the amount of food equal to 1 serving.

Note that the serving sizes listed in the descriptions of the food groups may be different from the serving sizes listed in the Food Section in this book or on food labels. The serving sizes used in the food groups are based on calories. For example, 1 average size slice of bread, which provides about 80 calories, is a serving in the food group list (page 35). Many of the serving sizes used by food manufacturers are larger than the serving sizes used in the food groups. For example, bread manufacturers often use a serving size of 2 slices on the label (to match more closely the FDA serving size of 1.75 ounces for bread).

Most of the food groups include a variety of foods; the Dairy Products group, for example, includes milk, cheese, and yogurt.

SERVINGS OF FOOD ACCORDING TO DAILY CALORIE LEVEL

Food Group	Daily Servings Allowed						
	1,200 Cal	1,400 Cal	1,600 Cal	1,800 Cal	2,000 Cal	2,200 Cal	2,500 Cal
Meat, poultry, fish	6 oz	6 oz	6 oz	6 oz	6 oz	6 oz	6 oz
Egg yolks	3/wk	3/wk	3/wk	3/wk	3/wk	3/wk	3/wk
Dairy products	2	2	3	3	3	4	4
Fats	3	3	4	5	6	7	8
Bread, cereals, pasta, starchy vegetables	3	4	4	6	7	7	10
Vegetables (nonstarchy)*	4+	4+	4+	4+	4+	4+	4+
Fruits	3	3	3	3	3	5	5
Sweets, alcohol†	0	100 cal	200 cal	200 cal	200 cal	200 cal	200 cal
Free foods	✓	✓	✓	✓	✓	✓	✓

Cal = calories; oz = ounces; wk = week.
* More nonstarchy vegetables may be included if desired.
† This food group is not usually included in a diabetic meal plan.
✓ = Not limited at any calorie level.

★ MEAT, POULTRY, AND FISH

Meat, poultry, and fish are a major source of fat, saturated fat, and cholesterol in the American diet. All meat should be very lean, and any visible fat should be trimmed off before cooking. Select red meat that has the least fat marbled through the muscle. Remove the skin before cooking poultry, and avoid self-basting poultry, which has had extra fat injected into it. Cook meat, poultry, and fish with little or no added fat. You will notice in the table above that the total amount of meat, poultry, and/or fish recommended for daily consumption does not exceed 6 ounces (cooked) at any calorie level; 3 ounces is about the size of a deck of playing cards.

One ounce of cooked lean meat, fish, or poultry provides about 60 calories, 3 grams of fat, 1 gram of saturated fat, and 25 milligrams of cholesterol.

★ EGGS

An average egg yolk contains 213 milligrams (mg) of cholesterol, making it one of the most concentrated sources of dietary cholesterol. A maximum of 3 eggs per week is recommended for an intake averaging less than 300 mg of cholesterol per day. Be sure to account for all the eggs you eat, including those used in cooking and baking. Egg whites may be eaten freely since they contain no cholesterol.

	Calories	Saturated Fat g	Fat g	Cholesterol mg	Sodium mg
Whole egg (1 large)	74	5	2	213	63
Egg white (1 large)	17	0	0	0	55
Egg yolk (1 large)	59	5	2	213	7

g = grams; mg = milligrams.

★ DAIRY PRODUCTS

Higher-fat dairy products represent a major source of saturated fat for children and adults. However, low-fat and fat-free dairy products, which provide about the same amount of calcium and protein as higher-fat dairy products, are widely available.

Dairy products have a variety of serving sizes. The following table lists serving sizes for common lower-fat dairy products.

One serving of lower-fat dairy products provides about 90 calories, 3 grams of fat, 2 grams of saturated fat, and 10 milligrams of cholesterol.

ONE SERVING OF LOWER-FAT DAIRY PRODUCTS

Dairy Product	Serving Size
Cheese with a maximum of 3 grams of fat per ounce	1 to 2 ounces*
Cottage cheese, low-fat or nonfat	1/2 cup
Frozen dairy dessert, low-fat or nonfat	1/3 to 1/2 cup*
Milk, skim, 1/2%, or 1% low-fat	1 cup
Yogurt, plain, nonfat (skim or fat-free), 1/2%, or 1% low-fat	1 cup

* Check the label; you may have to adjust the serving size because these low-fat products may vary in the amount it takes to equal 90 calories.

★ FATS

Much of the fat Americans eat is in the form of margarine, oil, mayonnaise, salad dressing, peanut butter, nuts, olives, avocado, and seeds. It is recommended that anyone following a cholesterol-lowering diet choose only those high-fat foods that are lower in saturated fat, such as the products listed in this book. All fats provide more than twice the calories of carbohydrate or protein; therefore, consuming a large amount of any type of fat means more calories and possible weight gain.

ONE SERVING OF FATS

Fat	Serving Size
Avocado	1/8 medium
Margarine	1 to 2 teaspoons*†
Mayonnaise	2 teaspoons*†
Nuts, chopped	1 tablespoon
Oil	1 teaspoon
Olives	10 small or 5 large
Peanut butter	2 teaspoons
Salad dressing	1 tablespoon*†
Seeds	1 tablespoon

* Check the label; you may have to adjust the serving size because lower-fat versions of these products may vary in the amount it takes to equal 45 calories.

† Foods for which 1 serving provides less than 20 calories may be considered free foods.

One serving of fats provides about 45 calories, 5 grams of fat, 1 gram of saturated fat, and little or no cholesterol.

★ BREAD, CEREALS, PASTA, AND STARCHY VEGETABLES

Low-fat diets emphasize using a higher proportion of complex carbohydrate foods — bread, cereals, pasta, and starchy vegetables (such as corn, peas, potato, and sweet potato). Most of these foods are naturally low in fat.

ONE SERVING OF BREAD, CEREALS, PASTA, AND STARCHY VEGETABLES

Bread, Cereal, Pasta, or Starchy Vegetable	Serving Size
Bagel, English muffin, or hamburger or hot dog bun	1/2
Bread, loaf	
Regular, average-size slice	1 slice
Diet or light (35 to 40 calories per slice)	2 slices
Bagel, English muffin, or hamburger or hot dog bun	1/2
Cereal, low-fat	
Cooked (measured after cooking)	1/2 cup
Ready-to-eat	1 ounce*
Pasta (measured after cooking)	1/2 cup
Rice (measured after cooking)	1/3 cup
Starchy vegetable	
Corn	1/2 cup
Peas, green	1/2 cup
Potato, white	
Baked	1 medium
Mashed	1/2 cup
Sweet potato (with no sugar added)	1/3 cup
Other starchy foods	
Crackers or pretzels	Amount equal to 80 calories
Graham crackers (2 1/2" squares)	3 squares
Popcorn, popped without fat	3 cups popped
Soup	3/4 to 1 cup

*Check the label; you may have to adjust the serving size because these low-fat products may vary in the amount it takes to equal 80 calories.

One serving of bread, cereal, pasta, or starchy vegetables provides about 80 calories, 1 gram of fat, and negligible amounts of saturated fat and cholesterol.

★ VEGETABLES

Nonstarchy vegetables (such as broccoli, cauliflower, carrots, tomatoes, and spinach) are an excellent choice in any low-fat, low-calorie eating plan. You may eat any number of servings of vegetables that contain less than 20 calories per cup. Eating a wide variety of vegetables is a good way to help ensure that you get an adequate supply of fiber and many vitamins and minerals.

Seasoning vegetables with fat or serving them with a sauce increases their fat content. You will need to account for any fat added to vegetables and subtract it from the servings of fat recommended for your calorie level. This is especially important when you are eating out. A good rule of thumb is to allow $1/2$ teaspoon of fat per $1/2$ cup of vegetables.

ONE SERVING OF NONSTARCHY VEGETABLES

Vegetables	Serving Size
Cooked vegetables	$1/2$ cup
Raw vegetables	1 cup
Vegetable juice	$1/2$ cup

> One serving of nonstarchy vegetables provides about 25 calories, negligible amounts of fat and saturated fat, and no cholesterol.

★ FRUITS

Fruits are good sources of vitamins and minerals and provide fiber. With the exception of avocados and olives, fruits do not naturally contain fat. Avocados and olives are high in fat but low in saturated fat; they are listed in the Fats section. Remember, adding whipped topping, sour cream, or nuts to fruit increases its fat content.

ONE SERVING OF FRUITS

Fruit	Serving Size
Canned fruit, unsweetened	$1/2$ cup
Dried fruit	2 tablespoons to $1/4$ cup
Fresh apple, peach, pear, orange, or kiwifruit	1 medium piece
Fresh banana, grapefruit, or mango	$1/2$ medium piece
Fresh strawberries (whole) or watermelon	$1 1/4$ cup
Fruit juice, unsweetened	$1/3$ to $1/2$ cup

One serving of fruits provides about 60 calories, negligible amounts of fat and saturated fat, and no cholesterol.

★ SWEETS AND ALCOHOL

The Sweets and Alcohol food group includes many of those sweet foods you enjoy but that are not part of the food groups described on the preceding pages. Many of the sweets are higher in calories than foods from the other food groups because they are prepared with fat (examples include cake, pie, candy, and cookies). Sweets are limited on a lower-calorie eating pattern because they provide calories without being important sources of nutrients.

Use the values for calories and fat in the Guide or on the Nutrition Facts portion of a food label to estimate the size portion that will provide about 100 or 200 calories (see page 32).

Alcoholic beverages are also included in this group. The recommendation is that people who do drink alcohol consume no more than 1 ounce of pure alcohol (about 2 drinks) per day. The following alcoholic beverages contain 1/2 ounce of alcohol, and each is considered 1 drink.

ONE ALCOHOLIC DRINK*

Alcoholic Drink	Serving Size
Beer, regular or light	12 fluid ounces
80-proof spirits, such as bourbon, gin, rum, scotch, or vodka	1 1/2 fluid ounces
100-proof spirits	1 fluid ounce
Table wine, red or white	5 fluid ounces
Fortified wine, such as sherry, port, marsala, or Madeira	3 fluid ounces

*Limit intake to no more than 2 drinks per day.

How many calories are contained in specific alcoholic beverages is shown on pages 59–60.

★ FREE FOODS

"Free" foods are those that contain very little or no fat, saturated fat, and cholesterol and are very low in calories. Free foods that contain less than 20 calories per serving do not have to be limited. A serving size is indicated for those free foods listed below that are slightly higher in calories.

FREE FOODS

Beverages
Bitters
Carbonated water, club soda, or carbonated soda, sugar-free*
Coffee or tea (no sugar or creamer)
Drink mixes and tonic water, sugar-free*

Condiments
Horseradish
Ketchup (1 tablespoon)
Mustard
Picante sauce
Pickles, dill, unsweetened
Soy sauce
Taco sauce
Worcestershire sauce

Fruits
Cranberries, unsweetened (1/2 cup)
Lemon
Lime
Rhubarb, unsweetened (1/2 cup)

Ingredients
Cocoa powder, unsweetened (1 tablespoon)

Flavoring essence (maple, vanilla, butter flavor, etc.)
Liquid smoke
Spices and herbs
Sugar substitutes*
Vinegar

Salad dressings
Salad dressing, oil-free

Soups
Bouillon, fat-free
Broth and consommé, fat-free

Sweets
Gelatin, sugar-free*
Jam or jelly, sugar-free* (2 teaspoons)
Pancake syrup, sugar-free*

Vegetables
Chinese cabbage
Lettuce, all varieties
Parsley
Radishes

* Subject to current warnings about sugar substitutes.

Chapter 4

Using *The Living Heart Brand Name Shopper's Guide* to Prevent or Treat High Blood Pressure

High blood pressure often has no symptoms, and it is possible to have elevated blood pressure for years without knowing it. Dietary changes and other lifestyle modifications to help prevent high blood pressure are especially important because many people sustain heart, brain, kidney, or eye damage before their high blood pressure is discovered. Dietary measures to lower blood pressure include weight reduction (when appropriate), a decrease in alcohol intake, and sodium restriction. The classifications of blood pressure for adults 18 years of age or older are shown in the following table.

If you have elevated blood pressure, consult a physician.

CLASSIFICATIONS OF BLOOD PRESSURE FOR ADULTS*

Category	Systolic mm Hg	Diastolic mm Hg
Normal	Less than 130	Less than 85
High normal	130–139	85–89
High blood pressure		
Mild	140–159	90–99
Moderate	160–179	100–109
Severe	180–209	110–119
Very severe	210 or greater	120 or greater

mm Hg = millimeters of mercury.

*In a blood pressure reading, systolic is the top number, diastolic is the bottom number. Elevated and unusually low readings need to be evaluated by a physician.

DIETARY CHANGES

The following lifestyle changes are proven effective in lowering blood pressure. They help in both *prevention* and *treatment*.

- Weight reduction (if overweight)
- Regular physical activity
- Reduction of alcohol intake
- Reduction of sodium intake

CONTROLLING WEIGHT

One of the most important factors in the prevention and treatment of high blood pressure is weight control. Losing weight helps lower blood pressure. You do not have to reach your desirable weight to benefit from weight loss; in many people, a sustained loss of 10 pounds or more can bring mildly or moderately elevated blood pressure levels to normal. Weight loss has the additional benefit of enhancing the effectiveness of medications to lower blood pressure. Methods of weight reduction are covered in more detail in Chapter 3 (pages 26 to 38).

REDUCING ALCOHOL

Reducing a high alcohol intake can lower blood pressure. People who do drink alcohol should not exceed 2 drinks per day. The amount of alcohol considered 1 drink is shown on page 37. The calories in different alcoholic beverages are shown on pages 59–60.

REDUCING SODIUM

There is a strong association between the amount of sodium consumed and blood pressure. A low-sodium diet reduces blood pressure in people with blood pressure in the normal range as well as in those with high blood pressure. Most of the sodium in the American diet comes from salt and other sodium-containing compounds used in food processing and preparation. The American Heart Association recommends consuming less than 3,000 milligrams (mg) of sodium per day. The National High Blood Pressure Education Program recommends a daily intake for everyone of no more than 2,400 mg of sodium (the amount in 1$\frac{1}{8}$ teaspoons of table salt). The Daily Value for sodium used by the Food and Drug Administration (FDA) on food labels is 2,400 mg per day (see page 13). There are two methods you can use to lower your sodium:

COUNT MILLIGRAMS OF SODIUM
First, write down all the foods and beverages you consume. Next, look up their sodium values. This book, which lists sodium values for about 5,500 foods, will

be helpful; you can also find sodium information on the Nutrition Facts portion of food labels. Finally, add up the milligrams of sodium you have consumed in a day and compare your total with the recommended levels.

SELECT FOODS LOW IN SODIUM

Reviewing the sodium column in each Food Section of the Guide will help you identify foods that are the lowest in sodium. For example, 1 serving of ready-to-eat cereal (pages 89 to 96) can range from 0 to 610 mg of sodium. You can see that shredded wheat, puffed wheat, and puffed rice are the lowest in sodium. A table of recipe substitutions to reduce the amount of sodium in the foods you cook appears on page 264 of the Appendix. *The Living Heart Guide to Eating Out,* another book by the same authors, lists more than 100 tips for choosing lower-sodium foods when eating away from home. The following table lists foods that are high in sodium; they should be limited on a low-sodium diet.

COMMON FOODS HIGH IN SODIUM

Anchovies	Meat, kosher
Bacon	Nuts, salted
Barbecue sauce	Olives
Bologna	Pastrami
Bread and rolls (several servings a day)	Pepperoni
	Pickles
Buttermilk	Pizza
Cereal, ready-to-eat	Pretzels, salted
Cheese	Salad dressing (regular and fat-free)
Chips, potato, corn, and other snack chips, salted	Salami
	Sauerkraut
Corned beef	Sausage
Crackers with salted tops	Seeds, salted
Frankfurters	Soup, commercial (all regular types)
Frozen entrées and dinners (check label)	Soy sauce
	Steak sauce
Ham	Wieners (beef, pork, chicken, and turkey)
Jerky	
Meat, canned or frozen in sauce	Worcestershire sauce
Meat, cured	

OTHER DIETARY CHANGES

Research suggests that minerals such as potassium and calcium also affect blood pressure. These minerals appear to have the opposite effect of sodium, and consumption of foods high in potassium and calcium is recommended.

INCREASING POTASSIUM

Some studies have suggested that a low intake of potassium in the diet is associated with higher blood pressure and that a high potassium intake helps protect against developing high blood pressure. It is important to get an adequate amount of potassium. There is no Recommended Dietary Allowance for potassium; the amount used for the Daily Value on food labels is 3,500 mg. As you can see in the table below, eating fruits, vegetables, and beans can easily provide adequate potassium.

POTASSIUM CONTENT OF SELECTED FOODS

Food	Potassium mg
White beans, cooked (3/4 cup)	750
Salt substitute containing potassium (1/4 teaspoon)	715
Potato, white, baked, medium (1)	610
Pinto beans, cooked (3/4 cup)	600
Yogurt, low-fat, plain (1 cup)	575
Baked beans, vegetarian, canned (3/4 cup)	565
Lentils, cooked (3/4 cup)	550
Lima beans, cooked (3/4 cup)	545
Kidney beans, cooked (3/4 cup)	535
Tomato juice, salt-free (1 cup)	535
Cantaloupe, cubed (1 cup)	495
Orange juice, frozen, reconstituted (1 cup)	475
Yogurt, low-fat, with fruit (1 cup)	475
Black beans, cooked (3/4 cup)	460
Honeydew melon, cubed (1 cup)	460
Tomatoes, unsalted, canned (3/4 cup)	460
Apricots, dried, uncooked (9 halves, or 1/4 cup)	450
Banana, large (1)	450
Milk, low-fat, protein-fortified (1 cup)	445
Spinach, frozen, cooked (3/4 cup)	425

Food	Potassium mg
Brussels sprouts, frozen, cooked (³/4 cup)	380
Grapefruit juice (1 cup)	380
Milk, low-fat (1 cup)	380
Pork, tenderloin, cooked (3 ounces)	370
Watermelon, cubed (2 cups)	370
Carrot juice (¹/2 cup)	360
Prune juice (¹/2 cup)	355
Prunes, dried, medium (5)	315
Avocado (¹/4 medium)	300
Apple juice (1 cup)	295
Flounder, cooked (3 ounces)	290
Nectarine (1)	290
Beef, round, cooked (3 ounces)	285
Blackberries (1 cup)	280
Pink salmon, unsalted, canned (3 ounces)	275
Beets, sliced, canned (³/4 cup)	260
Tomato, fresh (1 medium)	255
Strawberries, sliced (1 cup)	250
Carrot, raw (1)	235
Orange (1)	235
Cherries, sweet, raw (15)	230
Turkey, unprocessed, roasted (3 ounces)	225
Chicken, roasted (3 ounces)	205
Tuna, water-packed, unsalted (¹/2 cup)	200
Grapefruit, medium (¹/2)	165

Potassium values rounded to nearest 5; mg = milligrams.

*From *The New Living Heart Diet*, by DeBakey, M.E., Gotto, A.M., Scott, L.W., et al., Simon & Schuster, New York, 1996.

Calcium is the mineral present in the largest amount in the human body. It is vitally important in the structure of bone. Some studies have suggested that a low calcium intake contributes to high blood pressure.

Dairy products are the best sources of calcium. Other foods, such as broccoli, contain some calcium; however, the amount is much lower than that supplied by dairy products. The Recommended Dietary Allowance for calcium is 1,200 mg for both males and females 11 to 24 years of age and 800 mg for younger children and for adults 25 years of age and above. The FDA uses 1,000 mg of calcium for the Daily Value on food labels. The following table lists some good sources of calcium.

CALCIUM CONTENT OF SELECTED FOODS

Food	Calcium mg
Yogurt, nonfat, plain (8 ounces)	450
Yogurt, low-fat, with fruit (8 ounces)	385
Milk, skim (1 cup)	300
Tofu, raw, firm (1/2 cup)	260
Salmon, canned, with bones (3 ounces)	205
Cheese, fat-free (1 ounce)	200
Mozzarella cheese, part skim milk (1 ounce)	185
Rhubarb, cooked, sweetened (1/2 cup)	175
Molasses, blackstrap (2 tablespoons)	170
Frozen yogurt, nonfat, chocolate (1/2 cup)	155
Ice milk, hardened (1/2 cup)	90
Broccoli, fresh, cooked (1/2 cup)	90
Cottage cheese, 1% fat (1/2 cup)	70

Calcium values rounded to nearest 5; mg = milligrams.

*From *The New Living Heart Diet,* by DeBakey, M.E., Gotto, A.M., Scott, L.W., et al., Simon & Schuster, New York, 1996.

Using *The Living Heart Brand Name Shopper's Guide* to Manage Diabetes

Many people with diabetes mellitus are treated with lifestyle changes such as diet, weight control, and appropriate physical activity; others may also require oral medication or insulin injections. A diabetic eating plan is designed to control blood sugar levels and achieve and maintain a desirable body weight. Diabetes is a major independent risk factor for coronary heart disease; therefore, it is especially important for people with diabetes to control their levels of blood cholesterol and triglyceride. Reaching a desirable body weight and reducing total fat, saturated fat, and dietary cholesterol to control blood cholesterol and triglyceride levels are important goals in the nutritional management of diabetes.

CARBOHYDRATE

Total carbohydrate is also important in a diabetic eating plan because the amount of carbohydrate consumed affects blood glucose levels. The Food Sections in this book include values for carbohydrate. Individuals whose diabetic eating plan includes "counting grams of carbohydrate" should refer to the Food Sections to determine grams of carbohydrate for specific foods.

SUGARS IN FOOD

The "sugars" listed in the Nutrition Facts portion of food labels include all nutritive sweeteners (sweeteners providing calories) except the sugar alcohols (sorbitol, xylitol, and mannitol). Consumption of both sugars and sugar alcohols is restricted in diabetic eating plans. Check the list of ingredients to determine whether the food contains sugars or sugar alcohols. The following table lists the most common nutritive sweeteners.

COMMON NUTRITIVE SWEETENERS

Corn syrup
Dextrose (glucose)
Fructose
Fruit juice or fruit juice concentrate
High-fructose corn syrup
Honey
Maltose
Mannitol*
Maple syrup
Molasses
Sorbitol*
Sucrose (table sugar)
Sugar
Turbinado (partially refined cane sugar)
Xylitol*

* Sugar alcohols.

NUTRIENT CONTENT CLAIMS

The Food and Drug Administration allows the following Nutrient Content Claims regarding sugars in food. Check the list of ingredients on the food label because foods qualifying for the Nutrient Content Claims in this list may still contain sugar alcohols.

- "Sugar Free"—less than 0.5 gram of sugars per serving and with no ingredient that is sugar
- "Reduced/Less Sugar"—at least 25% less sugars per serving than reference food
- "No Added Sugar"—no sugar or ingredient containing sugar is added during processing

CONTROLLING WEIGHT

More than 80% of patients with type II diabetes (also known as non-insulin-dependent or late-onset diabetes) are overweight at the time their disease is diagnosed. For these people, reaching and maintaining a reasonable weight, which reduces blood glucose levels, is given high priority. Someone who is overweight and diabetic does not have to reach his or her desirable weight to benefit from weight loss; moderate weight loss can improve blood glucose levels. For more information on weight control, see Chapter 3.

FAT AND DIETARY CHOLESTEROL

It is important for someone with diabetes to control fat, saturated fat, and cholesterol intake to reduce elevated levels of blood cholesterol and triglyceride. Fat reduction may also result in the consumption of fewer calories, which can lead to weight reduction. For more information on a diet low in fat and cholesterol, see Chapter 2.

DETECTING DIABETES

It is important to be aware of the warning signs of diabetes since it is estimated that 6% of Americans have this disease. More than half of these people have had their disease diagnosed, but the others do not know that they are diabetic. You should see your physician if you experience two or more of the following symptoms:

- Blurred vision
- Dry skin or dry mouth
- Frequent urination
- Excessive thirst
- Extreme hunger
- Unexplained weight loss
- Irritability
- Weakness and fatigue
- Drowsiness
- Itching
- Tingling or numbness in hands and feet
- Recurring or hard-to-heal infections of the skin, gums, or bladder
- Nausea or vomiting

At present, diabetes is considered a disease that can be controlled but not cured. A combination of diet, exercise, weight control, glucose monitoring, and, when necessary, medication can be used to control blood glucose levels and may prevent the complications of diabetes.

Using *The Living Heart Brand Name Shopper's Guide* to Increase Fiber

In recent years there has been increased interest in fiber's role in a healthy diet and in the prevention of certain types of cancer. Cancer is the second leading killer of adults in America, exceeded only by cardiovascular diseases. A diet low in fat and high in fiber-containing grains, fruits, and vegetables has been linked to a reduced risk for cancer.

Fiber is a carbohydrate that has no calories because the body cannot digest it. There are two types of fiber—soluble and insoluble. Some studies have shown that the blood cholesterol lowering that results from an eating plan low in fat and saturated fat can be increased by a further 2% to 3% by the addition of 2 ounces of an oat cereal (oat bran or oatmeal), a source of soluble fiber. Insoluble fiber does not affect blood cholesterol levels; however, it aids in proper elimination.

It is difficult to assess with accuracy the fiber intake of Americans. It is estimated that the average intake is between 11 and 13 grams per day. The minimum fiber intake recommended is 11.5 grams per 1,000 calories consumed, or about 25 grams at the 2,000-calorie level. This is the amount used on food labels to determine the Daily Value (see page 50). Many Americans need at least to double their fiber intake to reach the recommended level. The Food and Drug Administration requires that all food labels include the grams of dietary fiber per serving. This value is listed under Total Carbohydrate on the label.

You can use the fiber column in the Food Sections of this book to estimate your fiber intake. You will notice that most dairy products, meat products, and sweets (desserts, cookies, cakes, candy) have very little if any fiber. The best sources of fiber, and the numbers of the pages where these foods are listed, are shown in the following table.

FIBER IN SELECTED FOODS

Food 1 serving*	Fiber g
Beans	
Canned (see page 249)	3–11
Dried (see page 257)	5–7
Bean soups (see page 228)	2–13
Bran breads (see page 76)	3–6
Bran cereals, ready-to-eat (see page 89)	3–15
Cooked cereals (see page 87)	1–7
Fresh fruit (see page 163)	1–6
Vegetables	
Canned (see page 248)	1–4
Fresh (see page 257)	1–8

g = grams.

* One serving as specified in this book for each food.

Chapter 7

Using Food Labels in
The Living Heart Brand Name Shopper's Guide

The Nutrition Facts section of each food label provides valuable information about the nutrient content of foods. Information that is a required part of each food label is shown in the sample on the following page.

More than 200 food manufacturers provided the values for calories, fat, saturated fat, carbohydrate, fiber, and sodium that were used to develop *The Living Heart Brand Name Shopper's Guide*. The only criteria used to evaluate foods for inclusion in the Guide were fat content and saturated fat content; the grams of fat and saturated fat in a serving of each food were carefully compared with the cutoff points described on pages 52–53.

DAILY VALUES

The Daily Value that appears in the Nutrition Facts portion of the food label provides a basis for comparing the food's nutrient content with a "standard" daily intake. The Daily Values for fat, saturated fat, carbohydrate, and dietary fiber are based on calorie intake; a reference level of 2,000 calories is used on food labels. Daily Values for these nutrients increase or decrease as the calorie intake increases or decreases. The reference values used on food labels are shown below:
- Fat based on 30% of 2,000 calories equals 65 grams
- Saturated fat based on 10% of 2,000 calories equals 20 grams
- Carbohydrate based on 60% of 2,000 calories equals 300 grams
- Dietary fiber based on 2,000 calories equals 25 grams

Serving sizes are stated in both household and metric measures. The serving sizes, which reflect the amounts people actually eat, are consistent across product lines.

The list of nutrients includes those of most importance to the health of consumers, most of whom need to avoid getting *too much* of certain nutrients (such as fat, and cholesterol) and *too little* of other nutrients (such as fiber and certain vitamins and minerals).

The label lists the number of calories per gram of fat, carbohydrates, and protein.

NUTRITION FACTS

Serving Size 1/2 cup (114g)

Servings Per Container 4

Amount Per Serving

Calories 90   Calories from Fat 30

	% Daily Value*
Total Fat 3g	**5%**
Saturated Fat 0g	**0%**
Cholesterol 0mg	**0%**
Sodium 300mg	**13%**
Total Carbohydrates 13g	**4%**
Dietary Fiber 3g	**12%**
Sugars 3g	
Protein 3g	

Vitamin A 80%	•	Vitamin C 60%
Calcium 4%	•	Iron 4%

*Percent Daily Values are based on a 2,000-calorie diet. Your daily values may be higher or lower depending on your calorie needs:

	Calories	2,000	2,500
Total Fat	Less than	65g	80g
Sat Fat	Less than	20g	25g
Cholesterol	Less than	300mg	300mg
Sodium	Less than	2,400mg	2,400mg
Total Carbohydrate		300g	375g
Fiber		25g	30g

Calories per gram:
Fat 9 • Carbohydrates 4 • Protein 4

Calories from fat are shown on the label to help consumers meet dietary guidelines that recommend people get no more than 30% of their calories from fat.

% Daily Value shows how a food fits into an overall daily diet at the 2,000-calorie level.

Most labels provide the grams of fat, saturated fat, carbohydrate, and fiber and the milligrams of cholesterol and sodium that represent the Daily Value at 2,000 calories; some labels also provide the Daily Values at the 2,500-calorie level.

People consuming more or less than 2,000 calories will need to adjust the Daily Values for fat, saturated fat, carbohydrate, and fiber to fit their own calorie intake. For example, many women who need to lose weight require about 1,200 calories. At this calorie level, the Daily Value is 40 grams for fat, 13 grams for saturated fat, 180 grams for carbohydrate, 30 grams for protein, and 14 grams for dietary fiber. Daily Values for dietary cholesterol (less than 300 milligrams) and sodium (less than 2,400 milligrams) are the same at all calorie levels.

For some nutrients, the Daily Value is the *uppermost* limit that is considered desirable. For example, it is recommended that healthy Americans with an intake of 2,000 calories consume *less than* the 65 grams of fat and *less than* the 20 grams of saturated fat listed above. Daily Values for carbohydrate and fiber are the *minimum* intake recommended — that is, the recommendation is for 300 grams *or more* of carbohydrate and for 25 grams *or more* of fiber at the 2,000-calorie level.

The percent Daily Values are intended to help consumers understand the part of a total day's intake provided by a serving of each food. For example, a food with 140 milligrams of sodium could be mistaken for a high-sodium food because 140 is a fairly large number. The information that 140 milligrams is in fact less than 6% of the Daily Value for sodium (2,400 milligrams per day) helps put the sodium content of the food into perspective. On the other hand, someone choosing 1/2 cup of rich ice cream containing 17 grams of fat might not realize how high in fat the food is until he or she sees that the 17 grams represents more than 25% of the Daily Value for fat.

CUTOFF POINTS FOR FOODS

Cutoff points for fat and saturated fat were used to evaluate foods for inclusion in the Guide. A cutoff point is the *upper limit* of fat or saturated fat that can be present in 1 serving of a food for it to be included in the Guide. The definition of a serving is on page 53. Some foods listed in the Guide may contain ingredients (egg yolk, butter, cream, palm kernel oil, coconut oil, beef fat, lard) that are high in fat and saturated fat. However, such small amounts of these ingredients are present that the food is still under the cutoff points for fat and saturated fat.

Most of the cutoff points used in the Guide are the same as the levels of fat and saturated fat established by the Food and Drug Administration (FDA) for the Nutrient Content Claims of "low fat" (3 grams of fat per serving) and "low saturated fat" (1 gram of fat per serving). The authors chose to make two exceptions:

1) dairy products and 2) foods high in fat that are low in saturated fat, such as oils, margarines, salad dressings, nuts, and seeds.

The dairy products listed in the Guide are low in fat; however, some of them are not low enough in saturated fat to meet the FDA definition of "low saturated fat." Dairy products are an excellent source of calcium. Limiting them to 1 gram of saturated fat per serving eliminates virtually all dairy products except those labeled "nonfat," "fat free," or "skim." Therefore, a cutoff point for saturated fat of 2 grams per serving was used for dairy products and milk-based frozen desserts (as shown in the table below).

Oils, margarines, salad dressings, nuts, and seeds that are high in fat but low in saturated fat have been included in the Guide because, in limited amounts, they can be part of a cholesterol-lowering eating plan. Therefore, no cutoff point was used for fat, and a cutoff point of 2 grams per serving was used for saturated fat in these higher-fat foods (as shown in the table below). Although all types of oil contain the same amount of fat and calories, oils differ in the amount of saturated fat they provide.

CUTOFF POINTS PER SERVING OF FOOD

Food	Fat g	Saturated Fat g
Meat		
"Lean" meat, poultry, fish, and game (3 oz cooked)	9	3
"Lean" luncheon meat (2 oz)	6	2
Dairy products (including milk-based frozen desserts)	3	2
Main dishes and meal-type products (per 100 g)*	3	1
Oil, margarine, salad dressing, nuts, and seeds	†	2
All other foods	3	1

g = grams; oz = ounces.

* A table on page 171 shows the amounts of fat and saturated fat to be used as cutoff points for various weights of main dishes and meal-type products.

† No cutoff point for fat; since oil, margarine, salad dressing, nuts, and seeds are naturally high in fat, the amount of saturated fat is used as the cutoff point.

SERVING SIZES

The amount of each brand name food listed in the Guide is 1 serving as indicated by the manufacturer. In most cases, these servings are the same as the standard servings established by the FDA and by the U.S. Department of Agriculture

(USDA) for use in food labeling. Although the serving sizes differ from one type of food to another (for example, frozen dessert has a different serving size than either cooked cereal or mustard), they are the same for all brands of the same food (all brands of frozen dessert have the same serving size). In cases in which the serving size on the label differed from the standard serving size, the amount of fat and saturated fat in 1 standard serving of the brand name food was calculated and compared with the cutoff points to determine whether the food could be listed in the Guide. For example, the cutoff points were applied to a standard 8-ounce serving of all brands of yogurt, even though manufacturers package yogurt in 4.4-ounce, 6-ounce, and 8-ounce containers. The serving size used by the manufacturer, which sometimes differs from the standard serving size, appears in the Guide.

PREPARATION OF FOOD PRODUCTS

Products listed in the Guide must meet the cutoff points 1) as purchased, 2) when prepared according to package directions, or 3) when prepared with ingredients listed next to that food in the Guide. As a rule, the Guide does not include products requiring preparation if the completed product produced by adding the ingredients in the package directions is not low enough in fat and saturated fat to meet the cutoff points. In a few cases, however, the Guide lists specific instructions for preparation. For example, the values for pudding printed in the Guide are for the dry mix combined with skim milk instead of the whole milk usually called for in the package directions.

ESTIMATED VALUES

Information from the manufacturers included values for calories, fat, carbohydrate, and sodium for every brand name food listed in the Guide. For a few foods, values for saturated fat and fiber were not available. These entries were handled in one of two ways. If possible, the missing values were estimated and listed in parentheses; if they could not be estimated, "NA" (not available) was noted.

BRAND NAME AND GENERIC FOODS

The food table contains both brand name and generic entries. For brand name products, the name is that on the food label. Generic entries are used in some sections of the food table when all the brand name foods in a section contain approximately the same amount of calories, fat, saturated fat, carbohydrate, fiber, and sodium. For example, specific brand names for coffee, plain low-fat cottage cheese, and skim milk are not used in the Guide because all brands have about the same nutrient content. The values for the generic entries came from the USDA Handbook No. 8 Series or the Nutrition Data System (University of Minnesota). These generic entries are indicated in one of two ways. Some sections such as fresh fruits, fresh vegetables, and fresh meats contain only generic entries; foods are simply listed in these sections. In sections that contain both generic and brand name foods, the generic entries are indicated as "Most Brands."

FOODS NOT APPEARING IN THE GUIDE

There are several possible reasons why a food may not appear in the Guide.

- Some foods have more fat and/or saturated fat in 1 serving than the cutoff points shown on page 53. Some mixes are not listed in the Guide because following the package directions results in a completed product too high in fat and/or saturated fat; these mixes might have qualified if some of the added ingredients were changed. For example, some cake mixes and pancake mixes are not listed in the Guide because they require the addition of eggs, oil, and whole milk in preparation. These ingredients make the completed product higher than the cutoff points for fat. However, decreasing the amount of oil and substituting egg white or egg substitute and skim milk for the ingredients listed on the package can result in a finished product that is lower in fat and cholesterol.
- The food manufacturer may not have supplied nutrition information or may not have given the authors permission to include the information in the Guide.
- Some foods are too new to have been evaluated by the authors.
- Some foods were simply missed. If you have a question about a food not in the Guide, compare the information on the Nutrition Facts portion of the label with the table on page 53 or the tables at the beginning of each of the Food Sections in this book.

FOOD SECTIONS

ABBREVIATIONS, SIGNS, AND SYMBOLS

The following abbreviations, signs, and symbols have been used in the Food Sections:

&	=	and
diam	=	diameter
env	=	envelope
fl oz	=	fluid ounce
g	=	gram
"	=	inch
<	=	less than
med	=	medium
mg	=	milligram
NA	=	not available
oz	=	ounce
pkg	=	package
pkt	=	packet
%	=	percent
prep w/	=	prepared with
prep w/o	=	prepared without
sm	=	small
tbsp	=	tablespoon
tsp	=	teaspoon
w/	=	with

Estimated values are in parentheses ( ).

BEVERAGES

Most of the beverages and beverage flavorings in this section of the Guide contain very little or no fat. These products were evaluated according to how they will be consumed—*as purchased, prepared according to package directions, or prepared with skim milk* (as indicated next to the individual food in the Guide). A serving of the foods in this section of the Guide contains a maximum of 3 grams of fat and 1 gram of saturated fat.

Alcoholic Beverage Mixes

	Calories	Fat g	Saturated Fat g	Carbohydrate g	Fiber g	Sodium mg
ALCOHOLIC BEVERAGE MIXES						
Bacardi Tropical Fruit Mixers, Margarita (8 fl oz)	100	0	0	25	0	0
Pina Colada (8 fl oz)	140	0	0	34	0	10
Rum Runner (8 fl oz)	140	0	0	35	0	10
Strawberry Daiquiri (8 fl oz)	140	0	0	35	0	0
V8 Bloody Mary Mix (11.5 oz container)	90	1	1	17	2	1,440
ALCOHOLIC BEVERAGES						
Higher-Fat						
Brandy Alexander (4 fl oz)	276	8	5	23	0	17
Eggnog w/Brandy (6 fl oz)	192	11	6	19	0	78
Grasshopper (4 fl oz)	299	8	5	36	0	17
Hot Buttered Rum (4 fl oz)	145	6	3	2	0	2
Irish Creme Liqueur (4 fl oz)	355	8	5	38	0	119
Pina Colada, not frozen (6 fl oz)	317	4	3	41	0	4
Russian Bear (8 fl oz)	252	4	2	18	0	14
Fat-Free						
Beer, Light (12 fl oz)	101	0	0	5	0	11

Alcoholic Beverages (continued)	Calories	Fat g	Saturated Fat g	Carbohydrate g	Fiber g	Sodium mg
Beer (continued)						
Malt Liquor (12 fl oz)	148	0	0	13	2	18
Near Beer (12 fl oz)	148	0	0	38	0	47
Regular (12 fl oz)	148	0	0	13	2	18
Liqueur, Coffee (1½ fl oz)	126	0	0	25	0	1
Creme de Menthe (1½ fl oz)	121	0	0	14	0	1
Liquor, Gin, Rum, Vodka or Whiskey (1½ fl oz)	96	0	0	0	0	0
Wine, Dessert (3 fl oz)	138	0	0	11	0	8
Red or White Table (5 fl oz)	103	0	0	2	0	12
BEVERAGE MEAL REPLACEMENTS						
Higher-Fat						
Chocolate Instant Breakfast, prep w/8 fl oz whole milk (8 fl oz)	280	9	6	35	1	255
Lower-Fat						
Carnation Instant Breakfasts, No Sugar Added, Classic Chocolate Malt, prep w/1 cup skim milk (9 fl oz)	160	2	1	24	1	240
Creamy Milk Chocolate, prep w/1 cup skim milk (9 fl oz)	160	1	1	24	1	216
French Vanilla or Strawberry Creme, prep w/1 cup skim milk (9 fl oz)	150	0	0	24	0	216
Carnation Instant Breakfasts, Cafe Mocha (10 fl oz can)	220	3	1	35	0	210
Cafe Mocha, prep w/1 cup skim milk (9 fl oz)	220	0	0	39	1	216
Classic Chocolate Malt, prep w/1 cup skim milk (9 fl oz)	220	2	1	39	1	240
Creamy Milk Chocolate (10 fl oz can)	220	3	1	37	1	230
Creamy Milk Chocolate, prep w/1 cup skim milk (9 fl oz)	220	1	1	39	1	240
French Vanilla, prep w/1 cup skim milk (9 fl oz)	220	0	0	39	0	240
Strawberry Creme, prep w/1 cup skim milk (9 fl oz)	220	0	0	39	0	288

Beverage Meal Replacements (continued)	Calories	Fat g	Saturated Fat g	Carbohydrate g	Fiber g	Sodium mg
Nestlé Sweet Success, Chocolate Mocha Supreme, Chocolate Raspberry Truffle, Dark Chocolate Fudge or Smooth Vanilla Creme (10 fl oz can)	200	3	1	38	6	220
Chocolate Mocha Supreme, prep w/1 cup skim milk (9 fl oz)	180	2	1	30	6	170
Chocolate Raspberry Truffle, prep w/1 cup skim milk (9 fl oz)	180	2	1	30	6	360
Creamy Milk Chocolate or Dark Chocolate Fudge, prep w/1 cup skim milk (9 fl oz)	180	2	1	30	6	336
Creamy Milk Chocolate or Rich Chocolate Almond (10 fl oz can)	200	3	1	38	6	240
Creamy Milk Chocolate, Dark Chocolate Fudge or Rich Chocolate Almond, refrigerated (12 fl oz)	220	2	1	45	6	300-310
Creamy Vanilla Delight, prep w/1 cup skim milk (9 fl oz)	180	0	1	33	6	312
Rich Chocolate Almond, prep w/1 cup skim milk (9 fl oz)	180	1	1	30	6	336
Pillsbury Instant Breakfasts, Chocolate or Variety Pack, prep w/1 cup skim milk (8 fl oz)	220	2	1	40	0	320
Sego Lite Chocolate (10 fl oz can)	150	3	0	21	0	400
Very Chocolate or Very Chocolate Malt (10 fl oz can)	240	2	0	44	0	310
Slim-Fast Chocolate Malt Flavored Powder, prep w/1 cup skim milk (8 oz)	190	1	1	32	2	230
Chocolate, Strawberry or Vanilla Flavored Powder, prep w/1 cup skim milk (8 oz)	190	1	1	32	2	236-256
Ultra Slim-Fast Apple-Cranberry-Raspberry (11.5 oz)	220	2	1	53	5	190
Cafe Mocha Flavored Powder, prep w/1 cup skim milk (8 oz)	200	1	1	38	6	280
Chocolate Malt Flavored Powder, prep w/1 cup skim milk (8 oz)	196	1	1	37	5	226
Chocolate Royale (11 oz can)	220	3	1	38	5	220

	Calories	Fat g	Saturated Fat g	Carbohydrate g	Fiber g	Sodium mg
Ultra Slim-Fast *(continued)*						
Chocolate Royale Flavored Powder, prep w/1 cup skim milk (8 oz)	200	1	1	37	5	226
Coffee (11 oz can)	200	3	1	37	5	300
Dutch Chocolate Flavored Water Mixable Powder, prep w/1 cup water (8 oz)	220	<1	0	40	5	260
French Vanilla (11 oz can)	230	3	1	38	5	250
French Vanilla or Strawberry Supreme Flavored Powder, prep w/1 cup skim milk (8 oz)	200	1	1	37	4	266
Fruit Juice Mixable Powder, prep w/1 cup juice (8 oz)	200	<1	0	44	6	30
Golden Apple (11.5 oz)	220	2	1	44	5	190
Milk Chocolate (11 oz can)	200	3	1	36	5	180
Orange-Pineapple (11.5 oz can)	220	2	1	54	5	190
Orange-Strawberry-Banana (11.5 oz can)	220	2	1	53	5	190
Strawberry Supreme (11 oz can)	230	3	1	42	5	250
Ultra Slim-Fast Plus Chocolate Fantasy Flavored Powder, prep w/1½ cups skim milk (12 oz)	250	2	(1)	50	8	330
CARBONATED BEVERAGES						
Most Brands, Club Soda (8 fl oz)	0	0	0	0	0	50
Cream Soda (8 fl oz)	101	0	0	26	0	32
Diet Cola, sweetened w/aspartame (8 fl oz)	0	0	0	0	0	16
Tonic Water (8 fl oz)	98	0	0	26	0	27
Cascadia Sparkling Water w/Juice, Pink Grapefruit, Raspberry Black Currant, Lemonade, Guava, Cherry Blackberry or Wild Berry (12.5 fl oz)	5	0	0	0	0	0
Coca-Cola Caffeine-free or Regular Coca-Cola Classic (8 fl oz)	97	0	0	27	0	9
Caffeine-free or Regular Diet Coke (8 fl oz)	1	0	0	0	0	4
Cherry Coca-Cola (8 fl oz)	104	0	0	28	0	4
Coke II (8 fl oz)	105	0	0	29	0	4
Diet Cherry Coca-Cola (8 fl oz)	1	0	0	0	0	4

Carbonated Beverages (continued)	Calories	Fat g	Saturated Fat g	Carbohydrate g	Fiber g	Sodium mg
Fanta Ginger Ale (8 fl oz)	86	0	0	23	0	4
Grape Soda (8 fl oz)	117	0	0	31	0	9
Orange Soda (8 fl oz)	118	0	0	32	0	9
Root Beer (8 fl oz)	111	0	0	29	0	4
Fresca Grapefruit Soda (8 fl oz)	3	0	0	0	0	1
Hansen's Natural Sodas, Cherry (12 oz)	130	0	0	35	0	0
Clear Cola (12 oz)	140	0	0	39	0	0
Clear Root Beer (12 oz)	140	0	0	40	0	0
Grapefruit or Kiwi Strawberry (12 oz)	130	0	0	38	0	0
Lemon-Lime, Mandarin Lime, Peach or Raspberry (12 oz)	130	0	0	37	0	0
Health Valley Ginger Ale, Old Fashioned Root Beer, Sarsaprilla Root Beer or Wild Berry Soda (12 fl oz)	160	0	0	40	0	0
Koala Springs Sparkling Mineral Water w/Essence of Lemon, w/Essence of Lime or Natural (8 fl oz)	0	0	0	0	0	0
Koala Springs Sparkling Mineral Water & Fruit Juice Flavor, Cranberry & Melon, Kiwi, Lime & Grapefruit, Raspberry & Guava or Wild Cherry (8 fl oz)	100	0	0	25	0	25
Lemon or Lime & Orange (8 fl oz)	100	0	0	23	0	25
Mandarin & Orange (8 fl oz)	90	0	0	22	0	25
Orange & Mango or Strawberry & Peach (8 fl oz)	100	0	0	24	0	25
Mello Yello Lemon-Lime Soda (8 fl oz)	119	0	0	32	0	9
Diet (8 fl oz)	4	0	0	0	0	0
Minute Maid Sodas, Berry or Raspberry (8 fl oz)	111	0	0	30	0	9
Black Cherry (8 fl oz)	110	0	0	29	0	11
Diet Orange (8 fl oz)	2	0	0	0	0	0
Fruit Punch (8 fl oz)	117	0	0	32	0	10
Grape (8 fl oz)	121	0	0	32	0	9
Grapefruit (8 fl oz)	108	0	0	29	0	9
Orange (8 fl oz)	118	0	0	32	0	0
Peach (8 fl oz)	110	0	0	29	0	9
Pineapple (8 fl oz)	109	0	0	30	0	9
Strawberry (8 fl oz)	122	0	0	33	0	9

	Calories	Fat g	Saturated Fat g	Carbohydrate g	Fiber g	Sodium mg
Carbonated Beverages (continued)						
Mountain Valley Spring America's Premium Mountain Valley Spring Water (8 fl oz)	0	0	0	0	0	0
Mr. Pibb Pepper-Type Cola (8 fl oz)	97	0	0	26	0	7
Diet (8 fl oz)	1	0	0	0	0	2
Royal Mistic All Natural Flavored Beverage w/Sparkling Water, Black Cherry (8 fl oz)	100	0	0	26	0	40
Peach Vanilla, Tangerine Orange or Tropical Supreme (8 fl oz)	100	0	0	26	0	10
Wild Berry (8 fl oz)	100	0	0	27	0	5
Natural Spring Water (8 fl oz)	0	0	0	0	0	0
Sprite Lemon-Lime Soda (8 fl oz)	100	0	0	26	0	31
Diet (8 fl oz)	3	0	0	0	0	0
Tab Diet Cola (8 fl oz)	1	0	0	0	0	4
COCOA MIXES						
Higher-Fat						
Cocoa Mix prep w/whole milk (8 fl oz)	224	9	6	31	1	164
Lower-Fat						
Alpine Light Cocoa Mixes, Irish Cream, Bavarian Chocolate Cream or Swiss Mocha (1 pouch = 6–8 fl oz)	60	2	1	8	1	160
Swiss Miss Hot Cocoa Mixes, Diet, prep w/water (6 oz)	20	<1	0	3	0	180
Double Rich, prep w/water (6 oz)	110	1	1	22	0	150
Lite, prep w/water (6 oz)	70	<1	0	17	0	160
Milk Chocolate, prep w/water (6 oz)	110	1	0	24	0	125
Sugar Free w/Sugar Free Marshmallows, prep w/water (6 oz)	50	<1	0	9	0	120
Sugar Free, prep w/water (6 oz)	60	<1	0	10	0	125
w/Mini Marshmallows, prep w/water (6 oz)	110	1	0	23	0	170
Weight Watchers Hot Cocoa Mixes, Plain or w/Marshmallows (1 env)	70	0	0	10	1	150-160

	Calories	Fat g	Saturated Fat g	Carbohydrate g	Fiber g	Sodium mg

COFFEES

Higher-Saturated Fat

	Calories	Fat g	Saturated Fat g	Carbohydrate g	Fiber g	Sodium mg
Suisse Mocha Flavored Instant Coffee, prep w/water (8 fl oz)	80	3	2	14	1	135

Lower-Saturated Fat

	Calories	Fat g	Saturated Fat g	Carbohydrate g	Fiber g	Sodium mg
Most Brands, Coffee, Brewed, decaffeinated, unsweetened (8 fl oz)	5	0	0	1	0	7
Regular, unsweetened (8 fl oz)	8	0	0	1	0	5
Most Brands, Coffee, Instant, decaffeinated or regular, prep w/water (8 fl oz)	5	0	0	1	0	7
Cafix All Natural Coffee Substitute (1.5 grams)	6	0	0	1	0	3
General Foods International Instant Coffees, Cafe Amaretto Flavored, prep w/water (8 fl oz)	60	3	1	8	0	105
Cafe Vienna Flavored, prep w/water (8 fl oz)	70	3	1	11	0	110
French Vanilla Cafe Flavored, prep w/water (8 fl oz)	60	3	1	10	0	55
Hazelnut Belgian Cafe Flavored, prep w/water (8 fl oz)	70	2	1	12	0	65
Italian Cappuccino Flavored, prep w/water (8 fl oz)	50	2	1	10	0	50
Kahlua Cafe Flavored, prep w/water (8 fl oz)	60	2	1	10	0	55
Orange Cappuccino Flavored, prep w/water (8 fl oz)	70	2	1	11	0	100
Suisse Mocha Flavored, prep w/water (8 fl oz)	60	3	1	8	0	50
Suisse Mocha Flavored, Decaffeinated, prep w/water (8 fl oz)	60	3	1	8	0	40
Viennese Chocolate Cafe Flavored, prep w/water (8 fl oz)	60	2	1	10	0	30
General Foods International Instant Coffees, Sugar Free Low Calorie, Cafe Vienna or Orange Cappuccino Flavored, prep w/water (8 fl oz)	30	2	1	3	0	75
French Vanilla Cafe Flavored, prep w/water (8 fl oz)	35	2	1	4	0	55

	Calories	Fat g	Saturated Fat g	Carbohydrate g	Fiber g	Sodium mg
General Foods International Instant Coffees *(continued)*						
Suisse Mocha Flavored, prep w/water (8 fl oz)	30	2	1	4	0	30
Suisse Mocha Flavored, Decaffeinated, prep w/water (8 fl oz)	30	2	1	4	0	35
Maxwell House Cinnamon Cappuccino, prep w/water (8 fl oz)	90	2	0	16	0	70
Coffee Cappuccino, prep w/water (8 fl oz)	90	1	0	18	0	65
Vanilla Cappuccino, prep w/water (8 fl oz)	90	1	0	19	0	65
Vanilla Cappuccino, Decaffeinated, prep w/water (8 fl oz)	90	1	0	19	0	65
Postum Coffee Flavor or Plain Instant Hot Beverage, prep w/water (8 fl oz)	10	0	0	3	0	0
FLAVORED MILK BEVERAGES						
Hershey's Banana Split, Chocolate Caramel, Chocolate Cherry, Chocolate Marshmallow, or Genuine Chocolate Flavored Drink (8 fl oz container)	160	3	0	29	1	115
Chocolate Milk Mix (2 tbsp)	70	0	0	17	0	30
Strawberry Drink (8 fl oz container)	140	2	0	26	0	90
Kraft Instant Malted Milks, Chocolate Flavored, prep w/skim milk (1 cup)	166	1	0	29	<1	166
Natural Flavored, prep w/skim milk (1 cup)	176	2	1	27	0	211
Weight Watchers Chocolate Yogurt Shake (7½ fl oz shake)	220	1	0	44	3	140
Weight Watchers Shake Mixes, Chocolate Fudge (.75 oz)	80	1	0	12	2	140
Orange (.75 oz)	70	0	0	12	NA	210
FRUIT-FLAVORED BEVERAGES (NONCARBONATED)						
Alpine Spiced Cider Drink Mixes, Regular (1 pkt = 6–8 fl oz)	80	0	0	19	0	20
Sugar Free (1 pkt = 6–8 fl oz)	15	0	0	4	0	25
America's Choice Grape Juice Cocktail, from frozen (8 fl oz)	130	0	0	33	0	10

Fruit-Flavored Beverages (continued)	Calories	Fat g	Saturated Fat g	Carbohydrate g	Fiber g	Sodium mg
Betty Crocker Squeezits, Chucklin' Cherry, Grumpy Grape, Mean Green Punch, Red Punch, Silly Billy Strawberry or Wildberry (6 2/3 fl oz bottle)	110	0	0	27	0	0
Smarty Arty Orange (6 2/3 fl oz bottle)	110	0	0	27	0	45
Bright & Early Beverages, Apple, Lemonade, Country Style Lemonade, Cranberry Lemonade, Pink Lemonade or Raspberry Lemonade, from frozen (8 fl oz)	120	0	0	30	0	0-10
Fruit Punch, from frozen (8 fl oz)	130	0	0	31	0	5
Grape, from frozen (8 fl oz)	140	0	0	34	0	5
Orange, from frozen or ready-to-drink (8 fl oz)	120	0	0	30	0	30
Tropical Punch (8 fl oz)	120	0	0	31	0	0
Capri Sun All Natural Juice Drinks, Fruit Punch, Mountain Cooler or Strawberry Cooler (6.75 fl oz)	100	0	0	26	0	20
Grape or Maui Punch (6.75 fl oz)	110	0	0	28	0	20
Orange (6.75 fl oz)	100	0	0	26	0	25
Pacific Cooler (6.75 fl oz)	110	0	0	29	0	20
Red Berry (6.75 fl oz)	100	0	0	28	0	20
Safari Punch (6.75 fl oz)	100	0	0	25	0	20
Surfer Cooler or Yo Yogi Berry (6.75 fl oz)	100	0	0	27	0	20
Wild Cherry (6.75 fl oz)	110	0	0	30	0	20
Country Time Sugar Free Low Calorie Drink Mixes, Lemonade or Pink Lemonade, prep w/water (8 fl oz)	5	0	0	0	0	0
Sugar Sweetened Drink Mixes, Lemonade Punch, prep w/water (8 fl oz)	70	0	0	16	0	10
Lemonade or Pink Lemonade, prep w/water (8 fl oz)	70	0	0	17	0	15
Crystal Light Low Calorie Soft Drink Mixes, Citrus Blend, Cranberry Breeze, Fruit Punch, Lemon-Lime, Lemonade, Pink Grapefruit or Raspberry Ice, prep w/water (8 fl oz)	5	0	0	0	0	0
Five Alive Berry Citrus or Citrus, from frozen (8 fl oz)	120	0	0	30	0	0
Citrus, ready-to-serve (8 fl oz)	120	0	0	30	0	25
Tropical Citrus, ready-to-serve (8 fl oz)	120	0	0	29	0	25

Fruit-Flavored Beverages (continued)	Calories	Fat g	Saturated Fat g	Carbohydrate g	Fiber g	Sodium mg
Hansen's Natural Juice Cocktails, California Paradise Punch (8 oz)	120	0	0	30	0	15
Strawberry Kiwi Melon (8 oz)	100	0	0	25	0	15
Tangerine Pineapple Passion Fruit (8 oz)	120	0	0	31	0	15
Old Fashioned Lemonade (8 oz)	100	0	0	26	0	15
Pink Lemonade (8 fl oz)	110	0	0	29	0	15
Strawberry Lemonade (8 oz)	100	0	0	27	0	15
Hi-C Boppin' Berry, Fruit Punch or Grape (8 fl oz)	130	0	0	32	0	30
Cherry (8 fl oz)	130	0	0	33	0	30
Double Fruit Cooler, Jammin' Apple or Stompin' Banana Berry (8 fl oz)	130	0	0	31	0	30
Ecto Cooler or Orange (8 fl oz)	130	0	0	32	0	25-30
Fruity Bubble Gum or Wild Berry (8 fl oz)	120	0	0	30	0	25-30
Hula Punch (8 fl oz)	120	0	0	29	0	30
Just Pik't All Natural, Frozen Cranberry Juice Cocktail, ready-to-serve (8 fl oz)	135	0	0	33	0	0
Frozen Fruit Punch, ready-to-serve (8 fl oz)	125	0	0	31	0	30
Frozen Lemonade, ready-to-serve (8 fl oz)	110	0	0	27	0	0
Koala Springs Fruit Juice Beverages, Kiwi, Lime & Grapefruit or Mandarin & Orange (8 fl oz)	110	0	0	29	0	0
Lemonade (8 fl oz)	100	0	0	25	0	0
Raspberry & Guava or Strawberry & Peach (8 fl oz)	120	0	0	34	0	0
Kool-Aid Bursts Soft Drinks, Cherry (6.75 fl oz)	100	0	0	25	0	35
Grape (6.75 fl oz)	100	0	0	25	0	30
Great Bluedini, Incrediberry, Orange Punch, Pink Swimmingo, Rock-A-Dile Red or Tropical Punch (6.75 fl oz)	100	0	0	24	0	30
Sugar Free Low Calorie Soft Drink Mixes, Cherry or Purplesaurus Rex, prep w/water (8 fl oz)	5	0	0	0	0	5

	Calories	Fat g	Saturated Fat g	Carbohydrate g	Fiber g	Sodium mg
Grape, Great Bluedini, Incrediberry, Lemonade, Pink Swimmingo or Rock-A-Dile Red, prep w/water (8 fl oz)	5	0	0	0	0	0
Tropical Punch, prep w/water (8 fl oz)	5	0	0	0	0	10
Sugar Sweetened Soft Drink Mixes, Cherry, Grape, Great Bluedini, Incrediberry, Orange, Pink Swimmingo, Purplesaurus Rex, Rock-a-Dile Red, Strawberry or Tropical Punch, prep w/water (8 fl oz)	60	0	0	16	0	0
Lemonade, prep w/water (8 fl oz)	70	0	0	17	0	0
Piña-Pineapple or Raspberry, prep w/water (8 fl oz)	60	0	0	17	0	0
Unsweetened Soft Drink Mixes, Black Cherry, Cherry, Grape, Great Bluedini, Incrediberry, Lemon-Lime, Lemonade, Orange, Piña-Pineapple, Pink Lemonade, Pink Swimmingo or Tropical Punch, prep w/sugar & water (8 fl oz)	100	0	0	25	0	10-20
Purplesaurus Rex, Raspberry, Rock-a-Dile Red or Strawberry, prep w/sugar & water (8 fl oz)	100	0	0	25	0	30-35
Mega Mistic All Natural Mango Mania (8 fl oz)	110	0	0	27	0	0
Minute Maid Berry Punch or Citrus Punch, ready-to-drink (8 fl oz)	130	0	0	31	0	25
Berry Punch, from frozen (8 fl oz)	130	0	0	31	0	35
Citrus Punch, from frozen (8 fl oz)	120	0	0	31	0	25
Concord Punch or Grape Punch, ready-to-drink (8 fl oz)	130	0	0	32	0	25
Country Style Lemonade, from frozen (8 fl oz)	120	0	0	30	0	0
Cranberry Apple Cocktail, ready-to-drink (8 fl oz)	170	0	0	42	0	25
Cranberry Lemonade or Fruit Punch, ready-to-drink (8 fl oz)	120	0	0	31	0	25
Fruit Punch, canned (8 fl oz)	119	0	0	32	0	5
Fruit Punch, from frozen (8 fl oz)	120	0	0	31	0	5
Grape Punch, from frozen (8 fl oz)	130	0	0	32	0	5

Fruit-Flavored Beverages (continued)	Calories	Fat g	Saturated Fat g	Carbohydrate g	Fiber g	Sodium mg
Minute Maid *(continued)*						
Lemonade, canned (8 fl oz)	106	0	0	28	0	0
Lemonade, from frozen or ready-to-serve (8 fl oz)	110	0	0	29	0	0
Limeade, from frozen (8 fl oz)	100	0	0	26	0	0
Orange Punch, ready-to-serve (8.45 fl oz)	130	0	0	33	0	0
Pink Grapefruit Juice Cocktail, ready-to-serve (8 fl oz)	110	0	0	27	0	25
Pink Lemonade, ready-to-serve (8 fl oz)	110	0	0	28	0	25
Raspberry Lemonade, ready-to-serve (8 fl oz)	120	0	0	30	0	0
Tropical Punch, ready-to-serve (8 fl oz)	120	0	0	31	0	5
Minute Maid Fruitopia, Citrus Consciousness or Raspberry Psychic Lemonade, ready-to-serve (8 fl oz)	120	0	0	30	0	25
Cranberry Lemonade Meditation, ready-to-serve (8 fl oz)	110	0	0	29	0	25
Fruit Integration, ready-to-serve (8 fl oz)	120	0	0	31	0	25
Grape Beyond, ready-to-serve (8 fl oz)	130	0	0	32	0	25
Lemonade Love, ready-to-serve (8 fl oz)	120	0	0	28	0	25
Pink Lemonade Euphoria, ready-to-serve (8 fl oz)	120	0	0	29	0	25
Strawberry Passion Awareness, ready-to-serve (8 fl oz)	120	0	0	31	0	30
Minute Maid Naturals, Apple Cranberry Medley, ready-to-serve (8 fl oz)	170	0	0	42	0	25
Concord Medley, ready-to-serve (8 fl oz)	130	0	0	32	0	25
Cranberry Lemonade, ready-to-serve (8 fl oz)	110	0	0	29	0	25
Fruit Medley or Tropical Medley, ready-to-serve (8 fl oz)	120	0	0	31	0	25
Lemonade, ready-to-serve (8 fl oz)	110	0	0	28	0	25
Orange Grape Blend, ready-to-serve (8 fl oz)	120	0	0	31	0	35
Raspberry Lemonade, ready-to-serve (8 fl oz)	120	0	0	29	0	25

Fruit-Flavored Beverages (continued)	Calories	Fat g	Saturated Fat g	Carbohydrate g	Fiber g	Sodium mg
Newman's Own Lemonade, ready-to-serve (8 fl oz)	110	0	0	27	0	40
Ocean Spray Drinks, Cranapple Cranberry Apple, ready-to-drink (8 fl oz)	160	0	0	41	<1	35
Cran-Blueberry Blueberry Cranberry, ready-to-serve (8 fl oz)	160	0	0	41	0	35
Cran-Cherry Cherry Cranberry, ready-to-serve (8 fl oz)	160	0	0	39	0	35
Cran-Grape Grape Cranberry, ready-to-serve (8 fl oz)	170	0	0	41	0	35
Cranicot Cranberry Apricot, ready-to-serve (8 fl oz)	160	0	0	40	0	35
Cran-Raspberry Raspberry Cranberry, ready-to-serve (8 fl oz)	140	0	0	36	0	35
Cran-Strawberry Cranberry Strawberry, ready-to-drink (8 fl oz)	140	0	0	36	<1	35
Fruit Punch, from frozen (8 fl oz)	130	0	0	32	0	35
Crantastic, ready-to-drink (8 fl oz)	150	0	0	37	0	35
Juice Cocktail, Cranberry, ready-to-serve (8 fl oz)	140	0	0	34	0	35
Pink Grapefruit, ready-to-drink (8 fl oz)	110	0	0	28	0	35
Juice Drinks, Ruby Red & Tangerine Grapefruit, from frozen (8 fl oz)	130	0	0	32	0	35
Ruby Red Grapefruit, from frozen (8 fl oz)	130	0	0	33	0	35
Lemonade from frozen (8 fl oz)	110	0	0	29	0	35
w/Cranberry Juice, from frozen (8 fl oz)	110	0	0	26	0	35
w/Raspberry Juice, from frozen (8 fl oz)	110	0	0	27	0	35
Lightstyle, Low Calorie Cran-Grape Grape Cranberry Juice Drink or Low Calorie Pink Grapefruit Juice Drink, ready-to-drink (8 fl oz)	40	0	0	9	0	35
Low Calorie Cran-Raspberry Raspberry Cranberry Juice Drink or Low Calorie Cranberry Juice Cocktail, ready-to-drink (8 fl oz)	40	0	0	10	0	35

	Calories	Fat g	Saturated Fat g	Carbohydrate g	Fiber g	Sodium mg
Ocean Spray *(continued)*						
Mauna La'i Fruit Juice Drinks, !Mango Mango! Mango & Hawaiian Guava, ready-to-drink (8 fl oz)	130	0	0	33	0	35
Island Guava Hawaiian Guava or Paradise Passion Hawaiian Guava & Passion Fruit Flavored, ready-to-drink (8 fl oz)	130	0	0	32	0	35
Reduced Calorie, Cranapple Apple Cranberry Drink, Cran-Raspberry Raspberry Cranberry Drink or Cranberry Juice Cocktail, from frozen (8 fl oz)	50	0	0	13	0	35
Refreshers Juice Drink, Citrus Cranberry, ready-to-drink (8 fl oz)	140	0	0	35	0	35
Citrus Peach, ready-to-drink (8 fl oz)	120	0	0	30	0	35
Orange Cranberry, ready-to-drink (8 fl oz)	130	0	0	33	0	35
Royal Mistic All Natural Flavored Beverages, Lemonade Limeade (8 fl oz)	100	0	0	28	0	45
Lime Tropical (8 fl oz)	100	0	0	26	0	0
Raspberry Guava or Watermelon Kiwi (8 fl oz)	110	0	0	27	0	0
Snapple Diet Kiwi Strawberry (16 fl oz)	13	0	0	3	0	10
Diet Mango Madness (16 fl oz)	13	0	0	1	0	10
Kiwi Strawberry (16 fl oz)	130	0	0	33	0	10
Mango Madness (16 fl oz)	110	0	0	29	0	10
Melon Berry Cocktail (16 fl oz)	120	0	0	29	0	10
Pink Lemonade (16 fl oz)	110	0	0	26	0	15
Tang Drink Mixes, Mango Flavored, prep w/water (8 fl oz)	100	0	0	25	0	0
Orange Flavored Sugar Free Low Calorie, prep w/water (8 fl oz)	5	0	0	1	0	0
Orange Flavored, prep w/water (8 fl oz)	100	0	0	24	0	0
Wyler's Fruit Flavored Drink Mixes, Black Cherry Blowout or Outrageous Orange, prep w/sugar & water (8 fl oz)	100	0	0	25	0	20
Blitzing Bananaberry, prep w/sugar & water (8 fl oz)	100	0	0	25	0	25

Fruit-Flavored Beverages (continued)	Calories	Fat g	Saturated Fat g	Carbohydrate g	Fiber g	Sodium mg
Cherry Charger, Lemon Landslide, Power Pink Lemonade or Radical Razzberry, prep w/sugar & water (8 fl oz)	100	0	0	25	0	15
Electric Grape, prep w/sugar & water (8 fl oz)	100	0	0	25	0	10
Fruit Punch, ready-to-drink (8 fl oz)	130	0	0	32	0	5
Lemonade, ready-to-serve (8 fl oz)	110	0	0	28	0	30
Lemon Lime Blitzer, Tropical Punch, Tutti Fruity or Watermelon Wipeout, prep w/sugar & water (8 fl oz)	100	0	0	25	0	0
Megaberry, prep w/sugar & water (8 fl oz)	100	0	0	25	0	30
Slam Dunk Strawberry, prep w/sugar & water (8 fl oz)	100	0	0	25	0	45
SPORTS DRINKS						
PowerAde Fruit Punch, Lemon-Lime or Orange (8 fl oz)	72	0	0	19	0	28
Grape (8 fl oz)	73	0	0	19	0	28
TEAS						
Country Time Sugar Sweetened Drink Mix, Iced Tea, prep w/water (8 fl oz)	70	0	0	17	0	0
Crystal Light Low Calorie Soft Drink Mixes, Iced Tea or Decaffeinated Iced Tea, prep w/water (8 fl oz)	5	0	0	0	0	0
Hansen's Natural Teas, Original w/Lemon, Tangerine or Tropical (8 oz)	70	0	0	21	0	15
Wildberry (8 oz)	70	0	0	22	0	15
Just Pik't Natural Lemon Flavor Frozen Iced Tea (8 fl oz)	75	0	0	19	0	0
Lipton Teas, Flavored Blends, Amaretto, Blackberry, Cinnamon, Earl Gray, English Blend, Honey & Orange, Orange & Spice, Peach or Raspberry (1 teabag)	0	0	0	0	0	0
Herbal Teas, Almond Pleasure, Gentle Orange, Golden Honey & Lime, Variety Pack, Mountain Berry Apple, Quietly Chamomile or Sweet Cinnamon Spice (1 teabag)	0	0	0	<1	0	0

	Calories	Fat g	Saturated Fat g	Carbohydrate g	Fiber g	Sodium mg
Lipton Herbal Teas *(continued)*						
Cinnamon Apple, Country Cranberry, Ginger Twist, Green, Iced Refresher, Lemon Mint Refresher, Lemon Soother, Moonlight Mint, Peppermint or Wildflowers & Honey (1 teabag)	0	0	0	0	0	0
Orange Refresher (1 teabag)	0	0	0	<1	0	0
Special Blends Variety Pack (1 teabag)	0	0	0	0	0	0
Lipton Iced Tea Mixes, Calorie Free or Decaffeinated (1 tsp)	0	0	0	0	0	0
Low Calorie or Sugar Free No Lemon (1 tsp)	0	0	0	0	0	0
Sugar No Lemon (1 tbsp)	80	0	0	19	0	0
w/Nutrasweet (1 tbsp)	5	0	0	1	0	0
Instant Herbals, Cinnamon Apple or Orange (1 env)	20	0	0	4	0	0
Instant Tea Mixes, Decaffeinated or Plain (1 tsp)	0	0	0	0	0	0
Lemon Flavored (2 tsp)	5	0	0	1	0	0
Sugar Free Iced Herbal Tea Mixes, Cran Raspberry or Lemon Cooler (8 fl oz)	10	0	0	2	0	0
Royal Mistic Iced Teas, All Natural, Naturally Lemon Flavored (8 fl oz)	90	0	0	24	0	20
Peach Flavored (8 fl oz)	90	0	0	30	0	5
Raspberry Flavored (8 fl oz)	90	0	0	25	0	25
Diet Natural Lemon Flavored (8 fl oz)	5	0	0	2	0	25
Red Herbal Strawberry Naturally Flavored (8 fl oz)	100	0	0	28	0	0
Snapple Diet Raspberry Tea (16 fl oz)	0	0	0	1	0	10
Raspberry Tea (16 fl oz)	120	0	0	29	0	10

BREAD AND BREAD PRODUCTS

Bread products included in this section of the Guide are low in fat and saturated fat *as purchased* or when *prepared according to package directions*. The levels of fat and saturated fat in a serving of these foods do not exceed the cutoff points of 3 grams of fat and 1 gram of saturated fat.

Bagels	Calories	Fat g	Saturated Fat g	Carbohydrate g	Fiber g	Sodium mg
BAGELS						
Most Brands, Plain (3" diam = 2 oz)	157	1	0	30	1	304
Lender's Bagelettes, Original (2 bagelettes)	140	1	0	28	1	260
Lender's Bagels, Blueberry (1 bagel)	200	2	0	38	2	330
Cinnamon Raisin (1 bagel)	200	2	0	39	2	290
Egg (1 bagel)	160	2	0	30	1	320
Garlic (1 bagel)	150	1	0	29	2	280
Oat Bran (1 bagel)	190	2	1	36	4	300
Onion (1 bagel)	170	2	0	30	2	300
Plain (1 bagel)	160	1	0	30	1	320
Big'n Crusty Bagels, Cinnamon Raisin (1 bagel)	240	3	0	47	2	330
Egg (1 bagel)	230	2	1	44	2	400
Onion (1 bagel)	220	2	0	43	3	410
Soft Bagels, Original (1 bagel)	210	4	1	37	2	330
S.B. Thomas' Bagels, Onion (1 bagel)	160	2	0	32	2	200
Plain (1 bagel)	170	2	0	32	2	220
Sara Lee Bagels, Cinnamon Raisin (1 bagel)	220	1	0	45	3	320
Plain (1 bagel)	210	1	0	43	2	510
Wolferman's Bagels, Egg (1 bagel)	250	2	0	48	0	450
Onion (1 bagel)	230	1	0	44	2	660
Original (1 bagel)	230	1	0	46	2	550

	Calories	Fat g	Saturated Fat g	Carbohydrate g	Fiber g	Sodium mg
BISCUITS						
Higher-Fat						
Baking Powder Biscuit, prep from mix (2 biscuits, 2" each)	249	14	4	27	1	265
Buttermilk Biscuits, refrigerated dough (3 sm)	197	8	2	27	1	685
Lower-Fat						
Ballard Extra Lights Ovenready Biscuits, Regular or Buttermilk (3 biscuits)	150	2	0	29	<1	490
Dunberry Toaster Biscuits (1 biscuit)	150	3	1	26	1	310
Pillsbury Biscuits, Butter, Buttermilk or Country (3 biscuits = 2¼ oz)	150	3	0	29	<1	490
BREAD MIXES						
Aunt Jemima Self-Rising Buttermilk White Corn Meal Mix (3 tbsp)	80	1	0	18	1	440
Bisquick Easy Breads Mix (¼ cup)	130	<1	0	26	<1	220
Reduced Fat Baking Mix (⅓ cup)	150	3	1	27	<1	460
Pioneer Low Fat Biscuit & Baking Mix (¼ cup)	150	1	0	40	<1	510
BREADS						
Higher-Fat						
Garlic Bread, "buttered" (1 med slice)	96	4	1	13	1	184
Lower-Fat						
Arnold Bakery Light Bread, Oatmeal (2 slices)	80	1	0	20	4	140
Wheat Bread (2 slices)	80	1	0	20	5	120
Arnold Bread, Bran'nola, Country Oat (1 slice)	90	3	1	18	3	115
Original (1 slice)	90	2	0	18	3	125
Brick Oven Bread, Wheat (2 slices)	110	3	0	21	3	170
White (2 slices)	130	3	0	25	1	230
Country Bread, Wheat (1 slice)	90	2	0	18	1	170
White (1 slice)	100	2	0	19	<1	190
Honey Wheat Berry (1 slice)	70	1	0	16	3	160
Raisin Cinnamon (1 slice)	70	1	0	14	0	90
Stoneground 100% Whole Wheat (2 slices)	100	2	0	20	3	170

Breads (continued)	Calories	Fat g	Saturated Fat g	Carbohydrate g	Fiber g	Sodium mg
B&M Brown Bread, Plain or Raisin (1/2" slice)	130	1	0	29	2	360-390
Beefsteak Bread, Hearty Rye or Hearty Wheat (1 slice)	70	1	0	13	1	160-170
Light Rye (2 slices)	70	1	0	17	5	250
Mild Rye (2 slices)	90	1	0	18	2	240
Pumpernickel or Soft Rye (1 slice)	70	1	0	13	1	180
Robust White or Soft Wheat (1 slice)	70	1	0	13	<1	140-150
Bread Du Jour Austrian Wheat (2 oz)	130	2	0	26	2	280
French (2 oz)	130	1	0	26	1	300
Brownberry Hearth Bread, Grain (1 slice)	90	2	0	17	2	190
Wheat (1 slice)	90	1	0	18	2	190
Brownberry Natural Bread, Caraway Rye (1 slice)	70	1	0	15	1	160
Oatmeal (1 slice)	70	1	0	13	1	135
Pumpernickel Rye (1 slice)	70	1	0	14	1	150
Wheat (2 slices)	80	1	0	16	2	200
White (2 slices)	120	2	0	24	1	160
Whole Bran (1 slices)	60	1	0	12	2	140
Dicarlo's Parisian French Bread (2 slices)	70	1	0	14	<1	150
Friend's Brown Bread, Plain or Raisin (1/2" slice)	130	1	0	29	2	360-390
Home Pride Bread, Hearty Bread, 100% Stoneground Whole Wheat (1 slice)	90	2	0	18	3	250
Buttermilk & Biscuit White (1 slice)	100	2	0	18	<1	280
Golden Honey Wheat (1 slice)	90	2	0	18	2	210
Honey Oats & Cracked Wheat (1 slice)	100	2	0	19	2	210
Seven Grain Multi Grain (1 slice)	100	2	0	17	2	200
Honey Wheat or Wheat (1 slice)	70	1	0	13	1	150-160
Lite Bread, Wheat or White (3 slices)	110	2	0	25	6	300-320
Seven Grain (1 slice)	60	1	0	12	1	130
White (1 slice)	70	1	0	13	0	160
White Grain (1 slice)	60	1	0	13	2	140
Lifestream Natural Foods Essene Sprouted Grain Loaf, 5 Seed (1 slice)	130	0	0	26	7	10
Carrot & Raisin or Whole Wheat (1 slice)	130	0	0	26	5	10-15
Date & Cinnamon (1 slice)	140	0	0	29	5	15

Breads (continued)	Calories	Fat g	Saturated Fat g	Carbohydrate g	Fiber g	Sodium mg
Lifestream Natural Foods Essene Sprouted Grain Loaf (continued)						
Fruit & Nut (1 slice)	150	2	0	29	6	10
Multigrain (1 slice)	140	0	0	27	6	15
Raisin (1 slice)	130	0	0	27	5	10
Whole Rye (1 slice)	140	0	0	32	5	10
Pillsbury Crusty French Loaf (¹/₅ of pkg = 2.2 oz)	150	1	0	28	<1	370
Pipin' Hot Loaf (1/6 of pkg=1.7 oz)	110	1	0	22	<1	350
Rubschlager Bread, 100% Stone Ground Honey Whole Wheat or German Style Kommissbrot (1 slice)	70	1	0	13	3	135-150
Bagel Bread (1 slice)	90	2	0	16	<1	180
Cocktail Bread, Honey Whole Grain or Pumpernickel (3 slices)	80	1	0	14	2	180
Rye (3 slices)	80	2	0	14	2	180
Danish Style Pumpernickel or Westphalian Style (1 slice)	70	1	0	14	2	135
European Style Whole Grain (1 slice)	70	1	0	14	3	135
Jewish Style Deli Rye (1 slice)	70	1	0	13	2	135
Marble Rye, Raisin Pumpernickel or Swedish Style Limpa (2 slices)	110	2	0	20	3	200
Pumpernickel or Rye (1 slice)	90	2	0	17	2	210
Stone-Ground Honey Wheat (1 slice)	90	2	0	17	2	180
Wolferman's Toasting Bread, Apple Strudel (1 slice)	80	1	0	16	2	150
Blueberry or Wheat (1 slice)	210	0	0	20	2	230
Cinnamon & Raisin (1 slice)	120	1	0	23	2	150
Heartland Harvest (1 slice)	80	0	0	22	2	230
Oatmeal Cinnamon (1 slice)	120	0	0	23	2	160
Original (1 slice)	80	0	0	15	1	166
Sourdough (1 slice)	80	0	0	16	1	205
Wonder Bread, 100% Soft Whole Wheat (2 slices)	110	2	0	21	1	240
100% Stoneground Whole Wheat (1 slice)	80	2	0	14	2	190
100% Whole Wheat (1 slice)	70	1	0	12	2	180
Cinnamon Raisin Bread (1 slice)	70	1	0	14	<1	100
Cracked Wheat (1 slice)	70	1	0	14	1	150

	Calories	Fat g	Saturated Fat g	Carbohydrate g	Fiber g	Sodium mg
Family Bread, Italian (1 slice)	70	1	0	13	<1	150
Wheat (1 slice)	70	1	0	13	<1	150
French Bread (1 slice)	80	2	0	15	<1	160
Granola (2 slices)	100	2	0	19	2	210
Iron Kids (1 slice)	60	1	0	12	2	130
Italian (1 slice)	80	1	0	15	<1	190
Light Bread, French, Italian or White (2 slices)	80	1	0	18	5	210-230
Honey Bran (2 slices)	80	1	0	18	6	190
Nine Grain (2 slices)	80	1	0	18	6	230
Oatmeal (2 slices)	90	1	0	19	4	230
Rye (2 slices)	70	1	0	17	5	220
Sourdough or White Calcium (2 slices)	80	1	0	18	5	250-260
Wheat or Wheat Calcium (2 slices)	80	1	0	18	6	230-240
Rye (1 slice)	70	1	0	13	1	170
Sourdough (1 slice)	90	2	0	17	<1	180
Vienna or White (1 slice)	70	1	0	13	<1	150-170
Wheat Golden Country Style (2 slices)	100	2	0	19	1	220
White Calcium (2 slices)	100	1	0	20	1	240
White w/Buttermilk (1 slice)	80	1	0	14	<1	180

BREADSTICKS

	Calories	Fat g	Saturated Fat g	Carbohydrate g	Fiber g	Sodium mg
Bread Du Jour Italian or Sourdough (1 breadstick)	130	1	0	25	1	280
Delicious Breadsticks, Cheese (1 breadstick)	40	1	0	7	0	85
Garlic or Italian (1 breadstick)	35	0	0	6	0	60-65
Sesame (1 breadstick)	35	1	0	6	0	60
Whole Wheat Sesame (1 breadstick)	30	0	0	5	0	50
Fattorie & Pandea Italian Breadsticks, Pizza (3 sticks)	60	1	0	12	0	105
Sesame (3 sticks)	60	2	0	12	0	110
Traditional (3 sticks)	60	1	0	11	0	115
Whole Wheat (3 sticks)	50	2	1	11	0	105
Forno Della Valle Italian Breadsticks, Garlic, Sesame or Traditional (5 sticks)	60	1	0	12	0	120
Lance Breadsticks, Cheese or Plain (4 pieces)	50	1	0	9	0	120-130
Garlic (4 pieces)	50	1	0	10	0	180
Sesame (4 pieces)	60	2	1	8	1	95

	Calories	Fat g	Saturated Fat g	Carbohydrate g	Fiber g	Sodium mg
Pepperidge Farm Crunchy Baked Thin Bread Sticks, Cheddar Cheese (7 sticks)	70	3	1	10	<1	120
Onion (7 sticks)	70	2	0	11	<1	115
Sesame (7 sticks)	60	2	0	11	<1	125
Stella D'Oro Breadsticks, Deli-Style, Garlic or Original (5 sticks)	60	0	0	12	<1	120-130
Grissini-Style, Original (3 sticks)	60	0	0	12	1	130
Italian Style, Onion (2 sticks)	80	2	0	13	<1	75
Sodium Free (2 sticks)	80	2	0	14	<1	0
Wheat (2 sticks)	80	3	0	13	1	40
Traditional, Sesame (2 sticks)	70	1	0	14	1	60
Wolferman's Breadsticks, Garlic Poppyseed (1 stick)	130	2	0	23	1	280

COFFEECAKES, DANISHES, AND SWEET ROLLS

Higher-Fat

	Calories	Fat g	Saturated Fat g	Carbohydrate g	Fiber g	Sodium mg
Coffeecake w/streusel topping (2 oz)	209	9	3	29	1	243
Danish Pastry w/frosting (3" diam)	245	14	7	28	1	71

Lower-Fat

	Calories	Fat g	Saturated Fat g	Carbohydrate g	Fiber g	Sodium mg
Entenmann's Buns, Apple (1 bun)	150	0	0	33	1	140
Blueberry Cheese (1 bun)	140	0	0	31	1	150
Cinnamon Raisin or Raspberry Cheese (1 bun)	160	0	0	36	1	125-135
Pineapple Cheese (1 bun)	140	0	0	30	<1	150
Coffee Cake, Cinnamon Apple (1/9 cake)	130	0	0	29	2	110
Pastries, Black Forest (1/9 Danish)	130	0	0	32	2	115
Raspberry Cheese (1/9 Danish)	140	0	0	32	1	110
Twists, Apricot Danish (1/8 Danish)	150	0	0	34	<1	110
Cinnamon Apple (1/8 Danish)	150	0	0	35	<1	110
Lemon (1/8 Danish)	130	0	0	31	1	140
Raspberry (1/8 Danish)	140	0	0	33	2	125
Hostess Crumb Cake Light (2 cakes)	150	1	0	35	<1	190
Pillsbury Date Quick Bread Mix, prep w/water, oil & egg substitute (1/12 bread)	160	3	<1	32	NA	150

	Calories	Fat g	Saturated Fat g	Carbohydrate g	Fiber g	Sodium mg
CORN MUFFINS AND CORNBREAD						
Higher-Fat						
Cornbread, prep from mix (3 1/2" x 2 1/2" x 3/4")	160	6	3	22	1	434
Lower-Fat						
Pepperidge Farms Wholesome Choice, Corn Muffins (1 muffin)	150	3	0	27	1	190
CRUMBS AND COATING MIXES						
Higher-Fat						
Bread Crumbs, "buttered" (2 3/4 tbsp = 1 oz)	166	11	2	14	1	282
Lower-Fat						
Most Brands, Graham Cracker Crumbs (1/3 cup)	118	3	1	22	1	169
Contadina Bread Crumbs (1/3 cup)	100	2	0	19	1	700
Kellogg's Corn Flake Crumbs (2 tbsp)	40	0	0	9	0	120
Krusteaz Mixes, Bake'N Fry (1/4 cup mix)	100	1	0	20	1	890
Tempura (1/4 cup mix)	110	1	0	23	0	200
Nabisco Honey Maid Graham Cracker Crumbs (1/8 of 9" pie shell)	70	2	0	13	<1	90
Nabisco Premium Fat Free Cracker Crumbs (1/4 cup)	100	0	0	23	1	0
Oven Fry Extra Crispy Recipe for Chicken (1/8 pkt)	60	1	0	10	0	420
Extra Crispy Recipe for Pork (1/8 pkt)	60	2	0	11	0	340
Home Style Flour Recipe for Chicken (1/8 pkt)	40	1	0	15	0	470
Progresso Bread Crumbs, Italian Style (1/4 cup)	110	2	0	20	1	430
Plain (1/4 cup)	100	2	0	19	1	210
Shake'N Bake Perfect Potatoes Herb & Garlic Seasoning Mix for Fresh Potatoes (1/6 pkt)	20	0	0	5	0	370
Shake'N Bake Seasoning & Coating Mixtures, Barbecue Chicken Glaze (1/8 pkt)	45	1	0	9	0	410
Barbecue Pork Glaze (1/8 pkt)	35	0	0	8	0	250
Honey Mustard (1/8 pkt)	45	1	0	9	0	290
Hot & Spicy Chicken (1/8 pkt)	40	1	0	7	0	190
Hot & Spicy Pork (1/8 pkt)	45	1	0	8	0	220

Crumbs and Coating Mixes (continued)	Calories	Fat g	Saturated Fat g	Carbohydrate g	Fiber g	Sodium mg
Shake 'N Bake Seasoning & Coating Mixtures *(continued)*						
Italian Herb Recipe (⅛ pkt)	40	1	0	7	0	300
Original Recipe for Chicken (⅛ pkt)	40	1	0	7	0	230
For Fish (¼ pkt)	70	2	0	14	1	420
For Pork (⅛ pkt)	40	0	0	9	0	320
Tangy Honey Glaze (⅛ pkt)	45	1	0	10	0	280
ENGLISH MUFFINS						
Amana English Muffin Slices, Almond Poppyseed (1 slice)	70	1	0	11	1	90
Apple-Cinnamon (1 slice)	80	0	0	15	1	120
Banana (1 slice)	70	0	0	12	1	80
Blueberry, Honey Wheat, Raisin Cinnamon, Regular or Sourdough (1 slice)	80	0	0	17	1	120-125
Cranberry-Apple (1 slice)	80	0	0	14	1	90
Dunberry Colossal English Muffins (1 muffin)	190	1	0	37	2	350
S.B. Thomas' English Muffins, Honey Wheat (1 muffin)	110	1	0	24	3	190
Raisin w/Cinnamon (1 muffin)	140	1	0	31	1	170
Regular (1 muffin)	120	1	0	25	1	200
Sun Maid Raisin English Muffins (1 muffin)	160	1	0	35	2	230
Wolferman's Crumpets, Blueberry (1 crumpet)	100	1	0	21	1	250
Brown Sugar (1 crumpet)	100	2	0	19	1	270
Buttermilk (1 crumpet)	90	1	0	18	1	260
Lemon Poppy Seed (1 crumpet)	90	1	0	19	2	280
Original (1 crumpet)	90	1	0	19	1	260
Whole Grain (1 crumpet)	100	1	0	19	2	310
Wolferman's English Muffins, Deluxe, Apple Strudel (1 muffin)	250	5	1	44	4	370
Blueberry (1 muffin)	220	1	1	46	3	300
Cinnamon Raisin (1 muffin)	240	2	1	48	6	310
Cranberry (1 muffin)	240	1	1	49	3	340
Golden Raisin (1 muffin)	250	2	(1)	51	NA	540
Heartland Harvest (1 muffin)	230	1	1	46	5	460
Honey Nut (1 muffin)	240	3	0	45	7	510

	Calories	Fat g	Saturated Fat g	Carbohydrate g	Fiber g	Sodium mg
Low Sodium (1 muffin)	220	1	1	44	2	430
Oatmeal Cinnamon (1 muffin)	250	1	1	48	4	330
Original (1 muffin)	220	1	0	45	3	410
Spicy Apple (1 muffin)	220	1	1	46	4	550
Wheat (1 muffin)	210	1	0	42	5	470
Mini English Muffins, Apple Strudel (1 mini muffin)	80	1	0	17	2	150
Blueberry (1 mini muffin)	80	<1	0	16	1	170
Cinnamon & Raisin (1 mini muffin)	80	1	0	16	2	100
Cranberry or Original (1 mini muffin)	70	0	0	15	1	135
Sourdough (1 mini muffin)	70	0	0	15	1	140
Wonder English Muffins, Regular or Sourdough (1 muffin)	120	1	0	25	1	290
Wonder Rounds Raisin (1 muffin)	150	2	0	30	2	240

FOCACCIA

	Calories	Fat g	Saturated Fat g	Carbohydrate g	Fiber g	Sodium mg
Dicarlo's Foccaccia (1/8 slice)	130	2	0	25	1	260

HAMBURGER AND HOT DOG BUNS

	Calories	Fat g	Saturated Fat g	Carbohydrate g	Fiber g	Sodium mg
Brownberry Wheat Sandwich Buns (1 bun)	130	2	0	24	2	210
Home Pride Potato Rolls Hamburger or Hot Dog Buns (1 bun)	130	2	0	27	2	270
Wonder Buns, Hamburger or Hot Dog, Enriched (1 bun)	110	2	0	21	<1	250
Light (1 bun)	80	2	0	13	5	210

PANCAKES AND WAFFLES

Higher-Fat

	Calories	Fat g	Saturated Fat g	Carbohydrate g	Fiber g	Sodium mg
Pancake Mix, prep w/whole milk, egg & shortening (3 pancakes, 4" each)	250	12	3	28	1	512
Waffles, frozen (2 large)	181	6	1	28	1	538

Lower-Fat

	Calories	Fat g	Saturated Fat g	Carbohydrate g	Fiber g	Sodium mg
Aunt Jemima, Buttermilk Complete Pancake & Waffle Mix (1/3 cup mix)	190	2	1	38	2	480
Complete Pancake & Waffle Mix (1/3 cup mix)	190	2	1	39	1	470
Low Fat Pancakes, frozen (3 pancakes)	130	2	0	33	8	580
Low Fat Waffles, frozen (2 waffles)	160	2	0	33	1	330

	Calories	Fat g	Saturated Fat g	Carbohydrate g	Fiber g	Sodium mg
Aunt Jemima *(continued)*						
Reduced Calorie Buttermilk Complete Pancake Mix (⅓ cup mix)	140	2	1	30	5	510
Betty Crocker Complete Pancake Mixes, Buttermilk (⅓ cup mix)	200	3	1	39	1	540
Original (⅓ cup mix)	210	3	1	40	1	540
Downyflake Waffles, Apple Cinnamon or Plain Crisp & Healthy (2 waffles)	160	2	1	32	1	350
Gold Medal Shake 'N Pour Pancake Mix, Buttermilk (3 pancakes)	200	3	1	38	1	680
Hungry Jack Pancake & Waffle Mixes, Buttermilk Complete, prep w/water (3 pancakes, 4" each)	160	2	0	32	<1	560
Extra Light & Fluffy Complete, prep w/water (3 pancakes, 4" each)	150	2	1	30	<1	600
Kellogg's Eggo Frozen Waffles, Special K (2 waffles)	140	0	0	29	0	250
Krusteaz Pancake Mixes, Buckwheat (½ cup mix = 3 pancakes, 4" each)	280	4	1	51	5	820
Buttermilk (½ cup mix = 3 pancakes, 4" each)	200	3	1	38	2	800
Harvest Apple Spice (½ cup mix = 3 pancakes, 4" each)	210	3	0	41	4	640
Imitation Blueberry (½ cup mix = 3 pancakes, 4" each)	210	3	1	40	2	750
Lite Oatbran (½ cup mix = 3 pancakes, 4" each)	140	1	0	35	7	390
Whole Wheat & Honey (½ cup mix = 3 pancakes, 4" each)	230	2	0	45	3	500
PITA BREADS						
Most Brands, White, Large (6½" pita)	165	1	0	33	2	322
White, Medium (5¼" pita)	124	1	0	25	1	241
White, Small (4" pita)	77	0	0	16	1	150
Whole Wheat, Large (6½" pita)	160	2	0	33	4	319
Whole Wheat, Medium (5¼" pita)	120	1	0	25	3	239
Whole Wheat, Small (4" pita)	74	1	0	15	2	149
S.B. Thomas' Sahara Regular Pita Bread, Oat Bran (1 loaf)	130	1	0	30	3	300

	Calories	Fat g	Saturated Fat g	Carbohydrate g	Fiber g	Sodium mg
Pita Breads (continued)						
White (1 loaf)	150	1	0	31	1	290
Whole Wheat (1 loaf)	130	1	0	28	5	310
PIZZA CRUSTS						
Appian Way Regular Crust Pizza Mix (1/3 pizza)	250	3	1	48	2	740
Pillsbury All Ready Pizza Crust (1/4 pkg = 2.5 oz)	180	3	1	33	1	390
Ragú Pizza Crust Mix (1/3 cup mix)	130	1	0	24	1	270
Robin Hood Pizza Crust Mix (1/4 crust)	160	2	<1	32	1	340
ROLLS						
Higher-Fat						
Croissant (5 1/2" long)	324	19	11	33	2	88
Lower-Fat						
Most Brands, Hard Rolls (3 1/2" roll)	146	2	0	27	2	272
Arnold Potato Dinner Rolls (2 rolls)	110	2	0	21	1	125
Bread Du Jour Rolls, Bavarian Cracked Wheat (1 roll)	90	1	0	17	1	190
Crusty Italian (1 roll)	80	1	0	16	<1	190
French Petite (1 roll)	230	2	0	47	2	530
Rye (1 roll)	90	2	0	16	1	230
Sourdough (1 roll)	140	2	0	29	2	230
Dicarlo's Rolls, Extra Sourdough (1 roll)	100	1	0	20	1	230
French (1 roll)	70	1	0	14	<1	150
Olof Sweden Crisp Four Grain Roll (1 Sweden crisp)	43	<1	0	8	NA	35
Wonder Rolls, Brown 'N Serve, Wheat or White (1 roll)	70	1	0	14	<1	135
Dinner Rolls, Light White (1 roll)	60	1	0	9	4	150
White Tea (1 roll)	80	1	0	19	5	210
SCONES						
Dunberry Scones, Blueberry Flavored (1 scone)	160	3	1	28	1	280
Cinnamon Raisin Flavored (1 scone)	150	3	1	27	1	300
TORTILLAS						
Most Brands, Corn (6 1/2" diam)	55	1	0	12	1	40
C & C Bakery Tortillas, Corn (2 tortillas)	120	2	0	22	3	15

Tortillas (continued)	Calories	Fat g	Saturated Fat g	Carbohydrate g	Fiber g	Sodium mg
C & C Bakery Tortillas *(continued)*						
Extra Thin Corn (3 tortillas)	130	2	0	25	3	15
Mission Tortillas,						
Extra Thin Corn (2 tortillas)	90	1	0	18	1	60
Light Flour (1 tortilla)	70	1	1	16	4	280
Soft Wraps Tortillas,						
Honey Wheat (1 tortilla)	120	2	0	24	1	280
Original (1 tortilla)	110	2	0	22	1	280
Valley Wraps (1 slice)	100	1	1	19	<1	125

CEREALS

Many cereals naturally contain a small amount of fat. Adding nuts, coconut, or seeds to cereal or spraying it with a fat-based coating to help it stay crisp increases the fat content. Cooked and ready-to-eat cereals included in this section of the Guide are low in fat and saturated fat *as purchased* or when *prepared according to package directions*. Cereal is usually eaten with milk; recommended types of milk are skim milk and 1/2% or 1% low-fat milk, which are low in fat and saturated fat. A serving of the cereals included in the Guide does not exceed the cutoff points of 3 grams of fat and 1 gram of saturated fat.

Cooked Cereals	Calories	Fat g	Saturated Fat g	Carbohydrate g	Fiber g	Sodium mg
COOKED CEREALS						
Higher-Fat						
Grits w/Cheese (1 cup cooked)	299	15	8	26	1	625
Lower-Fat						
Most Brands, cooked w/o fat or salt, Corn Grits, plain (1 cup cooked)	146	1	0	30	1	2
Farina (1 cup cooked)	134	1	0	28	1	4
Oat Bran (1 cup cooked)	90	3	1	24	5	3
Oatmeal (1 cup cooked)	145	2	0	25	4	3
Alber's Hominy Quick Grits (1/4 cup dry)	140	1	0	31	1	0
Arrowhead Mills Bear Mush (1/4 cup dry)	160	1	0	33	2	0
Arrowhead Mills Organically Produced Cereals, 7 Grain (1/3 cup dry)	140	2	0	25	5	0
Cracked Wheat (1/4 cup dry)	140	1	0	29	6	0
Oat Bran (1/3 cup dry)	150	3	0	23	7	0
Wheat Bran (1/4 cup dry)	30	1	0	7	6	0

	Calories	Fat g	Saturated Fat g	Carbohydrate g	Fiber g	Sodium mg
Erewhon Barley Plus (¼ cup dry)	170	1	0	37	4	0
Brown Rice Cream (¼ cup dry)	170	1	0	36	1	30
Instant Oatmeals, Apple Cinnamon (1 pkt)	130	2	1	24	3	100
Apple Raisin (1 pkt)	140	2	1	26	3	100
Maple Spice (1 pkt)	130	2	1	25	3	100
w/Added Bran (1 pkt)	130	3	1	25	4	0
General Mills Wheat Hearts (¼ cup dry)	130	1	0	26	2	0
Krusteaz Ala (⅓ cup dry)	150	1	0	32	8	5
Zoom (⅓ cup dry)	120	1	0	23	6	0
Mother's Instant Oatmeal (½ cup dry)	150	3	1	27	4	0
Multigrain Hot Cereal (½ cup dry)	130	2	0	29	5	10
Oat Bran (½ cup dry)	150	3	1	24	6	0
Whole Wheat Natural Cereal (½ cup dry)	130	1	0	30	4	0
Nabisco Cream of Rice (¼ cup dry)	170	0	0	38	<1	0
Cream of Wheat, Instant or Regular (3 tbsp dry)	120	0	0	26	1	0
Quick (3 tbsp dry)	120	0	0	25	1	85
Instant Cream of Wheat Hot Cereals, Burstin' Berry, Peachy Peach or Smashin' Strawberry (1 pkt)	130	0	0	30	1	170
Cinnamon Toast (1 pkt)	130	0	0	29	1	170
Original (1 pkt)	100	0	0	21	1	260
w/real Apple 'n Cinnamon (1 pkt)	130	0	0	29	1	300
w/real Brown Sugar Cinnamon (1 pkt)	130	0	0	29	1	220
Pillsbury Farina, prep w/water & salt (⅔ cup)	80	0	0	18	NA	270
Pritikin Hot Cereals, Apple Raisin Spice (1 pkt)	170	3	1	34	4	5
Multigrain (1 pkt)	160	2	0	34	4	0
Quaker Instant Grits, Original Flavor (1 pkt)	100	0	0	22	1	300
w/Bacon Bits (1 pkt)	100	1	0	22	1	340
w/Butter Flavor (1 pkt)	100	2	0	21	1	320
w/Red Eye Gravy & Ham (1 pkt)	90	1	0	21	1	530
w/Sausage Bits (1 pkt)	100	1	0	21	2	480
Instant Oatmeal, Cinnamon Toast Flavor (1 pkt)	130	2	0	27	2	160
Cinnamon-Spice (1 pkt)	170	2	0	36	3	290
Low Sodium (1 pkt)	130	3	1	22	3	95

Cooked Cereals (continued)

	Calories	Fat g	Saturated Fat g	Carbohydrate g	Fiber g	Sodium mg
Maple Brown Sugar (1 pkt)	160	2	1	33	3	240
Peaches & Cream or Strawberries & Cream (1 pkt)	130	2	1	27	2	150-160
Raisin Spice (1 pkt)	160	2	1	32	3	250
Strawberries 'N Stuff (1 pkt)	150	2	1	30	3	170
w/Apples & Cinnamon (1 pkt)	130	2	1	26	3	105
Oat Bran (1/2 cup dry)	150	3	1	24	6	0
Oats, Old Fashioned or Quick (1/2 cup dry)	150	3	1	27	4	0

READY-TO-EAT CEREALS

Higher-Fat

	Calories	Fat g	Saturated Fat g	Carbohydrate g	Fiber g	Sodium mg
Granola (1/2 cup)	251	10	7	38	3	179
Natural Cereal (1/2 cup)	244	11	8	33	4	22

Lower-Fat

	Calories	Fat g	Saturated Fat g	Carbohydrate g	Fiber g	Sodium mg
Most Brands, Toasted Wheat Germ (1/8 cup)	54	2	0	7	2	1
Arrowhead Mills Organically Produced Cereals, Barley Flakes (1/3 cup)	110	1	0	28	5	0
Kamut Flakes (1/3 cup)	130	1	0	29	<5	0
Nature O's (1 cup)	130	2	1	24	3	5
Oat Flakes (1/3 cup)	130	3	1	23	4	0
Rye Flakes (1/3 cup)	110	1	0	24	4	0
Wheat Flakes (1/3 cup)	110	1	0	24	5	0
Wheat Germ (3 tbsp)	50	1	0	10	2	0
Erewhon Apple Stroodles (3/4 cup)	110	1	0	25	1	15
Aztec (1 cup)	110	0	0	26	1	70
Banana-O's (3/4 cup)	110	0	0	26	2	15
Corn Flakes (1 1/4 cup)	210	3	0	45	3	100
Crispy Brown Rice (1 cup)	110	0	0	25	1	180
Crispy Brown Rice, No Salt Added (1 cup)	110	0	0	25	1	10
Fruit'n Wheat (3/4 cup)	170	2	0	39	5	105
Galaxy Grahams (3/4 cup)	100	1	0	23	2	60
Honey Crisp Corn (1 cup)	210	3	0	45	2	100
Kamut Flakes (2/3 cup)	110	0	0	25	4	75
Oat Bran w/Toasted Wheat Germ (1/3 cup)	170	3	1	31	5	0
Poppets (1 cup)	120	1	0	25	<1	10
Raisin Bran (1 cup)	160	1	0	40	6	100

	Calories	Fat g	Saturated Fat g	Carbohydrate g	Fiber g	Sodium mg
Erewhon *(continued)*						
Raisin Grahams (1 cup)	190	1	0	43	6	105
Super-O's (²/₃ cup)	110	0	0	26	1	60
Wheat Flakes (1 cup)	180	1	0	42	6	135
General Mills Basic 4 (1 cup)	210	3	0	42	3	310
Body Buddies, Natural Fruit Flavor (1 cup)	110	1	0	25	1	290
Boo Berry (1 cup)	120	1	0	26	<1	200
Cheerios (1 cup)	110	2	0	23	3	280
Honey Nut (1 cup)	120	2	0	24	2	270
Multi Grain (1 cup)	110	1	0	24	3	240
Cocoa Puffs or Count Chocula (1 cup)	120	1	0	26	0	190
Country Corn Flakes (1 cup)	120	1	0	26	<1	290
Crispy Wheats 'n Raisins (1 cup)	190	1	0	44	4	270
Fiber One (½ cup)	60	1	0	24	14	140
Frankenberry (1 cup)	120	1	0	26	<1	200
Golden Grahams (¾ cup)	120	1	0	25	1	280
Kaboom (1¼ cup)	120	2	0	24	1	280
Kix (1⅓ cup)	120	1	0	26	1	270
Berry Berry Kix (¾ cup)	120	2	0	25	1	180
Low Fat Granola, Cinnamon & Raisins (½ cup)	210	3	0	45	3	210
Lucky Charms (1 cup)	120	1	0	25	1	210
Oatmeal Crisp, w/Apples (1 cup)	210	3	0	44	3	350
w/Raisins (1 cup)	210	3	0	42	2	260
Reese's Peanut Butter Puffs (¾ cup)	130	3	1	24	0	180
Ripple Crisp Honey, Bran (1¼ cup)	190	1	0	48	5	410
Corn (¾ cup)	110	1	0	26	<1	290
S'mores Grahams (¾ cup)	120	2	1	25	<1	220
Sprinkle Spangles or Trix (1 cup)	120	2	0	26	0	125-140
Total (¾ cup)	110	1	0	24	3	200
Corn Flakes (1⅓ cup)	110	1	0	25	<1	210
Raisin Bran (1 cup)	180	1	0	43	5	240
Triples (1 cup)	120	1	0	25	<1	190
Wheaties Honey Gold (¾ cup)	110	1	0	26	1	200

	Calories	Fat g	Saturated Fat g	Carbohydrate g	Fiber g	Sodium mg
Health Valley Cereals, 10 Bran Apple Cinnamon ($^3/_4$ cup)	110	0	0	24	3	10
Almond Flavor, Apple Cinnamon or Honey Crunch Honey Clusters & Flakes ($^3/_4$ cup)	130	0	0	31	4	20
Amaranth Flakes, Fiber 7 Flakes or Oat Bran Flakes ($^3/_4$ cup)	100	0	0	23	4	10
Blue Corn Flakes ($^3/_4$ cup)	90	0	0	19	4	10
Crispy Brown Rice (1 cup)	110	0	0	30	1	0
Fat-Free Cereals, Almond, Apples & Cinnamon or Honey Crunch Granola O's ($^3/_4$ cup)	120	0	0	26	3	10
Date & Almond, Raisin Cinnamon or Tropical Fruit Granola ($^2/_3$ cup)	180	0	0	45	6	25
Healthy Fiber Flakes ($^3/_4$ cup)	100	0	0	23	4	10
Oat Bran Flakes w/Raisins ($^3/_4$ cup)	100	0	0	26	4	10
Oat Bran O's ($^3/_4$ cup)	110	0	0	25	3	10
Organic Bran, w/Apples & Cinnamon ($^3/_4$ cup)	170	0	0	39	7	10
w/Raisins ($^3/_4$ cup)	190	0	0	43	7	10
Puffed Corn (1 cup)	80	0	0	20	2	0
Raisin Bran ($1^1/_4$ cup)	200	0	0	46	6	20
Heartland Lowfat Granola ($^1/_2$ cup)	210	3	1	40	3	50
Kashi, Puffed (1 cup)	70	<1	0	19	2	0
Seven Whole Grains & Sesame, Honey Puffed (1 cup)	120	1	0	25	2	6
Medley O's, Nuggets, Granola, Puffs, Apples & Raisins ($^1/_2$ cup)	100	1	0	20	2	50
Kellogg's All-Bran ($^1/_2$ cup)	80	1	0	22	10	280
w/Extra Fiber ($^1/_2$ cup)	50	1	0	22	15	150
Apple Jacks (1 cup)	110	0	0	27	1	135
Apple Raisin Crisp (1 cup)	180	0	0	46	4	340
Bran Buds ($^1/_3$ cup)	70	1	0	24	11	210
Cinnamon Mini Buns ($^3/_4$ cup)	120	1	0	27	1	210
Cocoa Krispies ($^3/_4$ cup)	120	1	0	26	0	190
Common Sense Oat Bran ($^3/_4$ cup)	110	1	0	23	4	270
w/Raisins ($1^1/_4$ cup)	200	3	1	42	6	370

	Calories	Fat g	Saturated Fat g	Carbohydrate g	Fiber g	Sodium mg
Kellogg's *(continued)*						
Complete Bran Flakes (1 cup)	100	1	0	25	5	230
Complete Bran Flakes (1 box = 32 g)	100	1	0	26	5	250
Corn Flakes (1 cup)	110	0	0	26	1	330
Corn Pops (1 cup)	110	0	0	27	1	95
Crispix (1 cup)	110	0	0	26	1	230
Double Dip Crunch or Fruity Marshmallow Krispies (³/₄ cup)	110	0	0	27	0	160-180
Froot Loops (1 cup)	120	1	0	26	1	125
Frosted Bran (³/₄ cup)	100	0	0	26	3	200
Frosted Flakes (³/₄ cup)	120	0	0	28	0	200
Frosted Krispies (³/₄ cup)	110	0	0	27	0	230
Frosted Mini-Wheats or Frosted Mini-Wheats Bite Size (1 cup)	190	1	0	45	6	0
Fruitful Bran (1¹/₄ cup)	170	1	0	44	7	330
Healthy Choice, Multi-Grain Flakes (1 cup)	100	0	0	25	3	210
Multi-Grain Squares (1¹/₄ cup)	190	1	0	45	6	0
Multi-Grains, Raisins, Oat Clusters & Almonds (1¹/₄ cup)	200	2	0	45	5	250
Just Right, Fruit & Nut (1 cup)	200	2	0	46	3	250
w/Crunchy Nuggets (1 cup)	200	2	0	46	3	330
Kenmei Rice Bran (³/₄ cup)	110	1	0	25	1	250
Low Fat Granola (¹/₂ cup)	210	3	0	44	3	70
w/Raisins (²/₃ cup)	210	3	0	43	3	65
w/Raisins (1 box = 43 g)	160	3	1	33	3	105
Mueslix Crispy Blend (²/₃ cup)	200	3	0	42	4	190
Nut & Honey, Crunch (²/₃ cup)	120	2	0	25	0	200
Crunch O's (³/₄ cup)	120	3	0	23	2	200
Nutri-Grain, Almond Raisin (1¹/₄ cup)	200	3	0	44	4	330
Golden Wheat & Raisin (1¹/₄ cup)	180	1	0	45	6	310
Golden Wheat (³/₄ cup)	100	1	0	24	4	240
Product 19 (1 cup)	200	1	0	46	3	610
Product 19 (1 box = 23 g)	80	0	0	19	1	210
Raisin Bran (1 cup)	170	1	0	43	7	300
Raisin Bran (1 box = 39 g)	120	1	0	30	5	220
Rice Krispies (1¹/₄ cup)	110	0	0	26	1	360
Treats Cereal (³/₄ cup)	120	2	0	25	0	170

	Calories	Fat g	Saturated Fat g	Carbohydrate g	Fiber g	Sodium mg
Apple Cinnamon (³/₄ cup)	110	0	0	27	1	220
Shredded Wheat Miniatures (1 box = 28 g)	90	0	0	23	4	0
Smacks (³/₄ cup)	110	1	0	26	1	75
Special K (1 cup)	110	0	0	21	1	250
Squares, Apple Cinnamon (³/₄ cup)	180	1	0	44	5	15
Blueberry or Strawberry (1 cup)	180	1	0	44	5	10-15
Raisin (³/₄ cup)	180	1	0	44	5	0
Krusteaz Corn Flakes (1 cup)	130	0	0	28	<1	270
Crisp Rice Cereal (1 cup)	130	0	0	27	0	260
Frosted Flakes Cereal (³/₄ cup)	110	0	0	25	<1	170
Fruit Whirls (³/₄ cup)	120	1	0	25	1	120
Raisin Bran (³/₄ cup)	210	2	0	45	6	320
Toasted Oats (1 cup)	120	2	0	23	2	210
Apple Cinnamon (³/₄ cup)	130	2	0	25	1	150
Honey Nut (³/₄ cup)	120	2	0	23	1	220
Lifestream Natural Foods 8 Grain Flakes (1 cup)	210	0	0	46	6	20
Apple Cinnamon O's (³/₄ cup)	120	0	0	25	3	10
Multigrain Honey Puffs (³/₄ cup)	130	3	0	24	3	15
Malt-O-Meal Coco-Roos (³/₄ cup)	120	1	0	27	<1	190
Corn Flakes (1 cup)	100	0	0	23	1	280
Crispy Rice (1 cup)	120	0	0	26	<1	250
Frosted Flakes (³/₄ cup)	110	0	0	26	<1	190
Golden Sugar Puffs (³/₄ cup)	100	0	0	23	<1	25
Marshmallow Mateys (1 cup)	100	1	0	23	1	170
Puffed Rice (1 cup)	60	0	0	14	<1	0
Puffed Wheat (1 cup)	50	0	0	10	<1	0
Raisin Bran (1¹/₄ cup)	200	1	0	47	7	290
Toasty O's (1 cup)	100	2	0	19	2	220
Apple Cinnamon (³/₄ cup)	110	2	0	21	2	170
Honey & Nut (³/₄ cup)	100	1	0	20	1	170
Tootie Fruities (1 cup)	110	1	0	26	<1	130
Nabisco 100% Bran Cereal (¹/₃ cup)	80	1	0	23	8	120
Frosted Wheat Bites (1 cup)	190	1	0	44	5	10
Fruit Wheats, Blueberry or Strawberry (³/₄ cup)	170	1	0	41	4	15

	Calories	Fat g	Saturated Fat g	Carbohydrate g	Fiber g	Sodium mg
Nabisco Fruit Wheats *(continued)*						
Raspberry (³/₄ cup)	160	1	0	40	4	15
Shredded Wheat (2 biscuits)	160	1	0	38	5	0
Wheat'N Bran (1¹/₄ cups)	200	1	0	47	8	0
Spoon Size (1 cup)	170	1	0	41	5	0
Team Flakes (1¹/₄ cups)	220	0	0	49	1	360
Pacific Grain Products All Natural Nutty Rice Original Cereal (¹/₂ cup)	210	2	0	47	2	110
Post Alpha Bits (1 cup)	130	1	0	27	1	210
Marshmallow (1 cup)	120	1	0	25	1	160
Bran Flakes (²/₃ cup)	90	1	0	22	6	210
Bran'nola, Original (¹/₂ cup)	200	3	1	43	5	240
Raisin (¹/₂ cup)	200	3	1	44	5	220
Cocoa Pebbles (³/₄ cup)	120	1	1	25	<1	160
Fruit & Fibre, Dates, Raisins & Walnuts or Peaches, Raisins & Almonds (1 cup)	210	3	1	46	6	260-270
Fruity Pebbles (³/₄ cup)	110	1	1	24	0	150
Golden Crisp (³/₄ cup)	110	0	0	25	0	40
Grape-Nuts (¹/₂ cup)	200	1	0	47	5	350
Flakes (³/₄ cup)	100	1	0	24	3	140
Honey Bunches of Oats, Honey Roasted (³/₄ cup)	120	2	1	25	1	190
w/Almonds (³/₄ cup)	130	3	1	24	1	180
Honeycomb (1¹/₃ cups)	110	0	0	26	<1	190
Post Toasties (1 cup)	100	0	0	24	1	270
Raisin Bran (1 cup)	190	1	0	46	8	300
Quaker Cap'N Crunch (1 box = 25 g)	100	2	0	21	1	190
w/Crunchberries or Christmas Crunch (³/₄ cup)	100	2	0	22	1	190
Deep Sea Crunch (1 box = 25 g)	100	2	0	21	1	120
Peanut Butter Cereal (³/₄ cup)	110	3	1	21	1	210
Crunchy Bran (³/₄ cup)	90	1	0	23	5	250
Honey Crunch Wheat Germ (1²/₃ tbsp)	50	1	0	8	1	0
Honey Graham Oh!s (³/₄ cup)	110	2	1	23	1	180
Kids Favorites, Marshmallow Stars (³/₄ cup)	120	2	1	25	1	180

	Calories	Fat g	Saturated Fat g	Carbohydrate g	Fiber g	Sodium mg
Sugar Frosted Flakes (3/4 cup)	110	0	0	26	1	250
King Vitamin (1 1/2 cup)	120	1	0	26	1	260
Life (3/4 cup)	120	2	0	25	2	170
Oat Cinnamon (1 cup)	190	2	0	39	3	220
Oat Bran Cereal (1 1/4 cup)	210	3	1	41	7	210
Oat Squares (1 cup)	220	3	1	44	4	260
Cinnamon (1 cup)	230	3	1	48	5	260
Popeye, Cocoa Blasts (1 cup)	130	2	1	29	1	125
Fruit Curls (1 cup)	120	1	0	27	1	170
Popeye Jeepers Cereal (1 1/3 cup)	110	1	0	24	1	140
Crispy Corn Puffs Cereal (1 1/3 cup)	110	1	0	24	1	150
Popeye Oat'MMMS (1 cup)	120	2	1	25	2	300
Toasted Oat Cereal (1 cup)	110	2	0	22	2	160
Popeye Sweet Crunch or Quisp Cereal (1 cup)	110	2	1	23	1	190
Puffed Rice (1 box = 10 g)	40	0	0	9	0	0
Puffed Wheat (1 box = 9 g)	35	0	0	7	1	0
Shredded Wheat (3 biscuits)	110	2	1	50	7	0
Sweet Puffs (1 cup)	130	1	0	30	1	80
Toasted Oatmeal (1 pouch)	80	1	0	17	1	140
Honey Nut (1 pouch)	110	3	1	21	2	100
Toasted Wheat Bran (1/4 cup)	30	1	0	10	7	0
Unprocessed Bran (1/3 cup)	30	0	0	11	8	190
Wheat Germ (2 tbsp)	50	1	0	6	2	0
Ralston Almond Delight (1 cup)	210	3	0	41	4	410
Bran Flakes (3/4 cup)	110	1	0	24	5	220
Chex, Corn (1 1/4 cup)	110	0	0	26	<1	270
Double (1 1/4 cup)	120	0	0	27	0	230
Graham (1 cup)	210	2	0	45	1	340
Multi-Bran (1 1/4 cup)	220	2	0	46	7	320
Rice (1 cup)	120	0	0	27	0	230
Wheat (1 1/4 cup)	190	1	0	41	5	390
Cocoa Crispy Rice (1 cup)	200	1	0	45	<1	340
Cocoa Crunchies (3/4 cup)	120	1	0	26	0	170
Cookie Crisp (1 cup)	120	2	0	25	0	110
Corn Flakes (1 1/4 cups)	120	0	0	27	1	280
Crisp Crunch (3/4 cup)	120	1	0	26	1	240

	Calories	Fat g	Saturated Fat g	Carbohydrate g	Fiber g	Sodium mg
Ralston *(continued)*						
Crisp Rice (1¼ cups)	130	0	0	28	0	330
Frosted Flakes (¾ cup)	120	0	0	28	<1	180
Fruit Rings (¾ cup)	100	1	0	23	0	115
Magic Stars (¾ cup)	120	1	0	26	<1	160
Muesli, Cranberry (¾ cup)	200	3	0	40	4	180
Peach (¾ cup)	200	3	0	39	4	170
Raspberry (¾ cup)	220	3	0	44	4	170
Multi-Vitamin Whole Grain Flakes (1 cup)	120	1	0	25	3	300
Nutty Nuggets (½ cup)	180	2	0	38	5	220
Raisin Bran (¾ cup)	190	1	0	41	6	290
Tasteeos (1¼ cups)	130	3	0	22	3	260
Apple-Cinnamon (1 cup)	130	2	0	27	1	150
Honey Nut (1 cup)	130	2	0	28	1	250
Sun Belt Low Fat Granola (½ cup)	200	3	1	42	4	80
Muesli Five Whole Grains Cereal (½ cup)	210	2	1	44	3	70

CONDIMENTS

Most condiments contain little or no fat and are low in calories. The levels of fat and saturated fat in a serving of the foods listed in this section do not exceed the cutoff points of 3 grams of fat and 1 gram of saturated fat. Since the calories, fat, saturated fat, and sodium are similar in different brands of some types of condiments (such as regular ketchup, mustard, and dill pickles), "most brands" is used instead of individual brand names for many of these products. Olives are listed in the Fats section beginning on page 145.

Although many condiments are high in sodium, several low-sodium brands of ketchup, mustard, and pickles are included in the Guide for individuals trying to limit their sodium intake.

Capers	Calories	Fat g	Saturated Fat g	Carbohydrate g	Fiber g	Sodium mg
CAPERS						
Progresso Capers (1 tsp drained)	0	0	0	0	0	105
CHILI, PICANTE, SALSA, AND TACO SAUCES						
Chi-Chi's Pico De Gallo (2 tbsp)	10	0	0	2	0	170
Salsa Verde, Medium or Mild (2 tbsp)	15	0	0	3	0	180
Salsa, Hot (2 tbsp)	10	0	0	1	0	160
Medium or Mild (2 tbsp)	10	0	0	1	0	140-150
Taco Sauce, Thick & Chunky (1 tbsp)	10	0	0	1	0	75
Picante Sauce, Hot (2 tbsp)	10	0	0	2	0	270
Medium or Mild (2 tbsp)	10	0	0	2	0	200-210
Clemente Jacques Mexican Homestyle Salsa (2 tbsp)	10	0	0	2	0	240

Chili, Picante, Salsa, and Taco Sauces (continued)	Calories	Fat g	Saturated Fat g	Carbohydrate g	Fiber g	Sodium mg
Clemente Jacques (continued)						
Salsa Picante, Hot, Medium or Mild (2 tbsp)	10	0	0	2	<1	270
Salsa Verde (2 tbsp)	15	0	0		0	180
Del Monte Chili Sauce (1 tbsp)	20	0	0	5	0	480
Heinz Chili Sauce (1 tbsp)	15	0	0	4	0	230
Las Palmas Red Chile Sauce (1/4 cup)	15	1	0	2	1	310
Salsa Mexicana, Hot or Medium (2 tbsp)	10	0	0	2	0	75-85
Mild (2 tbsp)	10	0	0	1	0	90
Lawry's Chunky Taco Sauce (2 tbsp)	10	0	0	2	0	250
Taco Sauce N Seasoner (2 tbsp)	15	0	0	3	<1	320
Muir Glen Organic Fat Free Salsa (2 tbsp)	15	0	0	3	<1	75
Newman's Own Salsa, Hot (2 tbsp)	10	0	0	2	<1	150
Medium or Mild (2 tbsp)	10	0	0	2	<1	105
Old El Paso Green Chili Salsa, Medium (2 tbsp)	10	0	0	2	<1	110
Salsa Verde, Medium (2 tbsp)	10	0	0	2	0	95
Extra Chunky Taco Sauce, Mild or Medium (1 tbsp)	5	0	0	1	0	80
Homestyle Salsa, Medium or Mild (2 tbsp)	5	0	0	1	0	110
Picante Salsa, Hot, Medium or Mild (2 tbsp)	10	0	0	2	0	230
Pico de Gallo Salsa, Hot or Medium (2 tbsp)	5	0	0	2	<1	260
Taco Sauce, Hot (1 tbsp)	5	0	0	1	0	90
Medium (1 tbsp)	5	0	0	1	0	70
Mild or Regular (1 tbsp)	5	0	0	1	0	85
Thick 'n Chunky Picantes, Hot (2 tbsp)	10	0	0	2	0	160
Medium (2 tbsp)	10	0	0	2	0	140
Mild (2 tbsp)	10	0	0	2	0	130
Thick 'n Chunky Salsas, Hot (2 tbsp)	10	0	0	2	0	130
Medium or Mild (2 tbsp)	10	0	0	2	0	140
Ortega Garden Style Salsa, Medium or Mild (2 tbsp)	10	0	0	3	0	420
Thick & Chunky Salsas, Hot (2 tbsp)	10	0	0	2	0	370
Medium or Mild (2 tbsp)	10	0	0	2	0	320

	Calories	Fat g	Saturated Fat g	Carbohydrate g	Fiber g	Sodium mg
Thick & Smooth Taco Sauces, Hot, Medium or Mild (1 tbsp)	10	0	0	2	0	125
Pancho Villa Taco Sauce, Mild (2 tbsp)	15	0	0	3	0	170
Progresso Italian Salsa, Hot, Medium or Mild (2 tbsp)	10	0	0	2	<1	170
Smart Temptations Thick & Chunky Salsas, Hot, Medium or Mild (1 tbsp)	8	0	0	2	0	130
The Fat Free Gourmet Salsas, Hot (2 tbsp)	15	0	0	3	<1	88
Mild (2 tbsp)	15	0	0	3	<1	74
Tostitos Salsas, Hot or Medium (2 tbsp)	15	0	0	3	<1	260
Mild (2 tbsp)	15	0	0	3	1	230
COCKTAIL SAUCES						
Chelten House Seafood Cocktail Sauces, Hot or Regular (2 tbsp)	15	0	0	4	0	130
Del Monte Seafood Cocktail Sauce (1 tbsp)	25	0	0	6	0	210
Dockside Seafood Cocktail Sauces, Hot or Regular (2 tbsp)	15	0	0	4	0	130
Kraft Sauceworks Cocktail Sauce (1/4 cup)	60	1	0	13	<1	800
Silver Spring Cocktail Sauce (1/4 cup)	55	0	0	12	1	690
HORSERADISH AND HORSERADISH SAUCES						
Boar's Head Brand Horseradish (1 tsp)	0	0	0	0	0	30
Kraft Horseradishes, Cream Style or Prepared (1 tsp)	0	0	0	0	0	50
Sauceworks Horseradish Sauce (1 tsp)	20	2	0	<1	0	35
Silver Spring Horseradish Sauce (1 tsp)	15	1	0	1	0	40
Beet Style (1 tsp)	0	0	0	0	0	40
Cream Style or Prepared (1 tsp)	0	0	0	0	0	10
Miller (1 tsp)	0	0	0	0	0	0
HOT PEPPERS AND HOT SAUCES						
Most Brands, Hot Chili, canned (1 pepper)	10	0	0	2	0	469
Hot Chili, raw (1 pepper)	18	0	0	4	1	3
Jalapenos, canned (1/4 cup)	8	0	0	2	0	399

Hot Peppers and Hot Sauces (continued)	Calories	Fat g	Saturated Fat g	Carbohydrate g	Fiber g	Sodium mg
America's Choice Hot Cherry Peppers (1 oz = about 2 peppers)	10	0	0	2	0	480
Chi-Chi's Jalapenos Wheels, Green or Red (1 oz)	10	0	0	1	0	110
Whole Jalapenos, Green (1 oz)	10	0	0	2	0	110
Red (1 oz)	15	0	0	3	0	110
Clemente Jacques Jalapenos, Pickled Nacho Slices (about 17 slices)	10	0	0	2	<1	270
Pickled Peppers (about 2 peppers)	10	0	0	1	<1	290
Whole Peppers (about 2 peppers)	10	0	0	2	<1	270
Del Monte Hot Yellow Chili Peppers (4 peppers)	10	0	0	3	<1	610
Old El Paso Jalapenos, Peeled (3 jalapenos)	10	0	0	1	1	200
Pickled (2 jalapenos)	5	0	0	1	0	380
Pickled Slices (2 tbsp)	15	0	0	3	1	400
Progresso Peppers, Cherry (2 tbsp)	20	2	0	2	1	30
Hot Cherry (1 pepper)	15	0	0	3	0	250
Tuscan (3 peppers)	10	0	0	1	1	330
Tabasco brand Sauces, Jalapeno (1 tsp)	0	0	0	0	0	70
Pepper (1 tsp)	0	0	0	0	0	30
KETCHUPS						
Most Brands, Ketchup (1 tbsp)	16	0	0	4	0	178
Low Sodium (1 tbsp)	16	0	0	4	0	3
Del Monte Tomato Ketchup (1 tbsp)	15	0	0	4	0	190
Heinz Lite Ketchup (1 tbsp)	8	0	0	2	0	115
Hunt's Ketchups, No Salt Added (1 tbsp)	20	<1	0	5	<1	0
Tomato (1 tbsp)	15	<1	0	4	<1	160
McIlhenny Farms Spicy Ketchup (1 tbsp)	25	0	0	5	0	130
Weight Watchers Tomato Ketchup (1 tbsp)	8	0	0	2	0	115
MARINADES						
Adolph's Marinade Mix, Chicken (³/₄ tsp dry)	5	0	0	1	0	290
Chicken, Sodium Free (³/₄ tsp dry)	5	0	0	2	0	0
Meat (¹/₂ tsp dry)	0	0	0	1	0	390
Meat, Sodium Free (¹/₂ tsp dry)	5	0	0	2	0	0
Adolph's Marinade in Minutes, Barbecue (¹/₂ tsp dry)	5	0	0	1	0	310

Marinades (continued)	Calories	Fat g	Saturated Fat g	Carbohydrate g	Fiber g	Sodium mg
Cajun (1/2 tsp dry)	5	0	0	1	0	170
Garlic (1/2 tsp dry)	0	0	0	1	0	460
Garlic Dijon (3/4 tsp dry)	10	0	0	1	0	210
Hickory Grill (1 tbsp liquid)	20	1	0	4	0	200
Hot 'N Spicy (3/4 tsp dry)	5	0	0	1	0	130
Italian Herb (1/4 tsp dry)	0	0	0	1	0	270
Lemon Garlic (1 tbsp liquid)	20	3	0	2	0	80
Lemon Pepper (1/2 tsp dry)	10	0	0	2	0	180
Mesquite (1 tbsp liquid)	45	3	0	5	0	270
Mesquite or Parmesan Herb (3/4 tsp dry)	10	0	0	2	0	230
Steak Sauce (1/4 tsp dry)	0	0	0	1	0	350
Teriyaki (1 1/2 tsp dry)	15	0	0	3	<1	380
Teriyaki (1 tbsp liquid)	20	0	0	5	0	740
Adolph's Marinade in Minutes for Seafood, Lemon Herb (1/2 tsp dry)	10	0	0	2	0	170
Scampi (1/2 tsp dry)	10	0	0	2	0	240
House of Tsang Marinade, Mandarin (1 tbsp)	25	0	0	6	0	680
Lawry's Marinade, Hawaiian w/Tropical Fruit Juices (1 tbsp)	20	0	0	4	0	250
Lemon Pepper w/Lemon Juice (1 tbsp)	10	1	0	1	0	380
Red Wine w/Cabernet Sauvignon (1 tbsp)	5	0	0	1	0	270
MUSTARDS						
Most Brands, Chinese, Horseradish or Regular (1 tsp)	4	0	0	0	0	63
America's Choice Pure Prepared Mustards, All American, Horseradish Style or Spicy Brown (1 tsp)	0	0	0	0	0	60
Best Foods Dijonnaise Creamy Mustard Blend (1 tsp)	10	1	0	1	0	60
Boar's Head Brand Mustard Delicatessen Style (1 tsp)	0	0	0	0	0	40
Grey Poupon Mustards, Country Dijon or Dijon (1 tsp)	5	0	0	<1	0	120
Spicy Brown (1 tsp)	5	0	0	<1	0	60
Hellmann's Dijonnaise Creamy Mustard Blend (1 tsp)	10	1	0	1	0	60

Mustards *(continued)*	Calories	Fat g	Saturated Fat g	Carbohydrate g	Fiber g	Sodium mg
Ka-me Hot Mustard Sauce (Chinese style) (1 tsp)	0	0	0	1	0	80
Kraft Mustard, Horseradish or Pure Prepared (1 tsp)	0	0	0	0	0	55-60
Silver Spring Mustards, Beer 'N Brat (1 tsp)	0	0	0	0	0	55
Dijon (1 tsp)	0	0	0	0	0	100
Dill (1 tsp)	0	0	0	0	0	60
Jalapeno (1 tsp)	0	0	0	0	0	85
Polish (1 tsp)	10	0	0	0	0	70
Sweet 'N Hot (1 tsp)	5	0	0	1	0	45
PICKLED VEGETABLES						
Most Brands, Pickled Onions, Cocktail (1 onion)	1	0	0	0	0	5
Boar's Head Brand Sweet Vidalia Onions in Sauce (1 tbsp)	10	0	0	2	0	15
Claussen Tomato Halves (1 oz)	5	0	0	1	<1	320
PICKLES						
Most Brands, Bread & Butter (4 slices)	28	0	0	8	0	225
Dill (4" long)	24	0	0	6	2	1,731
Low Sodium (4" long)	24	0	0	6	2	24
Sour (3 3/4" long)	12	0	0	3	1	833
Sweet Gherkins (1 med)	18	0	0	5	0	141
Watermelon Rind (1 piece)	44	0	0	11	0	214
America's Choice Pickles, Bread & Butter Slices, No Salt Added (1 oz = about 5 slices)	30	0	0	7	NA	10
Dill Slices (1 oz = about 1/2 pickle)	0	0	0	0	0	390
Hamburger Dill Slices (about 7 slices)	0	0	0	0	0	390
Kosher Baby Dill or No Garlic Baby Dill (1 oz = about 1 pickle)	0	0	0	1	0	220
Kosher Dill Spears, No Garlic Dill Spears or Polish Dill Spears (1 oz = about 1 spear)	0	0	0	1	0	220
Kosher Dill or No Garlic Dill (1 oz = about 1/2 pickle)	0	0	0	1	0	220
Old Fashioned, Bread & Butter Slices (1 oz = about 3 slices)	30	0	0	7	NA	170
Kosher Dill (1 oz = about 1/2 pickle)	30	0	0	0	0	220

	Calories	Fat g	Saturated Fat g	Carbohydrate g	Fiber g	Sodium mg
Kosher Dill Spears (1 oz = about 1 spear)	0	0	0	1	0	340
Sweet (1 oz = about 1 pickle)	35	0	0	8	NA	180
Sweet Bread & Butter Slices (1 oz = about 5 slices)	30	0	0	7	NA	170
Sweet Cucumber Sticks (1 oz = about 1¼ spears)	30	0	0	7	NA	170
Sweet Gherkins (1 oz = about 1½ pickles)	35	0	0	8	NA	180
Sweet Midgets (1 oz = about 2 pickles)	35	0	0	8	NA	180
Sweet Mixed (1 oz = about 3 pieces)	35	0	0	8	NA	180
Sweet Salad Cubes (1 tbsp)	20	0	0	4	NA	140
Whole Dill (1 oz = ½ pickle)	0	0	0	0	0	390
Claussen Pickles, Bread'N Butter Chips (4 slices)	20	0	0	4	0	170
Hamburger Dill Slices/Chips (10 slices)	5	0	0	1	0	420
Kosher Dill Halves or Wholes (1 oz)	5	0	0	1	0	330
Kosher Dill Slices (4 slices)	5	0	0	1	0	320
Kosher Dill Spears (1 spear)	5	0	0	1	0	310
Kosher Mini Dills (1 pickle)	5	0	0	1	0	300
New York Deli Style Half Sours (1 oz)	5	0	0	1	0	260
Del Monte Pickles, Dill (1 pickle)	5	0	0	1	<1	590
Dill Hamburger Chips (5 chips)	5	0	0	<1	0	310
Tiny Kosher Dill (1 pickle)	5	0	0	<1	<1	200
Whole Sweet (1 pickle)	45	0	0	12	<1	230
Gedney Pickles, Dill Spears (1 oz = about 1 spear)	5	0	0	1	0	290
Hot & Sweet Snackers (1 oz = about 4 slices)	30	0	0	7	NA	180
Midget Dill (1 oz = about 1 med pickle)	5	0	0	1	0	290
Pantry Sweet (1 oz = about 5 slices)	30	0	0	8	NA	190
Sweet Gherkins (1 oz = about 2 pickles)	30	0	0	8	NA	180
Whole Dill (1 oz = about ½ large pickle)	5	0	0	1	0	290
State Fair Pickles, Bread & Butter, Regular or Hot (1 oz = about 9 slices)	35	0	0	7	NA	180
Dill or Kosher Midget Dill (1 oz = about 1 med pickle)	5	0	0	1	0	290

	Calories	Fat g	Saturated Fat g	Carbohydrate g	Fiber g	Sodium mg
Gedney State Fair Pickles *(continued)*						
Grandma's Baby-Baby Dill (1 oz = about 4 sm pickles)	5	0	0	1	0	290
Heinz Hamburger Dill Chips (8 slices)	0	0	0	1	0	370
McIlhenny Farms Hot 'N Sweet Sliced Pickles (about 5 slices)	40	0	0	10	0	30
Vlasic Pickles, Milwaukee Plain Dills (1 oz)	5	0	0	1	0	260
Sweet (1 oz)	40	0	0	10	0	170
PIMIENTOS						
Osage Pimientos (3/4 tsp)	0	0	0	0	0	0
RELISHES						
Most Brands, Chutney (1 tbsp)	21	0	0	5	0	9
Relishes, Corn (1 tbsp)	13	0	0	3	0	59
Cranberry-Orange (1/4 cup)	121	0	0	31	1	22
Hot Dog (1 tbsp)	19	0	0	5	0	122
Sour Pickle (1 tbsp)	1	0	0	0	0	242
Sweet Pickle (1 tbsp)	20	0	0	5	0	124
America's Choice Relish, Sweet (1 tbsp)	20	0	0	5	NA	140
Claussen Relish, Sweet Pickle (1 tbsp)	15	0	0	3	0	85
Del Monte Relishes, Hamburger (1 tbsp)	20	0	0	6	<1	220
Hot Dog (1 tbsp)	15	0	0	3	<1	140
Sweet Pickle (1 tbsp)	20	0	0	5	0	125
Gedney Relishes, Dill Pickle (1 tbsp)	0	0	0	<1	0	270
Hot Dog Pickle (1 tbsp)	18	0	0	4	NA	100
Green Giant Corn Relish (1 tbsp)	20	0	0	5	0	40
Heinz Relishes, Dill (1 tbsp)	0	0	0	0	0	220
Hot Dog (1 tbsp)	15	0	0	4	0	105
India (1 tbsp)	20	0	0	5	0	100
Sweet (1 tbsp)	15	0	0	4	0	90
Old El Paso Jalapeno Relish (1 tbsp)	5	0	0	1	0	110
Silver Spring Hot Dog Relish (1 tsp)	5	0	0	1	0	45
SOY SAUCES						
Chun King Soy Sauce (1 tbsp)	5	0	0	<1	0	1,050
Lite (1 tbsp)	5	0	0	<1	0	630
House of Tsang Soy Sauce (1 tbsp)	5	0	0	0	0	280
Dark (1 tbsp)	10	0	0	1	0	860

Soy Sauces (continued)	Calories	Fat g	Saturated Fat g	Carbohydrate g	Fiber g	Sodium mg
Ginger Flavored (1 tbsp)	20	0	0	4	0	730
Light (1 tbsp)	5	0	0	0	0	900
Low Sodium, Ginger or Mushroom Flavored (1 tbsp)	10	0	0	2	0	280
Ka-me Soy Sauces, Dark (Chinese) (1 tbsp)	10	0	0	3	0	1,020
Japanese (1 tbsp)	5	0	0	1	0	520
Light (Chinese) (1 tbsp)	5	0	0	1	0	1,170
Mild (1 tbsp)	5	0	0	0	0	490
La Choy Soy Sauce (1/2 tsp)	2	<1	0	<1	<1	230
STEAK SAUCES						
A-1 Steak Sauces, Bold (1 tbsp)	20	0	0	5	5	190
Regular (1 tbsp)	15	0	0	3	0	250
VINEGARS						
Ka-me Vinegars, Chinese Seasoned (1 tbsp)	5	0	0	1	0	60
Rice Wine (Chinese) (1 tbsp)	5	0	0	1	0	0
Rice Wine (Japanese) (1 tbsp)	0	0	0	1	0	0
Seasoned Rice (Japanese) (1 tbsp)	10	0	0	3	0	180
Progresso Vinegar, Garlic Flavored, Red or White Wine (1 tbsp)	0	0	0	0	0	0
WORCESTERSHIRE SAUCE						
Heinz Worcestershire Sauce (1 tsp)	0	0	0	0	0	55

CRACKERS

Crackers included in this section of the Guide are low in fat and saturated fat and do not exceed 3 grams of fat and 1 gram of saturated fat per serving. Many cracker labels specify the number of crackers equal to 1 serving, which is usually 1 ounce (oz) or ½ oz. If this information is not provided, you may need to weigh several crackers to determine the number equal to ½ oz or 1 oz.

Crackers	Calories	Fat g	Saturated Fat g	Carbohydrate g	Fiber g	Sodium mg
CRACKERS						
Higher-Fat						
Butter Crackers (10 round)	152	8	2	17	1	254
Cheese Crackers (30 sm square)	151	8	3	17	1	298
Cheese-Filled Cracker Sandwiches (4 sandwiches)	134	6	2	17	1	392
Peanut Butter-Filled Cracker Sandwiches (4 sandwiches)	137	7	1	16	1	264
Lower-Fat						
Ak-mak Original Sesame Cracker (5 crackers)	116	2	1	19	4	214
America's Choice Saltines (5 crackers)	60	0	0	13	0	135
Auburn Farms Fat Free 7-Grainers, Bite Size Multi-grain Crackers, Onion, Rye or Veggie (10 crackers)	60	0	0	12	1	105
Original (10 crackers)	60	0	0	12	1	110
Spicy Snack Crackers, Pesto & Dill or Sun Dried Tomato & Basil (20 crackers)	110	0	0	23	2	250
Pizza or Salsa & Hot Chipotle Pepper (20 crackers)	110	0	0	23	2	280

Crackers (continued)	Calories	Fat g	Saturated Fat g	Carbohydrate g	Fiber g	Sodium mg
Bremner Wafers (13 crackers)	130	3	1	22	2	200
Carr's Assorted Biscuits for Cheese (3 pieces)	80	3	1	13	<1	125
Croissant Crackers (3 pieces)	70	3	1	10	0	115
Table Water Crackers, Bite Size, w/Cracked Pepper or w/Sesame (5 pieces)	70	2	0	13	<1	95-100
King Size (2 pieces)	60	1	0	12	<1	90
Crispini, Fat Free (1/2 cup)	110	0	0	23	<1	400
Salt Free Stone Ground Wheat (5 crispini)	110	<1	<1	19	1	0
Seeds & Spice, Sesame or Sesame Garlic (5 crispini)	110	3	<1	18	1	120
Delicious Soup & Chili Crackers (80 pieces)	120	3	1	20	2	250
Edward & Sons Baked Brown Rice Snaps (5 crackers)	35	<1	0	7	NA	1
Finn Crisp Crispbread, Dark or Dark w/Caraway (3 pieces)	60	0	0	12	3	0
Health Valley Fat-Free Crackers, Cheese, Herb, Onion, Vegetable or Whole Wheat (7 crackers)	50	0	0	11	2	80
Vegetable, No Salt (5 crackers)	50	0	0	11	2	15
Fat-Free Fire Crackers, Hot 3 Chilies, Medium Jalapeno or Mild Chili (6 crackers)	50	0	0	11	2	80
Fat-Free Pizza Crackers, Garlic & Herb, Italiano or Spicy Cheese (6 crackers)	50	0	0	11	2	80
Jacobsen's Snack Toast, Cinnamon & Raisin (1 slice)	55	1	0	11	0	65
Cinnamon (1 slice)	50	1	0	11	0	75
Original (1 slice)	45	1	0	9	NA	65
Ka-me Rice Crunch Crackers, Cheese (16 pieces)	120	2	0	24	0	180
Onion (16 pieces)	120	1	0	25	0	75
Plain (16 pieces)	120	2	0	25	0	15
Seaweed (16 pieces)	120	2	0	25	0	100
Sesame (16 pieces)	120	2	0	24	0	85
Unsalted (16 pieces)	120	1	0	26	0	0

	Calories	Fat g	Saturated Fat g	Carbohydrate g	Fiber g	Sodium mg
Kavli All Natural Crispbread, 5 Grain (1 piece)	40	0	0	9	2	30
5 Grain Muesli (1 slice)	30	<1	0	7	2	35
Rye-Bran (2 wafers)	30	<1	0	6	2	35
All Natural Whole Grain Crispbread, Crispy Thin (3 pieces)	60	0	0	13	2	45
Hearty Thick (2 pieces)	70	1	0	15	3	55
Keebler Crackers, Club, 50% Reduced Sodium (4 crackers)	70	3	1	9	<1	80
Cheddar (4 crackers)	70	3	1	9	0	180
Club Partners Crackers, Garlic Bread Flavored (4 crackers)	70	3	1	9	0	140
Regular or Wheat (4 crackers)	70	3	1	9	<1	140-160
Toasteds, Reduced Fat Wheat (10 crackers)	120	3	1	20	<1	300
Town House, Reduced Fat (5 crackers)	70	2	1	11	<1	180
Zesta Saltines, 50% Reduced Sodium (5 crackers)	60	2	1	11	<1	95
Fat Free (5 crackers)	50	0	0	11	<1	90
Plain (5 crackers)	60	2	1	10	<1	190
Unsalted Tops (5 crackers)	70	2	1	10	<1	90
Krispy Crackers, Soup & Oyster (17 crackers)	60	2	0	11	<1	200
Saltines, Cracked Pepper or Plain (5 crackers)	60	2	0	10	<1	180
Fat Free (5 crackers)	60	0	0	12	<1	135
Mild Cheddar (5 crackers)	60	2	1	10	<1	180
Unsalted or Whole Wheat (5 crackers)	60	2	0	10	<1	120-130
Lance Crackers, Captain's Wafers, Very Low Sodium (4 crackers)	70	3	1	11	0	30
Multi-Grain (4 crackers)	70	3	1	10	<1	100
Oyster (1 pkg)	60	2	1	10	0	135
Saltines (6 crackers)	70	2	1	11	0	160
Sesame Twins (4 crackers)	70	2	1	12	1	125
Sour Dough (4 crackers)	70	3	1	10	0	100
Wheat Twins (4 crackers)	70	3	1	10	1	120
Wheatswafer (4 crackers)	60	3	1	9	1	100

	Calories	Fat g	Saturated Fat g	Carbohydrate g	Fiber g	Sodium mg
Lifestream Natural Foods Stoneground Wheat Crackers, Garden Vegetable (12 crackers)	120	2	0	22	4	210
Sesame Seed (12 crackers)	130	3	0	22	4	170
Wheat & Onion (12 crackers)	120	2	0	22	4	160
Manischewitz Egg 'n Onion Matzos (1 bread)	100	1	0	23	2	200
Mister Salty Pretzel Chips, Fat Free (16 chips)	100	0	0	22	1	620
Regular (16 chips)	110	3	0	21	<1	620
Nabisco Crackers, Crown Pilot (1 cracker)	70	2	0	13	<1	85
Mr. Phipp's Pretzel Chips, Fat Free Original (16 chips)	100	0	0	22	<1	630
Lower Sodium (16 chips)	120	3	0	21	<1	410
Original (16 chips)	120	3	0	21	<1	630
Oysterettes Soup & Oyster (19 crackers)	60	3	1	10	<1	150
Premium Soup & Oyster Crackers (23 crackers)	60	2	0	11	<1	230
Premium Saltines, Fat Free (5 crackers)	50	0	0	11	0	130
Low Sodium (5 crackers)	60	1	0	10	<1	35
Multigrain (5 crackers)	60	2	0	10	1	150
Original (5 crackers)	60	2	0	10	<1	180
Unsalted Tops (5 crackers)	60	2	0	10	<1	135
Ritz Crackers Reduced Fat (5 crackers)	70	3	1	10	0	135
Royal Lunch Milk (1 cracker)	50	2	0	3	0	65
Triscuit Wafers, Reduced Fat (8 wafers)	130	3	1	24	4	180
Uneeda Biscuit Unsalted Tops (2 crackers)	60	2	0	11	<1	110
Zwieback Teething Toast (1 toast)	35	1	1	5	<1	10
No-No 6 Grain Light Flat Breads, Cracked Pepper (3 pieces = 1 oz)	70	1	0	15	1	110
Garlic Salt (1 oz)	100	0	0	22	0	140
O.T.C. (Original Trenton Cracker) Crackers, Soup, Chowder & Oyster (3 pieces)	70	2	1	12	0	230
Old London Melba Snacks, Bacon Flavor, Garlic or White (5 pieces)	60	2	0	11	2	105-110
Mexicali Corn (5 pieces)	60	2	0	10	2	100
Onion (5 pieces)	60	2	0	11	2	140
Rye (5 pieces)	60	2	0	11	1	190

	Calories	Fat g	Saturated Fat g	Carbohydrate g	Fiber g	Sodium mg
Old London Melba Snacks *(continued)*						
Sesame (5 pieces)	60	3	1	9	1	110
Whole Grain (5 pieces)	60	2	0	11	2	120
Melba Toast, Onion (3 pieces)	50	1	0	11	1	140
Rye or White (3 pieces)	50	1	0	11	1	105
Sesame (3 pieces)	50	2	0	10	2	140
Unsalted (3 pieces)	50	2	0	10	2	0
Whole Grain (3 pieces)	45	1	0	11	2	120
Unsalted (3 pieces)	50	1	0	11	1	0
Pacific Grain Products No Fries Potato Snacks (34 pieces)	120	1	0	26	1	150
Au Gratin (30 pieces)	120	2	0	25	1	125
Bar-B-Que (30 pieces)	120	2	0	25	1	140
Sour Cream & Chives (30 pieces)	120	2	0	25	1	105
No Fries Tortilla Snacks (34 pieces)	120	1	0	26	1	55
Cheddar Jalapeno or Salsa & Sour Cream (30 pieces)	120	2	0	25	1	170
Ranch (30 pieces)	120	2	0	25	1	190
Pepperidge Farm Distinctive Crackers, Butter Thins (4 crackers)	70	3	1	10	0	95
Cracked Wheat (2 crackers)	70	3	1	9	<1	150
Sesame (3 crackers)	70	3	0	9	2	95
Three Cracker Assortment (4 crackers)	60	3	1	9	0	90
Pop Secret Pop Chips, Butter Flavor (1 oz = 31 chips)	120	3	1	21	1	380
Original (1 oz = 31 chips)	120	3	1	21	1	380
R.W. Frookie Fat Free Gourmet Crackers, Cracked Pepper (4 crackers)	35	0	0	7	NA	40
Garlic & Herb (4 crackers)	70	0	0	16	1	170
Water (4 crackers)	35	0	0	7	NA	60
Ry-Krisp Crackers, Original (2 crackers)	60	0	0	13	4	75
Seasoned (2 crackers)	60	2	0	10	3	90
Wheat Krisp (2 crackers)	70	2	0	12	2	150
Ryvita Crispbread, Flavorful Fiber (2 slices)	50	1	0	14	3	20
Tasty Dark Rye (2 slices)	60	1	0	14	3	35
Tasty Light Rye (2 slices)	60	0	0	15	3	20
Toasted Sesame Rye (2 slices)	70	2	0	14	2	35

Crackers (continued)	Calories	Fat g	Saturated Fat g	Carbohydrate g	Fiber g	Sodium mg
SnackWell's Fat Free Crackers, Cracked Pepper (7 crackers)	60	0	0	13	<1	150
Wheat (5 crackers)	60	0	0	12	1	170
Reduced Fat Crackers, Cheese (38 crackers)	130	2	1	23	1	340
Classic Golden (6 crackers)	60	1	0	11	0	140
French Onion (32 crackers)	120	2	0	23	1	290
Zesty Cheese (32 crackers)	120	2	1	23	1	350
The House of Aulsebrooks Water Crackers, Cracked Pepper (5 crackers)	60	1	0	11	1	90
Sesame (5 crackers)	70	2	0	10	<1	85
The Original JJ Flats Breadflat, Flavorall or Sesame (1 piece)	50	1	0	1	1	130
Poppy (1 piece)	50	1	0	1	<1	130
Valley Lahvosh, 15" Rounds (1.8 oz)	190	2	0	37	1	250
15" Wheat Rounds (1.8 oz)	190	2	0	37	3	250
2" or 3" Rounds or Hearts (1 oz)	110	1	0	21	<1	140
3" Wheat Rounds (1 oz)	110	1	0	20	2	140
5" Rounds (1.2 oz)	140	2	0	26	<1	180
5" Wheat Rounds (1.2 oz)	130	2	0	26	2	180
Sweetheart Crispies (1 oz)	120	3	1	22	<1	130
Venus Crackers, Fat Free, Cracked Pepper or Garlic & Herb (22 crackers)	110	0	0	24	<1	120
Garden Vegetable (10 crackers)	110	0	0	24	<1	150
Multi-Grain (10 crackers)	110	0	0	24	1	170
Stoned Wheat, Salt Free (10 crackers)	120	3	1	22	2	0
Venus Wafers, Bran, Salt Free (10 wafers)	120	2	1	22	3	0
Wasa Crisp'N Light Crackerbread, Wheat (1 slice)	20	<1	0	4	<1	38
Wasa Original Crispbread, Fiber Plus (1 slice)	35	0	0	5	3	60
Golden Rye (1 slice)	36	0	0	7	2	50
Hearty Rye (1 slice)	45	0	0	9	3	40
Sesame Rye (1 slice)	30	1	0	5	3	55
Sesame Wheat (1 slice)	50	2	0	8	1	75

	Calories	Fat g	Saturated Fat g	Carbohydrate g	Fiber g	Sodium mg
POPCORN, RICE, AND OTHER GRAIN CAKES						
Lifestream Natural Foods Toasted Whole Brown Rice Cakes, Multigrain, Original or Sesame (2 cakes)	110	1	0	23	0	25-35
Original Unsalted or Sesame Unsalted (2 cakes)	110	1	0	23	0	5
Mother's Mini Rice Cakes, Apple, Caramel or Cinnamon (5 mini cakes)	50	0	0	12	0	40
Plain, Unsalted (7 mini cakes)	60	0	0	12	0	0
Popped Corn Cakes, Unsalted (1 cake)	35	0	0	8	0	0
Unsalted Butter Flavor (1 cake)	35	0	0	7	0	0
Rice Cakes, Multigrain, Lightly Salted (1 cake)	35	0	0	7	0	30
Wheat Cakes, Unsalted (1 cake)	35	0	0	7	1	0
Pritikin Mini Rice Cakes, Apple Crisp (5 cakes)	50	0	0	12	0	20
Caramel Nut Flavor (5 cakes)	50	0	0	12	0	45
Rice Cakes, Multigrain, Plain or Sesame, Low Sodium (1 cake)	35	0	0	7	0	20
Unsalted Rice Cakes, Multigrain, Plain or Sesame (1 cake)	35	0	0	7	0	0
Quaker Corn Cakes, Caramel Flavored (1 cake)	50	0	0	12	0	30
Mild White Cheddar (1 cake)	40	0	0	8	0	100
Nacho (1 cake)	40	0	0	8	0	80
Quaker Mini Rice Cakes, Buttered Popcorn (6 mini cakes)	50	0	0	12	0	120
Caramel Corn, Cinnamon Crunch or Honey Nut (5 mini cakes)	50	0	0	12	0	25
White Cheddar (6 mini cakes)	50	0	0	11	0	120
Rice Cakes, Apple Cinnamon (1 cake)	50	0	0	11	0	0
Cinnamon Crunch (1 cake)	50	0	0	11	0	25
Wheat Cakes (1 cake)	35	0	0	7	1	45
Snack Lovers Popped Corn Cakes, Natural Butter Flavor or Natural White Cheddar Flavor (1 cake)	50	0	0	11	0	45-55
Natural Caramel Flavor (1 cake)	60	0	0	13	0	10

DAIRY PRODUCTS AND DAIRY SUBSTITUTES

The butterfat in "regular" dairy products is a major source of saturated fat in the typical American diet. A cutoff point for saturated fat of 2 grams has been used for dairy products instead of the 1 gram used for the dairy substitutes in this section and for most other products in the Guide. Although almost two-thirds of the fat in dairy products is saturated, many of these foods are excellent sources of calcium and protein. Using a cutoff point of 2 grams of saturated fat in a serving of dairy products allows inclusion in the Guide of a greater variety of calcium-rich foods, which are important to health. A serving of the dairy products and dairy substitutes included in this section of the Guide does not exceed the cutoff points shown below.

CUTOFF POINTS FOR
DAIRY PRODUCTS AND DAIRY SUBSTITUTES

	Fat g	Saturated Fat g
Dairy Products	3	2
Dairy Substitutes	3	1

Cheeses

Cheeses	Calories	Fat g	Saturated Fat g	Carbohydrate g	Fiber g	Sodium mg
CHEESES						
Higher-Fat						
American Process Cheese (1 oz)	113	9	6	0	0	429
Brie Cheese (1 oz)	90	7	5	0	0	253
Camembert Cheese (1 oz)	90	7	5	0	0	253
Cheddar Cheese (1 oz)	121	10	6	0	0	186
Mozzarella Cheese, made w/whole milk (1 oz)	96	7	5	1	0	124
Swiss Cheese, Natural (1 oz)	113	8	5	1	0	78

	Calories	Fat g	Saturated Fat g	Carbohydrate g	Fiber g	Sodium mg
Lower-Fat						
Alpine Lace Fat Free Pasteurized Process Skim Milk Cheese Products, American, Cheddar or Mozzarella, deli-cut (1 oz)	45	0	0	2	0	280
American, singles (²/₃ oz)	25	0	0	<1	0	280
Cheddar or Mozzarella, chunk (1 oz = ¹/₆ bar)	45	0	0	2	0	280
Shredded (¹/₄ cup)	45	0	0	2	0	280
Di Giorno 100% Parmesan Cheese, grated (2 tsp)	20	2	1	0	0	85
Shredded (2 tsp)	20	2	1	0	0	75
100% Romano Cheese, grated (2 tsp)	20	2	1	0	0	90
Shredded (2 tsp)	20	2	1	0	0	70
Parmesan Cheese (2 tsp)	20	1	1	0	0	55
Romano Cheese (2 tsp)	20	2	1	0	0	75
Formägg Cheese Alternatives, Cheddar, shredded (1 oz)	60	3	0	1	0	190
Mozzarella, shredded (1 oz)	60	3	0	1	0	140
Parmesan, grated (2 tsp)	15	1	0	<1	<1	80
Frigo Truly Lite Cheese, Reduced Fat Low Moisture Part Skim Mozzarella, chunk (1 oz = 1" piece)	60	3	2	<1	0	200
Shredded (¹/₄ cup)	60	3	2	<1	0	200
String (1 oz)	60	3	2	<1	0	200
Romano, shredded (1 tbsp)	25	2	1	0	0	115
Healthy Choice Cheeses, Cheddar or Mozzarella, shredded (¹/₄ cup)	45	0	0	2	0	200
Cheddar, Mozzarella or Pizza, fancy shredded (¹/₄ cup)	45	0	0	2	0	200
Mexican, shredded (¹/₄ cup)	45	0	0	2	<1	200
Mozzarella Ball (1" cube)	45	0	0	1	<1	200
Process Loaf (1" cube)	35	0	0	3	<1	390
String Cheeses, Mozzarella or Pizza (1 stick)	45	0	0	1	0	200
White or Yellow American Singles (³/₄ oz slice)	30	0	0	2	<1	290
Yellow American Singles (²/₃ oz slice)	25	0	0	2	<1	270

Cheeses (continued)	Calories	Fat g	Saturated Fat g	Carbohydrate g	Fiber g	Sodium mg
Healthy Farms Antioxidant Fortified Fat Free Cheeses, Cheddar, Salsa Cheddar, Sharp Cheddar or Swiss (1 oz)	40	0	0	1	0	220
Heart Beat Foods Smart Beat Fat Free Non-Dairy Slices, American Flavor, American Flavor Lactose Free or Mellow Cheddar Flavor (1 slice)	25	0	0	3	0	180
Sharp Cheddar Flavor (1 slice)	25	0	0	3	0	230
Low-Sodium Reduced Calorie Slices, American Flavor (1 slice)	35	2	<1	2	0	90
Kraft 100% Parmesan Cheese, dry or fresh, grated (2 tsp)	25	2	1	0	0	85-90
100% Parmesan Cheese, shredded (2 tsp)	20	2	1	0	0	75
American Cheese Food, grated (1 tbsp)	25	2	1	1	0	135
Cheez Whiz Light Pasteurized Process Cheese Product (2 tbsp)	80	3	2	6	0	540
Harvest Moon American Flavor Pasteurized Process Cheese Product (2/3 oz)	50	3	2	1	0	280
Healthy Favorites Fat-Free Natural Non-Fat Cheeses, Cheddar, shredded (1/4 cup)	45	0	0	1	0	220
Mozzarella, shredded (1/4 cup)	50	0	0	2	<1	280
House Italian (1/3 Less Fat), grated (2 tsp)	25	1	1	1	0	115
Italian Blend, grated (2 tsp)	25	2	1	0	0	95
Light N' Lively Pasteurized Process Cheese Products, American Flavor (50% Less Fat), Yellow or White (3/4 oz)	50	3	2	2	0	280-300
Pasteurized Process Cheese Product (1/3 Less Fat) Singles, American Flavor, Yellow or White (3/4 oz)	50	3	2	2	0	330
Cheddar Flavor (3/4 oz)	50	3	2	2	0	300
Swiss Flavor (3/4 oz)	50	3	2	2	0	270
Kraft Free Nonfat Pasteurized Process Cheese Slice Singles, Sharp Cheddar or Swiss, Artificially Flavored (3/4 oz)	30	0	0	3	0	290
Yellow or White (3/4 oz)	30	0	0	3	0	320
Lifetime Fat Free Cheese, Cheddar, Garden Vegetable, Mild Mexican, Monterey Jack, Sharp Cheddar or Swiss (1 oz)	40	0	0	1	0	220

	Calories	Fat g	Saturated Fat g	Carbohydrate g	Fiber g	Sodium mg
Miceli's Fat Free Ricotta (¹/₄ cup)	50	0	0	5	0	65
Sargento Natural Light Ricotta Cheese (¹/₄ cup)	60	3	2	3	0	55
Preferred Light Natural Reduced Fat Low-Moisture Mozzarella Cheese, fancy shredded (¹/₄ cup)	70	3	2	<1	0	140
Swiss Knight Light (1 oz)	45	3	1	0	0	270
The Laughing Cow Light Pasteurized Process Cheese Spread (1 oz piece)	50	3	2	1	0	370
Velveeta Light Pasteurized Process Cheese Product (1 oz)	60	3	2	3	0	420
Weight Watchers Fat Free Parmesan Italian Topping, grated (1 tbsp)	15	0	0	2	0	45
Fat Free Cheese Slices, Sharp Cheddar, White or Yellow (³/₄ oz)	30	0	0	2	0	310
Swiss (³/₄ oz)	30	0	0	2	0	280
Low Sodium Cheese Slices, White or Yellow (³/₄ oz)	50	2	1	2	0	110

COTTAGE CHEESES

Higher-Fat

	Calories	Fat g	Saturated Fat g	Carbohydrate g	Fiber g	Sodium mg
Cottage Cheese, made from whole milk (¹/₂ cup)	109	5	3	3	0	425

Lower-Fat

	Calories	Fat g	Saturated Fat g	Carbohydrate g	Fiber g	Sodium mg
Breakstone's Cottage Cheeses, Dry Curd (Less than ¹/₂% Milk Fat w/Added Skim Milk) (¹/₄ cup)	45	0	0	3	0	25
Low Fat Large Curd or Small Curd (2% Milkfat) (¹/₂ cup)	90	3	2	4	0	380
Cabot No Fat Cottage Cheese (¹/₂ cup)	70	0	0	5	0	410
Crowley Nonfat Cottage Cheese, Plain (¹/₂ cup)	90	0	0	7	0	500
w/Aspartame Sweetened Peach or Pear (¹/₂ cup)	90	0	0	8	0	410
w/Aspartame Sweetened Pineapple (¹/₂ cup)	90	0	0	10	0	440
w/Aspartame Sweetened Spiced Apple (¹/₂ cup)	90	0	0	9	0	420
Knudsen Free Nonfat Cottage Cheese (¹/₂ cup)	80	0	0	4	0	370

	Calories	Fat g	Saturated Fat g	Carbohydrate g	Fiber g	Sodium mg
Lowfat Cottage Cheese (1.5% Milkfat),						
& Peach (4 oz)	110	2	1	12	0	290
& Pineapple (4 oz)	110	2	1	11	0	290
& Strawberry (4 oz)	110	2	1	12	0	280
& Tropical Fruit (4 oz)	120	2	2	15	0	300
Lowfat Cottage Cheese, Small Curd (2% Milkfat) (1/2 cup)	100	3	2	3	0	400
Kraft Light N' Lively Free Nonfat Cottage Cheese (1/2 cup)	80	0	0	5	0	440
Lowfat Cottage Cheese (1% Milkfat), Plain (1/2 cup)	80	2	1	4	0	380
W/Garden Salad (1/2 cup)	90	2	1	5	0	410
W/Peach & Pineapple (1/2 cup)	120	1	1	14	0	350
Nancy's Lowfat Cottage Cheese (1/2 cup)	80	1	1	3	0	460
Sealtest Lowfat Small Curd Cottage Cheese (2% Milkfat) (1/2 cup)	90	3	2	4	0	380
Weight Watchers 1% Cottage Cheese (1/2 cup)	90	1	1	4	0	460
CREAM CHEESES						
Higher-Fat						
Cream Cheese, regular (1 oz)	105	10	7	1	0	89
Lower-Fat						
Alpine Lace Fat Free Cream Cheeses, Plain, w/Garden Vegetables, Garlic & Herb or Mexican Nacho (2 tbsp)	30	0	0	1	0	165
America's Choice Fat Free Cream Cheese (2 tbsp)	30	0	0	3	0	150
Healthy Choice Cream Cheeses, Herbs & Garlic or Plain (2 tbsp)	25	0	0	2	<1	200
Strawberry (2 tbsp)	35	0	0	2	<1	200
Kraft Philadelphia Brand Free Fat Free Cream Cheeses, Brick (1 oz)	25	0	0	2	0	135
Soft (2 tbsp)	30	0	0	2	0	160
Weight Watchers Cream Cheese (1 oz)	35	2	1	1	0	40
CREAMERS						
Carnation Coffee-mate Fat Free Non-Dairy Creamer, refrigerated (1 tbsp)	10	0	0	0	0	5

	Calories	Fat g	Saturated Fat g	Carbohydrate g	Fiber g	Sodium mg
Carnation Coffee-mate Fat Free Non-Dairy Creamers *(continued)*						
Butter Rum, French Vanilla, Hazelnut or Irish Creme, refrigerated (1 tbsp)	25	0	0	6	0	20
Non-Dairy Creamer, Amaretto or Irish Creme, refrigerated (1 tbsp)	40	2	0	5	0	5
Lite, refrigerated (1 tbsp)	10	1	0	1	0	5
International Delight Gourmet Non-Dairy Creamer, Amaretto or Irish Creme, refrigerated (1 tbsp)	45	2	0	7	0	5
No Fat Non-Dairy Creamer, Amaretto, French Vanilla Royale, Hawaiian Macadamia or Irish Creme, refrigerated (1 tbsp)	30	0	0	7	0	5
Mocha Mix Non-Dairy Creamer, Fat Free, refrigerated (1 tbsp)	10	0	0	1	0	0
Original, refrigerated (1 tbsp)	20	2	0	1	0	5
N-Rich Coffee Creamer (1 tsp dry)	10	<1	0	1	0	0
Weight Watchers Dairy Creamer Instant Nonfat Milk (1 pkt)	10	0	0	1	0	15
MILK SUBSTITUTES						
A&A Amazing Foods Vegelicious Beverage Mix, prep w/water (8 oz)	90	3	0	17	0	115
Fat Free Beverages, Chocolate, ready-to-serve (8 oz)	140	0	0	35	1	200
Regular, ready-to-serve (8 oz)	90	0	0	21	0	100
EdenBlend (8 fl oz)	120	3	1	16	0	85
EdenRice (8 fl oz)	110	3	0	21	0	85
Edensoy Extra Vanilla (8 fl oz)	140	3	0	23	0	90
Vanilla (8 fl oz)	150	3	0	23	0	90
Health Valley Fat-Free Soy Moo (1 cup)	110	0	0	22	1	60
A Taste of Thai Lite Coconut Milk (1 tbsp)	15	1	1	1	0	5
MILKS AND BUTTERMILKS						
Higher-Fat						
Milk, 2% fat (8 fl oz)	121	5	3	12	0	122
Whole (8 fl oz)	150	8	5	11	0	120
Lower-Fat						
Most Brands, 1% Fat (1 cup)	102	2	2	12	0	123

Milks and Buttermilks (continued)	Calories	Fat g	Saturated Fat g	Carbohydrate g	Fiber g	Sodium mg
½% Fat (1 cup)	92	1	1	12	0	125
Buttermilk, lowfat (1 cup)	99	2	1	12	0	257
Evaporated Skim (2 tbsp)	25	0	0	4	0	37
Nonfat Instant Dry (¼ cup)	61	0	0	16	0	93
Nonfat or Skim (1 cup)	86	0	0	12	0	126
Borden Fat Free Skim Milk w/Solids Added (1 cup)	90	0	0	13	0	125
Low Fat Sweetened Condensed Milk (2 tbsp)	120	2	1	23	0	40
Carnation Nonfat Dry Milk (⅓ cup)	80	0	0	12	0	125
Evaporated Milks, Lowfat (2 tbsp)	25	1	0	3	0	35
Skimmed (2 tbsp)	25	0	0	4	0	40
Golden Jersey Fat Free Cholesterol Free Milks, Chocolate, No Sugar Added (1 cup)	110	0	0	16	0	155
Plain (1 cup)	100	0	0	14	0	120
Horizon Organic Nonfat Milk (1 cup)	90	0	0	13	0	130
Oak Farms Lowfat Eggnog (½ cup)	140	3	2	13	0	85
Pet Evaporated Skim Milk (2 tbsp)	25	0	0	3	0	35
Robinson ½% Plus Lowfat Milk (1 cup)	90	1	1	12	0	125
Saco Cultured Buttermilk Blend (4 tbsp dry)	80	1	0	13	0	166
Mix 'n Drink Pure Skim Milk (⅓ cup dry)	80	0	0	12	0	125
Sanalac Nonfat Dry Milk, prep w/water (8 oz)	80	<1	0	12	0	125

SOUR CREAMS

Higher-Fat

	Calories	Fat g	Saturated Fat g	Carbohydrate g	Fiber g	Sodium mg
Sour Cream, Regular (2 tbsp)	57	6	3	1	0	11

Lower-Fat

	Calories	Fat g	Saturated Fat g	Carbohydrate g	Fiber g	Sodium mg
Breakstone Free Fat Free Sour Cream (2 tbsp)	35	0	0	6	0	25
Crowley Nonfat Sour Cream (2 tbsp)	20	0	0	3	0	45
Daisy Sour Cream, Light (2 tbsp)	30	3	2	1	1	10
No Fat (2 tbsp)	20	0	0	1	0	15
Knudsen Free Fat Free Sour Cream (2 tbsp)	35	0	0	6	0	25
Light Sour Cream (2 tbsp)	40	3	2	2	0	20
Land O'Lakes Sour Cream, Light (2 tbsp)	35	2	2	4	0	30
No Fat (2 tbsp)	30	0	0	5	0	40

	Calories	Fat g	Saturated Fat g	Carbohydrate g	Fiber g	Sodium mg
Sour Creams (continued)						
Naturally Yours Real Dairy No Fat Sour Cream (2 tbsp)	20	0	0	4	<1	25
Sealtest Free Fat Free Sour Cream (2 tbsp)	35	0	0	6	0	25
Light Sour Cream (2 tbsp)	40	3	2	2	0	20
Weight Watchers Light Sour Cream (1 oz)	35	2	1	2	0	40
WHIPPED TOPPINGS						
Cool Whip Lite Whipped Topping (2 tbsp)	20	1	1	2	0	0
D-Zerta Reduced Calorie Whipped Topping Mix (2 tbsp)	10	1	1	1	0	10
Dream Whip Whipped Topping Mix, prep w/skim milk (2 tbsp)	18	1	1	2	0	10
Kraft Toppings, Real Cream (2 tbsp)	20	2	1	1	0	0
Whipped (2 tbsp)	20	2	1	1	0	0
YOGURT DRINKS						
Nancy's Nonfat Yogurt Drinks, Blueberry (1 cup)	180	0	0	35	1	150
Boysenberry or Raspberry (1 cup)	180	0	0	34	1	140
Cherry (1 cup)	190	0	0	36	1	140
Strawberry (1 cup)	170	0	0	32	1	140
YOGURTS						
Higher-Fat						
Yogurt, Whole Milk, Plain (1 cup)	150	8	5	11	0	114
Lower-Fat						
Borden Fat Free Swiss Style Yogurt, Blueberry, Mixed Berry, Peach, Raspberry, Strawberry or Strawberry-Banana (8 oz container)	100	0	0	17	0	105
Breyers Lowfat Yogurt (1% Milkfat), Black Cherry (8 oz)	260	3	2	50	0	110
Blueberry, Mixed Berry or Peach (8 oz)	250	3	2	48	0	110
Pineapple (8 oz)	250	3	2	49	0	110
Red Raspberry (8 oz)	250	3	2	48	2	110
Strawberry (8 oz)	250	3	2	47	0	110
Strawberry Banana (8 oz)	250	3	2	50	<1	115
Lowfat Yogurt (1.5% Milkfat), Coffee (8 oz)	250	3	2	38	0	135

	Calories	Fat g	Saturated Fat g	Carbohydrate g	Fiber g	Sodium mg
Creamy Lemon or Vanilla (8 oz)	220	3	2	38	0	135-140
Plain (8 oz)	130	3	2	15	0	150
Cabot No Fat Yogurt, Black Cherry, Blueberry, French Vanilla, Lemon, Peach, Raspberry, Strawberry or Very Berry (1 cup)	130	0	0	24	0	115
Plain (1 cup)	100	0	0	19	0	135
Strawberry Banana (1 cup)	130	0	.0	24	0	120
Crowley All Natural Nonfat Yogurt, Plain (1 cup)	140	0	0	21	0	220
Raspberry (1 cup)	230	0	0	42	0	220
Strawberry (1 cup)	220	0	0	41	0	220
Strawberry Banana (1 cup)	230	0	0	40	0	220
Vanilla (1 cup)	220	0	0	40	<1	220
Nonfat Swiss Aspartame Yogurt, Black Cherry, Blueberry, Cappuccino, Cherry Vanilla, Chocolate, Lemon, Mixed Berry, Peach, Raspberry, Strawberry Banana, Strawberry or Vanilla (8 oz container)	100	0	0	17	0	130
Dannon Blended Fat Free Yogurt, Blueberry (6 oz container)	160	0	0	33	0	105
French Vanilla or Peach (6 oz container)	150	0	0	31	0	100
Lemon Chiffon (6 oz container)	150	0	0	31	0	110
Raspberry (6 oz container)	150	0	0	32	0	100
Strawberry or Strawberry/Banana (6 oz container)	160	0	0	31	0	105
Fruit on the Bottom Lowfat Yogurt, Apple Cinnamon, Blueberry, Cherry or Strawberry (8 oz container)	240	3	2	46	1	135-140
Boysenberry, Mixed Berries or Raspberry (8 oz container)	240	3	2	45	1	150
Orange or Pear (8 oz container)	240	3	2	45	0	135
Peach (8 oz container)	240	3	2	45	1	140
Plum (8 oz container)	240	3	2	45	0	160
Strawberry/Banana (8 oz container)	230	3	2	43	1	140
Light 'N Crunchy 99% Fat Free Yogurt, Cappuccino w/Chocolate Crunchies (8 oz container)	150	1	0	27	0	160
Vanilla w/Chocolate Crunchies (8 oz container)	150	1	0	26	0	160

	Calories	Fat g	Saturated Fat g	Carbohydrate g	Fiber g	Sodium mg
Dannon *(continued)*						
Light 'N Crunchy Nonfat Yogurt, Lemon Chiffon or Vanilla w/Blueberry Crunchies (8 oz container)	140	0	0	26	0	150
Raspberry w/Granola Crunchies (8 oz container)	150	0	0	27	1	135
Light Nonfat Yogurt w/Aspartame, Banana Cream Pie or Creme Caramel (8 oz container)	100	0	0	15	0	125
Blueberry or Cherry Vanilla (8 oz container)	100	0	0	20	0	140
Cappuccino, Lemon Chiffon or Vanilla (8 oz container)	100	0	0	17	0	140
Peach, Strawberry, Strawberry Fruit Cup or Strawberry/Banana (8 oz container)	100	0	0	18	0	140
Raspberry (8 oz container)	100	0	0	18	1	150
Tropical Fruit (8 oz container)	100	0	0	19	0	140
Lowfat Yogurt, Coffee, Lemon or Vanilla (8 oz container)	210	3	2	36	0	160
Cran/Raspberry (8 oz container)	200	3	2	35	0	150
Nonfat Yogurt, Plain (8 oz container)	110	0	0	16	0	150
Tropifruta Nonfat Yogurt, Guava (6 oz container)	150	0	0	29	0	105
Mango, Strawberry or Strawberry-Banana (6 oz container)	150	0	0	31	0	105
Papaya-Pineapple or Pina Colada (6 oz container)	150	0	0	30	0	105
Horizon Organic Yogurt, Blueberry, Cherry or Peach (3/4 cup)	130	0	0	23	1	110-115
Cappuccino (3/4 cup)	110	0	0	19	2	125
Plain (3/4 cup)	80	0	0	11	0	115
Raspberry (3/4 cup)	120	0	0	23	1	115
Strawberry (3/4 cup)	120	0	0	22	1	105
Vanilla (3/4 cup)	120	0	0	21	1	125
Knudsen Cal 70 Nonfat Yogurt w/Aspartame Sweetener, Black Cherry or Blueberry (6 oz)	70	0	0	12	0	80-85
Lemon (6 oz)	70	0	0	11	<1	100

Yogurts (continued)	Calories	Fat g	Saturated Fat g	Carbohydrate g	Fiber g	Sodium mg
Peach (6 oz)	70	0	0	11	<1	80
Pineapple, Red Raspberry or Vanilla (6 oz)	70	0	0	11	0	75-80
Red Raspberry (6 oz)	70	0	0	11	0	75
Strawberry Banana, Strawberry Fruit Basket or Strawberry (6 oz)	70	0	0	11	0	85-90
Knudsen Free Nonfat Yogurt, Lemon (6 oz)	160	0	0	33	0	105
Mixed Berry or Peach (6 oz)	170	0	0	33	0	105
Red Raspberry (6 oz)	160	0	0	31	0	105
Strawberry (6 oz)	160	0	0	32	0	105
Vanilla (6 oz)	170	0	0	32	0	100
Kraft Light N'Lively Free 50 Calories Nonfat Yogurt w/Aspartame, Blueberry, Red Raspberry, Strawberry, Strawberry Banana or Strawberry Fruit Cup (4.4 oz)	50	0	0	8	0	60
Peach (4.4 oz)	50	0	0	9	0	60
Light N'Lively Free 70 Calories Nonfat Yogurt w/Aspartame, Black Cherry, Blueberry, Red Raspberry, Strawberry, Strawberry Banana or Strawberry Fruit Cup (6 oz)	70	0	0	11	0	80-85
Lemon (6 oz)	70	0	0	12	0	120
Peach (6 oz)	70	0	0	12	0	80
Light N'Lively Free Nonfat Yogurt, Blueberry (6 oz)	190	0	0	38	0	105
Lemon Flavored, Peach or Strawberry Fruit Cup (6 oz)	170	0	0	35	0	105
Mixed Berry (6 oz)	170	0	0	34	0	105
Red Raspberry or Strawberry (6 oz)	180	0	0	36	0	105
Vanilla (6 oz)	160	0	0	32	0	105
Light N'Lively Kidpack Lowfat Yogurt (1% Milkfat), Banana Berry, Grape or Red Raspberry (4.4 oz)	130	1	1	24	0	65
Berry Blue (4.4 oz)	150	1	1	30	0	65
Cherry, Wild Berry or Wild Strawberry (4.4 oz)	140	1	1	27	0	65
Outrageous Orange (4.4 oz)	150	1	1	29	0	65
Tropical Punch (4.4 oz)	140	1	1	28	0	65

	Calories	Fat g	Saturated Fat g	Carbohydrate g	Fiber g	Sodium mg
Kraft *(continued)*						
Light N'Lively Lowfat Yogurt Multipack (1% Milkfat), Blueberry, Peach, Pineapple or Strawberry Fruit Cup (4.4 oz)	140	1	1	27	0	60-65
Strawberry (4.4 oz)	140	1	1	26	0	65
Strawberry Banana (4.4 oz)	140	1	1	28	0	60
Nancy's Lowfat Yogurt, Blueberry (1 cup)	180	3	2	28	1	150
Maple (1 cup)	180	3	2	26	0	160
Peach (1 cup)	170	3	2	26	0	150
Raspberry (1 cup)	180	3	2	29	1	150
Strawberry (1 cup)	170	3	2	26	1	150
Vanilla (1 cup)	140	3	2	15	0	160
Nonfat Yogurt, & Fruit Cup (9.5 oz)	175	0	0	29	0	180
Plain (1 cup)	120	0	0	17	0	180
"TCBY" Traditional Style Lowfat Yogurts, Blueberry, Cherry Vanilla or Raspberry (8 oz container)	220	2	2	42	0	150
Blueberry, Cherry Vanilla, Strawberry or Strawberry Banana (6 oz container)	180	2	2	34	0	110-115
Peach (6 oz container)	170	2	2	31	0	130
Peach (8 oz container)	200	2	2	38	0	150
Raspberry (6 oz container)	180	2	2	33	0	120
Traditional Style Nonfat Yogurts, Black Cherry or Strawberry (6 oz container)	80	0	0	12	0	125-130
Black Cherry or Strawberry (8 oz container)	100	0	0	16	0	170
Blueberry or Strawberry-Banana (6 oz container)	80	0	0	12	0	140
Blueberry or Strawberry-Banana (8 oz container)	100	0	0	16	0	180-190
Cherry Vanilla (6 oz container)	80	0	0	12	0	110
Cherry Vanilla (8 oz container)	100	0	0	16	0	150
Raspberry (6 oz container)	80	0	0	12	0	160
Raspberry (8 oz container)	100	0	0	16	0	220
Twosomes, Vanilla Yogurt w/Granola Topping (5 oz container)	190	2	1	35	0	75

	Calories	Fat g	Saturated Fat g	Carbohydrate g	Fiber g	Sodium mg
Vanilla Yogurt w/Strawberry Topping or w/Blueberry Topping (6 oz container)	150	2	1	28	0	90
Viva Fat Free Swiss Style Yogurt, Blueberry, Mixed Berry, Peach, Raspberry, Strawberry or Strawberry-Banana (8 oz container)	100	0	0	17	0	105
Weight Watchers Ultimate 90, Blueberries 'n Creme (1 cup)	90	0	0	14	3	140
Cappuccino, Cherry Jubilee, Cranberry Raspberry, Lemon Chiffon, Peach, Raspberries 'n Creme or Vanilla (1 cup)	90	0	0	14	0	140
Plain (1 cup)	90	0	0	14	0	150
Strawberry or Strawberry/Banana (1 cup)	90	0	0	14	2	140
Wells' Blue Bunny Lite 85 Nonfat Yogurt, Black Cherry, Blueberry, Cherry Vanilla, Orange, Peach, Pina Colada, Pineapple, Raspberry, Strawberry Banana or Strawberry (6 oz cup)	80	0	0	14	0	130
Lemon (6 oz cup)	80	0	0	13	0	160
Mixed Berry (6 oz cup)	80	0	0	14	0	140
Plain (1 cup)	110	0	0	16	0	170
Vanilla (6 oz cup)	80	0	0	14	0	130
Yoplait Breakfast Lowfat Yogurt, Mixed Berry (6 oz)	200	2	1	38	2	125
Strawberry Banana (6 oz)	200	2	1	39	2	115
Tropical Fruit (6 oz)	210	3	1	41	2	125
Crunch 'n Yogurt, Peach w/Granola (7 oz)	220	2	0	43	<1	115
Strawberry or Vanilla w/Granola (7 oz)	220	2	0	42	<1	115-120
Strawberry w/Cereal Nuggets (7 oz)	200	1	0	42	2	160
Vanilla w/Chocolate Flavor Crunchies (7 oz)	220	2	1	42	<1	180
Crunch 'n Yogurt Light, Cappucino w/Chocolate Nuggets (7 oz)	130	2	0	22	0	150
Cherry Cheesecake w/Graham Crunch (7 oz)	130	1	0	23	0	115
Strawberry or Raspberry w/Granola (7 oz)	130	1	0	25	4	115

	Calories	Fat g	Saturated Fat g	Carbohydrate g	Fiber g	Sodium mg
Yoplait *(continued)*						
Fruit on the Bottom Fat Free Yogurt, Blueberry, Cherry, Peach, Raspberry, Strawberry or Strawberry/Banana (6 oz)	160	0	0	33	0	105
Light Custard Style Yogurt, Cherry Vanilla, Peach, Strawberry or Vanilla (6 oz)	90	0	0	14	0	85
Light Yogurt, Blueberry, Cherry, Peach, Raspberry, Strawberry or Strawberry/Banana (6 oz)	90	0	0	16	0	85
Multi-Pack, all flavors (4 oz)	60	0	0	10	0	55
Nonfat Yogurt, Plain (1 cup)	140	0	0	21	0	190
Vanilla (1 cup)	210	0	0	41	0	160
Original 99% Fat Free Yogurt, Blueberry, Boysenberry, Cherry, Lemon, Mixed Berry, Orange, Peach, Pina Colada, Pineapple, Raspberry, Spiced Apple, Strawberry, Strawberry-Rhubarb or Strawberry/Banana (6 oz)	170	2	1	30	0	105
Multi-Pack (4 oz)	110	1	1	20	0	70
Vanilla (6 oz)	170	2	1	30	0	140
Original Nonfat Yogurt, Plain (6 oz)	100	0	0	16	0	140

DESSERTS

The desserts included in this section of the Guide are low in fat and saturated fat *as purchased,* when *prepared according to package directions,* or *when prepared with skim milk.* The levels of fat and saturated fat in a serving of these foods do not exceed the cutoff points of 3 grams of fat and 1 gram of saturated fat.

Analysis of each product as it will be eaten was used to determine if it qualified for the Guide. For example, a product such as cake mix or muffin mix that requires preparation qualifies for the Guide only if the dry mix plus the added ingredients do not exceed the cutoff points. Some package directions list the addition of an ingredient, such as whole milk, that is high in fat. For some of these products, simply substituting skim for whole milk allows the product to qualify for the Guide. In these cases, "prepared with skim milk" is clearly indicated next to the food in the Guide.

Brownies

	Calories	Fat g	Saturated Fat g	Carbohydrate g	Fiber g	Sodium mg
BROWNIES						
Higher-Fat						
Chocolate Brownie w/Nuts (2"x 2"x 1")	220	14	5	24	1	100
Butterscotch Brownie w/Nuts (2"x 2"x 1")	207	9	2	30	1	168
Lower-Fat						
Auburn Farms Jammers Fat Free Brownies, Butterscotch (1 brownie)	100	0	0	22	2	65
Cappuccino Fudge (1 brownie)	100	0	0	22	2	90
Chocolate Fudge or Raspberry Fudge (1 brownie)	90	0	0	22	2	95
Entenmann's Fudge Brownies (¹/₁₀ strip)	110	0	0	27	1	140

	Calories	Fat g	Saturated Fat g	Carbohydrate g	Fiber g	Sodium mg
Formägg Cream Cheese Fudgy Brownie (1 brownie)	130	3	0	27	0	30
Greenfield Healthy Foods Fat Free Brownie (1 bar)	120	0	0	29	<1	65
Fat Free Blondies, Apple Spice or Chocolate Chip (1 bar)	120	0	0	29	<1	65
Health Valley Fat Free Brownies, Caramel, Cherry, Fudge, Raspberry or Strawberry (1 bar)	110	0	0	26	4	30
Weight Watchers Brownies, Chocolate Frosted (1 brownie)	100	3	1	22	3	135
Mint Frosted (1 brownie)	100	2	0	22	3	130
Swiss Mocha Fudge (1 brownie)	90	2	0	18	2	140

CAKES AND CUPCAKES

Higher-Fat

	Calories	Fat g	Saturated Fat g	Carbohydrate g	Fiber g	Sodium mg
Carrot Cake w/Cream Cheese Frosting (3"x 3"x 1³/₄")	481	18	7	76	0	376
Cheesecake w/Graham Cracker Crust, Plain (¹/₉ of 9" diam, 1¹/₃" high)	495	35	20	39	0	320
German Chocolate Cake w/Coconut & Pecan Frosting (¹/₁₀ of 9" diam, 2¹/₂" high)	579	35	14	63	3	516
Pound Cake, White, w/o Frosting (3¹/₄"x 3¹/₄" x 1¹/₈")	370	22	10	38	1	72

Lower-Fat

	Calories	Fat g	Saturated Fat g	Carbohydrate g	Fiber g	Sodium mg
Betty Crocker Angel Food Cake Mixes, Chocolate Swirl (¹/₁₂ of pkg)	150	0	0	34	0	280
Confetti (¹/₁₂ of pkg)	150	0	0	34	0	300
Lemon Custard (¹/₁₂ of pkg)	140	0	0	33	0	290
One Step (¹/₁₂ of pkg)	140	0	0	32	0	280
Traditional (¹/₁₂ of pkg)	130	0	0	30	0	160
Entenmann's Cakes, Carrot (¹/₈ cake)	170	0	0	40	1	230
Fudge Iced Chocolate (¹/₆ cake)	210	0	0	51	2	270
Fudge Iced Golden (¹/₆ cake)	220	0	0	52	2	200
Mocha Iced Chocolate (¹/₆ cake)	200	0	0	46	1	270
Crumb Cakes, Apple Spice (¹/₈ cake)	130	0	0	30	2	140
Golden French (¹/₈ cake)	140	0	0	35	2	150
Banana (¹/₈ cake)	140	0	0	33	2	150

Cakes and Cupcakes (continued)

	Calories	Fat g	Saturated Fat g	Carbohydrate g	Fiber g	Sodium mg
Crunch Cakes, Blueberry (1/8 cake)	140	0	0	32	2	200
Chocolate (1/8 cake)	130	0	0	32	2	170
Louisiana (1/6 cake)	220	0	0	51	<1	220
Loaf Cakes, Banana (1/8 loaf)	150	0	0	34	1	190
Chocolate (1/8 loaf)	130	0	0	30	1	250
Golden (1/8 loaf)	120	0	0	28	<1	160
Golden Chocolatey Chip (1/8 loaf)	130	0	0	31	1	220
Marble (1/8 loaf)	130	0	0	29	1	190
Raisin (1/8 loaf)	140	0	0	33	1	150
Hostess Chocolate Cup Cakes Light (1 cake)	120	2	0	26	<1	170
Twinkie Lights (1 cake)	120	2	0	24	0	200
Pillsbury Plus Cake Mix, Angel Food, prep w/water (1/10 of cake)	150	0	0	34	0	360
Sweet'N Low Cake Mixes, Banana, Chocolate, Lemon, White or Yellow (1/6 of cake)	150	3	1	30	1	30

COOKIES

Higher-Fat

	Calories	Fat g	Saturated Fat g	Carbohydrate g	Fiber g	Sodium mg
Chocolate Chip Cookies w/nuts (3 cookies, 2 1/4" each)	139	6	2	19	1	95
Peanut Butter Cookies (2 med)	134	6	3	20	1	61
Butter Cookies (2 med)	151	7	2	19	0	136
Chocolate Sandwich Cookie (3 med)	133	6	1	20	1	150

Lower-Fat

	Calories	Fat g	Saturated Fat g	Carbohydrate g	Fiber g	Sodium mg
Almondina Cookies, Choconut (3 cookies)	80	1	0	12	1	10
America's Choice Fig Bars (2 fig bars)	120	3	0	23	1	55
Archway Cookies, Apple Filled Oatmeal (1 cookie)	110	3	1	18	0	105
Cookie Jar Hermits (1 cookie)	110	3	1	19	<1	160
Old Fashioned Molasses (1 cookie)	120	3	1	20	0	150
Pfeffernusse (2 cookies)	140	1	0	32	<1	100
Auburn Farms Jammers Cookies, Apple Spice (2 cookies)	80	0	0	18	2	90
Chewy Chocolate or Devil's Food (2 cookies)	80	0	0	20	2	80
Chocolate Mint (2 cookies)	90	0	0	20	2	95
Cinnamon Graham (2 cookies)	90	0	0	20	1	85

	Calories	Fat g	Saturated Fat g	Carbohydrate g	Fiber g	Sodium mg
Auburn Farms Jammers Cookies *(continued)*						
Molasses (2 cookies)	80	0	0	19	2	40
Oatmeal Raisin (2 cookies)	80	1	0	19	2	70
P'Nutty Crisp (2 cookies)	90	1	0	19	2	90
Bakery Wagon Fat Free Chewy Fruit Cookies, Apple Cobbler (1 cookie)	70	0	0	16	0	50
Cranberry Apple or Raspberry Cobbler (1 cookie)	70	0	0	16	1	60
Mixed Fruit Cobbler (1 cookie)	70	0	0	16	1	65
Peach Apricot Cobbler (1 cookie)	70	0	0	16	0	60
Strawberry Cobbler (1 cookie)	70	0	0	17	0	60
Bursting w/Fruit Fruity Chewy Cookies, Apple (1 cookie)	50	0	0	12	<1	70
Fig Bars (1 cookie)	60	0	0	13	<1	50
Peach Apricot (1 cookie)	60	0	0	13	0	60
Delicious Cookies, Ginger Snaps (4 cookies)	130	3	1	23	<1	170
Vanilla Wafers (8 cookies)	110	2	1	24	<1	90
Entenmann's Cookies, Chocolate Brownie (2 cookies)	80	0	0	20	1	90
Oatmeal Chocolatey Chip (2 cookies)	80	0	0	19	1	110
Oatmeal Raisin (2 cookies)	80	0	0	18	<1	120
Estee Low Fat Fig Bars (2 bars)	100	1	0	23	3	20
Apple (2 bars)	100	1	0	22	3	25
Cranberry (2 bars)	100	1	0	22	3	20
Famous Amos Fat Free Fruit Bars, Apple or Strawberry (2 cookies)	100	0	0	21	1	60
Fig (2 cookies)	100	0	0	21	1	70
Fig Bars (2 cookies)	120	3	1	23	1	95
Formägg Cookies, Chocolate Cheese Cake Chocolate Chip (1 cookie)	110	3	0	18	0	50
Cream Cheese Cookies, Fudgy Brownie (1 cookie)	100	2	0	20	0	30
Oatmeal Cranberry (1 cookie)	100	2	0	21	1	80
Oatmeal Raisin (1 cookie)	100	2	0	21	<1	80
Health Valley Fat Free Bakes, Apple, Date or Raisin (1 bar)	70	0	0	18	2	30

	Calories	Fat g	Saturated Fat g	Carbohydrate g	Fiber g	Sodium mg
Blueberry Apple, Raspberry or Strawberry (1 bar)	110	0	0	26	3	25
Fat Free Chocolate Cookies w/Caramel, w/Cherry, w/Fudge, w/Mint Fudge, w/Raspberry or w/Strawberry Centers (2 cookies)	70	0	0	17	3	20
Fat Free Cookies, Apple Spice, Apricot Delight, Date Delight, Hawaiian Fruit, or Raisin Oatmeal (3 cookies)	100	0	0	24	3	50
Double Chocolate, Old Fashioned or Original Healthy Chip (3 cookies)	100	0	0	24	4	20
Fat Free Fruit Center Cookies, Apple, Apricot, Date, Raisin Apple, Raspberry or Tropical (1 cookie)	70	0	0	18	2	20
Fat Free Graham Crackers, Amaranth or Oat Bran (8 crackers)	100	0	0	23	3	30
Fat Free Jumbo Cookies, Apple-Raisin, Raisin-Raisin or Raspberry (1 cookie)	80	0	0	19	3	35
Fat Free Mini Fruit Center Cookies, Apple-Cinnamon, Orange-Pineapple, Peach-Apricot, Raspberry-Apple or Strawberry (2 cookies)	70	0	0	19	2	25
Interbake Low-Fat Devil's Food Chocolate Cookie Cakes (2 cookies)	120	1	0	26	0	80
Keebler Elfin Delights Reduced Fat Sandwich Cookies, Chocolate w/Fudge Creme or w/Vanilla Creme (2 cookies)	110	3	1	19	<1	100-120
Creme (2 cookies)	110	3	1	19	0	90
Fat Free Devils Food Cookies (1 cookie)	70	0	0	14	0	80
Fig Bar (1 bar)	60	2	1	11	<1	70
Low Fat Cinnamon Crisp (8 crackers)	110	2	1	24	1	190
Low Fat Honey Graham Cracker (9 crackers)	120	2	1	25	1	210
Original Graham Selects Old Fashioned Graham Crackers (8 crackers)	130	3	1	23	<1	135
La Choy Fortune Cookies (1 cookie)	15	<1	0	4	<1	1
Lance Fat Free Bars, Apple (6 bars = 1½ oz)	140	0	0	33	<1	75
Cranberry (6 bars = 1½ oz)	140	0	0	33	1	45
Fat Free Fig Cake (½ of 2⅛ oz cake)	100	0	0	22	1	85

Cookies (continued)	Calories	Fat g	Saturated Fat g	Carbohydrate g	Fiber g	Sodium mg
Lance (continued)						
Fig Bar (1/2 of 2 oz bar)	100	2	1	20	1	85
Fig Cake (1/2 of 2 1/8 oz cake)	110	2	1	21	1	70
Nabisco Old Fashion						
Ginger Snaps (4 cookies)	120	3	1	22	<1	170
Fat Free Newtons, Apple (2 cookies)	100	0	0	24	1	60
Cranberry (2 cookies)	100	0	0	23	1	95
Fig (2 cookies)	100	0	0	22	2	115
Raspberry or Strawberry (2 cookies)	100	0	0	23	<1	115
Grahams (8 crackers)	120	3	1	22	1	180
Honey Maid Grahams, Cinnamon (10 crackers)	140	3	1	26	1	210
Honey (8 crackers)	120	3	1	22	1	180
Newtons, Fig (2 cookies)	110	3	1	20	1	120
Natural Lady Foods Lites Cookies, Cinnamon (1 cookie)	90	1	0	18	1	65
Oatmeal Date (1 cookie)	80	1	0	19	2	80
No-No All Natural Fat Free Biscotti, Almond, Cherry Vanilla or Coconut (1 oz = 6 cookies)	110	1	0	25	0	55
Free Ladyfingers, Almond Crisp, Coconut Flavor or Cinnamon Cappuccino Crisp (1 oz)	80	1	0	19	0	140
SnackWell's Fat Free Cookies, Cinnamon Graham Snacks (20 pieces)	110	0	0	26	1	90
Devil's Food Cookie Cakes (1 cookie)	50	0	0	13	<1	25
Double Fudge Cookie Cakes (1 cookie)	50	0	0	12	<1	70
Reduced Fat Cookies, Chocolate Sandwich w/Chocolate Creme (2 cookies)	100	3	1	20	1	190
Oatmeal w/Raisins (2 cookies)	110	3	0	20	1	135
Vanilla Creme Sandwich w/Vanilla Creme (2 cookies)	110	3	1	21	1	95
Sun Belt Fruit Boosters Snack Bars, Apple or Strawberry (1 bar)	130	2	0	27	0	60
Blueberry (1 bar)	130	2	0	27	1	60
Sunshine Fig Bars (2 cookies)	110	3	1	20	1	60
Golden Fruit, Apple (1 cookie)	80	2	0	15	<1	55
Cranberry (1 cookie)	70	1	0	15	<1	55

	Calories	Fat g	Saturated Fat g	Carbohydrate g	Fiber g	Sodium mg
Cookies *(continued)*						
Raisin (1 cookie)	80	2	0	15	<1	40
Weight Watchers Apple Fruit Filled Cookie (.7 oz)	70	0	0	15	0	40
Apple Raisin Bar (1 oz)	100	3	1	18	2	115
Smart Snackers Cookies, Oatmeal Raisin (.7 oz)	120	2	0	22	1	90
Vanilla Sandwich (1.06 oz)	140	3	1	25	1	80
Fruit Filled Cookies, Fig or Raspberry (.7 oz)	70	0	0	16	0	45-50

CREAM PIE FILLINGS, CUSTARDS, MOUSSES, AND PUDDINGS

	Calories	Fat g	Saturated Fat g	Carbohydrate g	Fiber g	Sodium mg
Higher-Fat						
Bread Pudding w/Raisins, prep w/whole milk & margarine (1/2 cup)	217	9	3	31	1	272
Chocolate Instant Pudding prep w/whole milk (1/2 cup)	145	4	2	24	1	368
Chocolate Mousse, prep w/half & half (1/2 cup)	222	12	6	28	2	45
Lower-Fat						
D-Zerta Chocolate Reduced Calorie Pudding, prep w/skim milk (1/2 cup)	60	0	0	11	<1	65
Del Monte Fat Free Pudding Cup, Chocolate (4 oz cup)	100	0	0	23	0	170
Vanilla (4 oz cup)	100	0	0	22	0	160
Light Pudding, Chocolate (4 oz container)	100	1	0	19	0	140
Vanilla (4 oz container)	90	1	0	18	0	190
Hershey's Fat Free Pudding, Chocolate or Kiss (4 oz)	100	0	0	22	<1	170-180
Special Dark (4 oz)	100	0	0	22	1	170
Tapioca (4 oz)	90	0	0	21	0	190
Vanilla (4 oz)	100	0	0	21	<1	230
Hunt's Snack Pack Light Pudding, Chocolate (4 oz)	100	2	0	20	0	120
Tapioca (4 oz)	100	2	0	18	0	105
Jell-O Americana Custard Dessert Mix, prep w/skim milk (1/2 cup)	123	0	0	25	0	193

Cream Pie Fillings, Custards, Mousses, and Puddings (continued)	Calories	Fat g	Saturated Fat g	Carbohydrate g	Fiber g	Sodium mg
Jell-O *(continued)*						
Americana Pudding Mixes, Rice, prep w/skim milk ($^1/_2$ cup)	143	0	0	30	0	163
Tapioca, prep w/skim milk ($^1/_2$ cup)	123	0	0	26	0	168
Cook & Serve Pudding & Pie Filling, Banana Cream, prep w/skim milk ($^1/_2$ cup)	123	0	0	26	0	243
Butterscotch, prep w/skim milk ($^1/_2$ cup)	133	0	0	30	0	193
Chocolate Fudge, prep w/skim milk ($^1/_2$ cup)	133	0	0	28	1	178
Chocolate, prep w/skim milk ($^1/_2$ cup)	133	0	0	28	<1	173
Flan, prep w/skim milk ($^1/_2$ cup)	123	0	0	26	0	68
Milk Chocolate, prep w/skim milk ($^1/_2$ cup)	133	0	0	28	<1	178
Vanilla, prep w/skim milk ($^1/_2$ cup)	123	0	0	26	0	198
Fat Free Sugar Free Instant Reduced Calorie Pudding & Pie Filling, Banana, Butterscotch or Vanilla, prep w/skim milk ($^1/_2$ cup)	70	0	0	12	0	400-410
Chocolate or Chocolate Fudge, prep w/skim milk ($^1/_2$ cup)	80	0	0	14	<1	390
Pistachio, prep w/skim milk ($^1/_2$ cup)	70	0	0	12	0	380
Instant Pudding & Pie Filling, Banana Cream, French Vanilla or Vanilla, prep w/skim milk ($^1/_2$ cup)	133	0	0	29	0	413
Butter Pecan, prep w/skim milk ($^1/_2$ cup)	143	1	1	29	0	413
Butterscotch, prep w/skim milk ($^1/_2$ cup)	133	0	0	29	0	453
Chocolate Fudge, prep w/skim milk ($^1/_2$ cup)	143	0	0	31	<1	443
Chocolate, prep w/skim milk ($^1/_2$ cup)	143	0	0	31	<1	473
Lemon, prep w/skim milk ($^1/_2$ cup)	133	0	0	30	0	363
Milk Chocolate, prep w/skim milk ($^1/_2$ cup)	143	1	0	31	<1	463
Pistachio, prep w/skim milk ($^1/_2$ cup)	143	1	0	29	0	413
Sugar Free Reduced Calorie Cook & Serve Pudding & Pie Filling, Chocolate, prep w/skim milk ($^1/_2$ cup)	73	0	0	13	<1	173

Cream Pie Fillings, Custards, Mousses, and Puddings (continued)	Calories	Fat g	Saturated Fat g	Carbohydrate g	Fiber g	Sodium mg
Vanilla, prep w/skim milk (1/2 cup)	63	0	0	11	0	178
Jell-O Free Fat Free Pudding Snacks, Chocolate (4 oz snack)	100	0	0	23	0	190
Chocolate-Vanilla Swirl or Vanilla-Chocolate Swirl (4 oz snack)	100	0	0	23	0	210-220
Vanilla (4 oz snack)	100	0	0	23	0	240
My*T*Fine Pudding, Butterscotch, prep w/skim milk (1/2 cup)	133	0	0	28	0	253
Chocolate Almond, prep w/skim milk (1/2 cup)	133	1	0	27	<1	198
Chocolate Fudge, prep w/skim milk (1/2 cup)	133	0	0	27	1	203
Chocolate, prep w/skim milk (1/2 cup)	133	0	0	28	<1	203
Vanilla Tapioca, prep w/skim milk (1/2 cup)	123	0	0	26	0	223
Vanilla, prep w/skim milk (1/2 cup)	123	0	0	26	0	178
Pudding & Pie Filling, Lemon Flavored, prep w/skim milk (1/6 of filling)	93	0	0	19	0	178
Royal Instant Pudding & Pie Filling, Banana Cream, prep w/skim milk (1/2 cup)	133	0	0	28	0	463
Butterscotch, prep w/skim milk (1/2 cup)	133	0	0	28	0	443
Chocolate Almond, prep w/skim milk (1/2 cup)	143	1	0	29	1	493
Chocolate, prep w/skim milk (1/2 cup)	143	0	0	30	0	453
Dark 'n Sweet Chocolate, prep w/skim milk (1/2 cup)	143	0	0	30	<1	513
Lemon, prep w/skim milk (1/2 cup)	133	0	0	29	0	393
Pistachio, prep w/skim milk (1/2 cup)	133	1	0	28	0	413
Vanilla, prep w/skim milk (1/2 cup)	133	0	0	28	0	383
Pie Filling, Key Lime or Lemon, prep w/skim milk (1/6 of filling)	93	0	0	19	0	183
Pudding, Vanilla Tapioca, prep w/skim milk (1/2 cup)	123	0	0	26	<1	123
Pudding & Pie Filling, Banana Cream, prep w/skim milk (1/2 cup)	123	0	0	26	<1	173
Butterscotch, prep w/skim milk (1/2 cup)	133	0	0	29	<1	243

Cream Pie Fillings, Custards, Mousses, and Puddings 135

Cream Pie Fillings, Custards, Mousses, and Puddings (continued)	Calories	Fat g	Saturated Fat g	Carbohydrate g	Fiber g	Sodium mg
Royal Pudding and Pie Fillings *(continued)*						
Chocolate, prep w/skim milk (1/2 cup)	133	0	0	28	<1	143
Dark 'n Sweet Chocolate, prep w/skim milk (1/2 cup)	133	0	0	28	<1	163
Flan Caramel Custard, prep w/skim milk (1/2 cup)	123	0	0	26	<1	88
Vanilla, prep w/skim milk (1/2 cup)	123	0	0	26	<1	223
Sugar Free Instant Pudding & Pie Filling, Banana Cream, Butterscotch or Vanilla, prep w/skim milk (1/2 cup)	83	0	0	16	0	473
Chocolate, prep w/skim milk (1/2 cup)	88	0	0	18	1	493
Pistachio, prep w/skim milk (1/2 cup)	83	0	0	15	0	473
Sans Sucre de Paris Mousse Mixes, Cheesecake, prep w/skim milk (1/2 cup)	73	2	1	10	0	105
Chocolate Cheesecake, prep w/skim milk (1/2 cup)	75	2	1	10	0	105
Chocolate, prep w/skim milk (1/2 cup)	76	3	1	8	0	45
Lemon, prep w/skim milk (1/2 cup)	70	3	1	9	NA	50
Strawberry, prep w/skim milk (1/2 cup)	70	2	1	9	0	45
Swiss Miss Light Pudding, Chocolate or Chocolate Fudge (4 oz)	100	1	0	20	0	120
Vanilla or Vanilla/Chocolate Parfait (4 oz)	100	1	0	20	0	105-110
Ultra Slim-Fast Pudding Snacks, Butterscotch (4 oz)	100	<1	0	21	2	230
Chocolate (4 oz)	100	<1	0	21	2	240
Weight Watchers Instant Pudding, Chocolate, prep w/skim milk (1/2 cup)	90	1	0	18	1	420
Vanilla, prep w/skim milk (1/2 cup)	90	0	0	17	1	510
Mousse Mix, White Chocolate Almond, prep w/skim milk (1/2 cup)	70	3	1	7	1	105
FRUIT PIE FILLINGS						
Most Brands, Apple Pie Filling (1/2 cup)	159	0	0	40	3	3
Pumpkin, canned (1/2 cup)	42	0	0	10	1	6
Libby's Pumpkin Pie Mix (1/2 cup)	100	0	0	25	2	150
Marie's Creamy Glaze for Bananas or Glaze for Strawberries (2 tbsp)	40	0	0	9	0	30
Glaze for Blueberries (2 tbsp)	40	0	0	10	0	30
Glaze for Peaches (2 tbsp)	40	0	0	10	0	50

Gelatins	Calories	Fat g	Saturated Fat g	Carbohydrate g	Fiber g	Sodium mg

GELATINS

	Calories	Fat g	Saturated Fat g	Carbohydrate g	Fiber g	Sodium mg
Most Brands, Gelatin, Sweetened w/aspartame, all flavors, prep w/water (1/2 cup)	8	0	0	1	0	56
Sweetened w/saccharin, all flavors, prep w/water (1/2 cup)	8	0	0	1	0	2
Sweetened w/sugar, all flavors, prep w/water (1/2 cup)	80	0	0	19	0	57
Betty Crocker GELOOZE, Berry Blue, Cherry, Orange or Strawberry (7.5 oz bottle)	130	0	0	32	0	65
D-Zerta Low Calorie Gelatin, Strawberry, prep w/water (1/2 cup)	10	0	0	0	0	5
Del Monte Gel Cup, Blue Berry, Cherry, Grape, Orange, Raspberry or Strawberry (3.5 oz can)	90	0	0	23	<1	80
Jell-O 1-2-3, Strawberry Gelatin, prep w/water (2/3 cup)	130	2	1	26	0	45
Gelatin, Apricot, Berry Blue, Black Cherry, Blackberry, Mixed Fruit, Orange, Peach, Raspberry, Strawberry Banana, Strawberry or Watermelon, prep w/water (1/2 cup)	80	0	0	19	0	50
Black Raspberry, prep w/water (1/2 cup)	80	0	0	20	0	35
Cherry or Cranberry, prep w/water (1/2 cup)	80	0	0	19	0	70
Grape, Mango, Pineapple or Tropical Punch, prep w/water (1/2 cup)	80	0	0	19	0	45
Lemon or Wild Strawberry, prep w/water (1/2 cup)	80	0	0	19	0	75
Lime, prep w/water (1/2 cup)	80	0	0	19	0	60
Orange Pineapple, prep w/water (1/2 cup)	80	0	0	19	0	65
Gelatin Snacks, Berry Blue, Cherry, Grape, Orange, Raspberry, Strawberry or Strawberry-Banana (3.5 oz snack)	80	0	0	18	0	45
Sugar Free Low Calorie Gelatin, Berry Blue or Lime, prep w/water (1/2 cup)	10	0	0	0	0	60

	Calories	Fat g	Saturated Fat g	Carbohydrate g	Fiber g	Sodium mg
Cherry, prep w/water (1/2 cup)	10	0	0	0	0	70
Grape, Hawaiian Pineapple, Mixed Fruit, Strawberry Banana or Triple Berry, prep w/water (1/2 cup)	10	0	0	0	0	50
Lemon, Raspberry, Strawberry or Watermelon, prep w/water (1/2 cup)	10	0	0	0	0	55
Orange, prep w/water (1/2 cup)	10	0	0	0	0	65
Sugar Free Low Calorie Gelatin Snacks, Cherry, Orange, Raspberry or Strawberry (3.25 oz snack)	10	0	0	0	0	50
Kraft Handi-Snacks Gel Snacks, Blue Raspberry, Cherry or Orange (3.5 oz snack)	80	0	0	20	0	40
Strawberry (3.5 oz snack)	80	0	0	20	0	45

MUFFINS

Higher-Fat

	Calories	Fat g	Saturated Fat g	Carbohydrate g	Fiber g	Sodium mg
Blueberry Muffin Mix, prep w/egg & whole milk (2 2/3" diam x 1 1/4" high = about 2 oz)	186	9	4	25	1	166
Chocolate Chip Muffin (2 2/3" diam x 1 1/3" high = about 2 oz)	181	7	3	26	1	160

Lower-Fat

	Calories	Fat g	Saturated Fat g	Carbohydrate g	Fiber g	Sodium mg
Entenmann's Muffins, Blueberry (1 muffin)	120	0	0	26	<1	220
Health Valley Fat-Free Muffins, Apple Spice or Banana (1 muffin)	170	0	0	38	5	55
Krusteaz Fat Free Muffin Mixes, Apple Cinnamon (1/4 cup mix/fruit = 1 muffin)	130	0	0	28	2	310
Blueberry (1/4 cup mix/fruit = 1 muffin)	130	0	0	30	1	260
Muffin-A-Day, Carrot, Blueberry Bran or Apple Bran (1 muffin = 2.8 oz)	120	0	0	31	9	140
Pepperidge Farms Wholesome Choice Muffins, Blueberry (1 muffin)	140	3	0	27	2	190

PIES

Higher-Fat

	Calories	Fat g	Saturated Fat g	Carbohydrate g	Fiber g	Sodium mg
Cherry Snack Pie (1 individual = 4 1/4 oz)	379	19	3	51	2	449
Coconut Cream Pie, prep w/whole milk (1/8 of 8" diam, 1 1/8" high)	321	18	8	35	1	314

	Calories	Fat g	Saturated Fat g	Carbohydrate g	Fiber g	Sodium mg
Pies (continued)						
Lower-Fat						
Entenmann's Beehive Pies,						
Apple (1/5 pie)	270	0	0	65	2	330
Cherry (1/5 pie)	270	0	0	64	1	310
TOASTER PASTRIES						
Higher-Fat						
Toaster Pastry (1 pastry)	204	5	1	37	1	218
Lower-Fat						
Auburn Farms Toast 'N Jammers **Fat Free Toaster Pastries, Apple-Cinnamon, Blueberry, Raspberry or Strawberry (1 pastry)**	180	0	0	42	4	200

EGGS AND EGG SUBSTITUTES

The egg substitutes included in this section of the Guide are low in fat and saturated fat. A serving of these foods does not exceed the cutoff points of 3 grams of fat and 1 gram of saturated fat.

Eggs and Egg Substitutes	Calories	Fat g	Saturated Fat g	Carbohydrate g	Fiber g	Sodium mg
Higher-Fat						
Whole Egg, raw (1 large)	74	5	2	1	0	63
Lower-Fat						
Most Brands, Egg White, raw (1 large)	17	0	0	0	0	55
America's Choice						
99% Egg Product (¼ cup)	30	0	0	1	0	80
Fleischmann's Egg Beaters, frozen or refrigerated (¼ cup)	30	0	0	1	0	100
Healthy Choice Cholesterol Free Egg Product (¼ cup)	25	0	0	<1	0	95
Morningstar Farms						
Better 'n Eggs, frozen (¼ cup)	20	0	0	0	0	90
Scramblers, frozen (¼ cup)	35	0	0	2	0	95
Second Nature Real Egg Product, No Cholesterol (¼ cup)	60	2	0	3	0	110
No Fat (¼ cup)	40	0	0	3	0	115

FATS

Foods that are high in total fat but that are low in saturated fat can be included (in limited amounts) in a cholesterol-lowering diet, described in *The Living Heart Diet* (another book by the same authors). Therefore, the level of saturated fat was used as the only cutoff point to evaluate avocado, margarine, nuts and nut butters, oils, olives, and seeds; a cutoff point for fat was not used. Since these foods are naturally high in fat, the quantity eaten needs to be limited.

This section of the Guide also includes margarine and cooking sprays. To be listed in the Guide, a serving of these products, as specified by the manufacturer, does not exceed the cutoff points listed below.

Salad dressing, another food that can be high in fat and low in saturated fat, is included in the Salad Dressings and Sandwich Spreads section beginning on page 200.

CUTOFF POINTS FOR FATS

	Fat g	Saturated Fat g
Avocado, Margarine, Nuts, Nut Butters, Oil, Olives, and Seeds	*	2
Butter Substitutes, Margarine, and Cooking Sprays	3	1

* No cutoff point; these foods are naturally high in fat.

Fats	Calories	Fat g	Saturated Fat g	Carbohydrate g	Fiber g	Sodium mg
AVOCADOS						
Avocado, California (2 tbsp mashed)	48	5	1	2	1	3

	Calories	Fat g	Saturated Fat g	Carbohydrate g	Fiber g	Sodium mg
BUTTER						
Higher-Saturated Fat						
Butter (1 tbsp)	102	12	7	0	0	76
COOKING SPRAYS						
Mazola No Stick Cooking Spray (0.2 gram)	0	0	0	0	0	0
Weight Watchers Buttery Spray or Cooking Spray (1 second spray)	0	0	0	0	0	0
Wesson Lite Cooking Spray (.27 g)	0	0	0	0	0	0
FAT SUBSTITUTES						
Butter Buds Butter Flavored Mix, dry (1 tsp)	5	0	0	2	0	75
Sprinkles, dry (1 tsp)	5	0	0	2	0	120
Molly McButter Sprinkles, Natural Butter (1 tsp)	5	0	0	1	0	180
Natural Cheese (1 tsp)	5	0	0	1	0	125
Natural Garlic & Herb (1 tsp)	5	0	0	1	0	130
Natural Sour Cream (1 tsp)	5	0	0	1	0	115
MARGARINES						
Blue Bonnet Light Taste, stick (1 tbsp)	70	8	2	0	0	105
Pure Vegetable Oil Spread, stick (1 tbsp)	80	10	2	0	0	110
Tub (1 tbsp)	80	10	2	0	0	80
Canola Sunrise Margarine, stick (1 tbsp)	100	11	1	0	0	95
Spread, tub (1 tbsp)	70	7	1	0	0	95
Fleischmann's Fat Free Low Calorie Spread (1 tbsp)	5	0	0	1	0	125
Light Taste, stick (1 tbsp)	70	8	2	0	0	90
Canola Choice, stick or tub (1 tbsp)	70	8	1	0	0	90
Lower Fat Margarine, stick (1 tbsp)	50	6	1	0	0	60
Tub (1 tbsp)	40	5	0	0	0	55
Margarine, sweet, unsalted, stick (1 tbsp)	100	11	2	0	0	0
Heart-Beat Foods Nucanola 52% Spread, tub (1 tbsp)	70	7	<1	0	0	90
Smart Beat Margarine, Light, unsalted, tub (1 tbsp)	25	3	0	0	0	0
Super Light, tub (1 tbsp)	20	2	0	0	0	105
Kraft Chiffon Margarine, Soft, tub (1 tbsp)	100	11	2	0	0	105
Whipped, tub (1 tbsp)	70	7	2	0	0	70

Margarines (continued)

	Calories	Fat g	Saturated Fat g	Carbohydrate g	Fiber g	Sodium mg
Parkay Margarine, Soft Diet, tub (1 tbsp)	50	6	1	0	0	110
Soft, tub (1 tbsp)	100	11	2	0	0	105
Whipped, tub (1 tbsp)	70	7	2	0	0	70
Parkay Spread, 50% Vegetable Oil, stick (1 tbsp)	60	7	2	0	0	110
53% Vegetable Oil (1/3 Less Fat), tub (1 tbsp)	70	7	2	0	0	120
64% Vegetable Oil, squeeze (1 tbsp)	80	9	2	<1	0	120
70% Vegetable Oil, tub (1 tbsp)	90	10	2	0	0	110
Light, 40% Vegetable Oil, tub (1 tbsp)	50	6	1	0	0	120
Touch of Butter, 47% Vegetable Oil & Dairy Spread, stick (1 tbsp)	60	7	2	0	0	110
64% Vegetable Oil & Dairy Spread, squeeze (1 tbsp)	80	9	2	0	0	115
70% Vegetable Oil & Dairy Spread, tub (1 tbsp)	90	10	2	0	0	110
Land O'Lakes Country Morning Blend, tub (1 tbsp)	100	11	2	0	0	80
Spread w/Sweet Cream, stick, salted (1 tbsp)	90	10	2	0	0	95
Stick, unsalted (1 tbsp)	90	10	2	0	0	0
Tub (1 tbsp)	80	8	2	0	0	70
Mazola Margarine, Diet Reduced Calorie, tub (1 tbsp)	50	6	1	0	0	130
Stick (1 tbsp)	100	11	2	0	0	100
Unsalted (1 tbsp)	100	11	2	0	0	0
Spread, Extra Light, tub (1 tbsp)	50	6	1	0	0	100
Move Over Butter, stick (1 tbsp)	90	10	2	0	0	100
Weight Watchers Spread, Extra Light, tub (1 tbsp)	45	4	1	2	0	75
Unsalted, tub (1 tbsp)	45	4	1	2	0	0
Light, stick (1 tbsp)	60	7	1	0	0	130

NUT BUTTERS

Higher-Saturated Fat

	Calories	Fat g	Saturated Fat g	Carbohydrate g	Fiber g	Sodium mg
Cashew Butter (2 tbsp)	188	16	3	9	1	197
Peanut Butter (2 tbsp)	191	16	3	6	2	151

	Calories	Fat g	Saturated Fat g	Carbohydrate g	Fiber g	Sodium mg
Lower-Saturated Fat						
Almond Butter, salted (2 tbsp)	203	19	2	7	3	144
Unsalted (2 tbsp)	203	19	2	7	3	4
Peanut Butter, reduced fat (2 tbsp)	188	12	2	13	1	203
NUTS AND SEEDS						
Higher-Saturated Fat						
Cashews, dry roasted, salted (about 19)	172	14	3	9	2	187
Brazil Nuts, salted (about 8)	213	22	5	4	2	278
Macadamia Nuts, unsalted (about 12)	217	23	3	4	2	2
Lower-Saturated Fat						
Most Brands, Almonds, dry roasted, salted (1 oz = about 23 nuts)	182	17	2	5	3	230
Honey roasted (1 oz = about 21 nuts)	172	15	1	8	3	204
Chestnuts, roasted (1 oz = about 4 nuts)	78	1	0	16	2	8
Filberts or Hazelnuts, dry roasted, salted (1 oz = about 21 nuts)	188	19	1	5	2	232
Unsalted (1 oz = about 21 nuts)	188	19	1	5	2	1
Peanuts, dry roasted, salted (1 oz = about 30)	176	15	2	6	2	132
Pecans, dry roasted, salted (1 oz = about 33 halves)	207	22	2	5	2	228
Unsalted (1 oz = about 33 halves)	201	20	2	6	2	0
Pistachio Nuts, dry roasted, salted (1 oz = about 50 nuts)	182	16	2	8	3	234
Unsalted (1 oz = about 50 nuts)	173	15	2	7	3	2
Sunflower Seed Kernels, salted (1 oz = ¼ cup)	182	16	2	6	2	250
Unsalted (1 oz = ¼ cup)	182	16	2	6	2	1
Walnuts, unsalted (1 oz = 15 halves)	195	19	2	4	1	3
Diamond of California Walnuts, unsalted (1 oz)	215	20	2	3	3	3
Lance Almonds, Smoked (¾ oz)	130	10	1	4	3	125
Pistachios (1⅛ oz)	90	7	1	4	2	105
OILS						
Higher-Saturated Fat						
Cottonseed Oil (1 tbsp)	120	14	4	0	0	0

	Calories	Fat g	Saturated Fat g	Carbohydrate g	Fiber g	Sodium mg
Lower-Saturated Fat						
Most Brands, Canola (1 tbsp)	120	14	1	0	0	0
Corn (1 tbsp)	120	14	2	0	0	0
Olive (1 tbsp)	119	14	2	0	0	0
Peanut (1 tbsp)	119	14	2	0	0	0
Safflower (1 tbsp)	120	14	1	0	0	0
Sesame (1 tbsp)	120	14	2	0	0	0
Soybean (1 tbsp)	120	14	2	0	0	0
Sunflower (1 tbsp)	120	14	1	0	0	0
America's Choice Pure Canola Oil (1 tbsp)	130	14	1	0	0	0
Crisco Canola & Corn Oil Blend (1 tbsp)	120	14	2	0	0	0
Puritan Canola Oil (1 tbsp)	120	14	1	0	0	0
Heart-Beat Foods Smart Beat Canola Oil (1 tbsp)	120	14	1	0	0	0
Ka-me Oil, Hot Chili (1 tbsp)	130	14	2	0	0	0
Sesame (1 tbsp)	130	14	2	0	0	0
Mazola Corn Oil (1 tbsp)	120	14	2	0	0	0
Orville Redenbacher's Gourmet Popping & Topping Oils (1 tbsp)	120	14	2	0	0	0
Progresso Olive Oils, Extra Mild, Extra Virgin or Riviera Blend (1 tbsp)	120	14	2	0	0	0
Wesson Oil, Canola (1 tbsp)	120	14	1	0	0	0
Corn (1 tbsp)	120	14	2	0	0	0
Olive (1 tbsp)	120	14	2	0	0	0
Sunflower (1 tbsp)	120	14	2	0	0	0
Vegetable (1 tbsp)	120	14	2	0	0	0
OLIVES						
Most Brands, Green (about 4 med)	19	2	0	0	0	384
Ripe (about 4 med)	18	2	0	1	1	140
America's Choice Ripe Pitted Olives, Colossal (2 olives)	20	2	0	1	0	110
Extra Large (3 olives)	25	3	0	1	0	110
Jumbo (3 olives)	25	2	0	1	0	135
Large (4 olives)	25	3	0	1	0	115
Medium (5 olives)	25	3	0	1	0	115
Small (6 olives)	25	3	0	1	0	115
Super Colossal (1 olive)	15	1	0	1	0	75

	Calories	Fat g	Saturated Fat g	Carbohydrate g	Fiber g	Sodium mg
Olives (continued)						
Progresso Oil Cured Olives (6 olives)	80	6	1	3	1	330
Olive Salad (2 tbsp)	25	3	0	1	1	360
OTHER COOKING FATS						
Higher-Saturated Fat						
Butter (1 tbsp)	102	12	7	0	0	76
Lard (1 tbsp)	116	13	5	0	0	0
All Vegetable Shortening (1 tbsp)	113	13	3	0	0	0

FROZEN DESSERTS

Many of the low-fat products that are included in this section of the Guide have been developed as substitutes for ice cream. For example, ice milk and frozen yogurt are much lower in fat and saturated fat than ice cream. Note that the cutoff point for saturated fat for frozen desserts that are primarily milk based, such as frozen yogurt, is 2 grams. Frozen desserts that are not milk based, such as sorbet, have a cutoff point for saturated fat of 1 gram, the same used for most foods in the Guide. Values for fat and saturated fat in 1 serving of the foods included in this section of the Guide do not exceed the cutoff points listed below.

CUTOFF POINTS FOR FROZEN DESSERTS

	Fat g	Saturated Fat g
Milk-Based Frozen Desserts	3	2
Not Milk-Based Desserts	3	1

Bars and Pops

	Calories	Fat g	Saturated Fat g	Carbohydrate g	Fiber g	Sodium mg
BARS AND POPS						
Higher-Fat						
Ice Cream Bar, Chocolate Coated (4 fl oz)	237	17	12	19	0	38
Ice Cream Sandwich (4 fl oz)	219	8	5	34	2	69
Lower-Fat						
Blue Bell Big Red (1 bar)	90	0	0	22	0	5
Big Shot (1 bar)	140	0	0	36	0	15
Buried Treasure or Rainbow Freeze (1 bar)	110	0	0	28	0	10
Cherry Freeze Bar or Snow Cone (1 bar)	70	0	0	18	0	5
Cream Bars, Cherry (1 bar)	110	2	1	21	0	20

	Calories	Fat g	Saturated Fat g	Carbohydrate g	Fiber g	Sodium mg
Blue Bell Cream Bars *(continued)*						
Orange (1 bar)	100	2	1	19	0	25
Flintstone Pushup (1 bar)	90	1	1	19	0	20
Frostbite (1 bar)	80	0	0	21	0	10
Rainbow Fruiti Freeze (1 bar)	120	0	0	30	0	10
Twin Pop (1 bar)	80	0	0	20	0	5
Delicious Tube Freeze Pops, Box (1.5 oz stick)	30	0	0	7	0	0
Box (5 oz stick)	110	0	0	26	0	15
Giant (1 stick)	150	0	0	35	0	20
Dole Frozen Fruit Juice Bars No Sugar Added Variety Pack (raspberry, grape, strawberry) (1 bar)	25	0	0	6	0	5
Strawberry Fruit 'N Juice Frozen Fruit Ice (1 bar)	70	0	0	17	0	5
Frozfruit Chunky Frozen Fruit Bars, Cantaloupe (1 bar)	60	0	0	15	0	5
Cherry (1 bar)	70	0	0	18	1	0
Orange (1 bar)	90	0	0	21	0	15
Pineapple (1 bar)	80	0	0	19	0	0
Raspberry (1 bar)	80	0	0	20	1	5
Strawberry (1 bar)	80	0	0	20	1	20
Watermelon (1 bar)	50	0	0	13	0	0
Fat-Free Frozen Fruit & Yogurt Bars, Peach or Strawberry (1 bar)	100	0	0	22	0	85-95
Strawberry Banana (1 bar)	100	0	0	21	1	85
Frozen Fruit Bars, Double Lemon (1 bar)	90	0	0	22	0	10
Double Lime (1 bar)	90	0	0	21	0	10
Good Humor Frozen Yogurt Creamsicle (1 piece)	60	1	1	14	0	15
Popsicle Ice Pops, Regular or Rainbow (1 piece)	45	0	0	11	0	0
Sugar Free (1 piece)	15	0	0	3	0	0
Popsicle Twister (1 piece)	45	0	0	10	0	0
Fudgesicle Fudge Pops, Sugar Free (1 piece)	40	1	0	8	<1	35
Fudgesicle, The Original Fudge Bar (1 piece)	90	1	1	17	1	55

Bars and Pops (continued)	Calories	Fat g	Saturated Fat g	Carbohydrate g	Fiber g	Sodium mg
Häagen-Dazs Frozen Yogurt Bars, Peach (1 bar)	90	1	1	19	0	20
Piña Colada (1 bar)	100	1	1	19	0	45
Raspberry & Vanilla (1 bar)	90	1	0	19	0	25
Strawberry Daiquiri (1 bar)	90	1	1	18	0	20
Tropical Orange Passion (1 bar)	100	1	1	20	0	20
Just Pik't Orange Juice Bars (1 bar)	60	0	0	16	0	5
Mr. Freeze Freezer Bars, Assorted (2 oz bar)	35	0	0	9	0	15
Assorted or Tropical (3 bars, each 1 oz, or 2 bars, each 1.5 oz)	50	0	0	14	0	20
Sugar Free (3 bars, each 1 oz, or 2 bars, each 1.5 oz)	20	0	0	5	0	45
Weight Watchers Mousse Bars, Berries 'N Creme (3.5 fl oz)	70	2	0	7	1	75
Berries 'N Creme Sugar Free (1 bar)	30	<1	<1	7	NA	40
Chocolate (1 bar)	70	1	1	18	4	80
Treat Bars, Chocolate (1 bar)	100	1	0	21	1	150
Orange Vanilla (2 bars)	70	1	1	17	3	80
Wells' Blue Bunny Frozen Nonfat Yogurt & Fruit Snacks, Burgundy Cherry, Peach or Strawberry Flavors (2 bars)	90	0	0	22	0	50
Sweet Freedom (No Added Sugar) Bars, Assorted Pops (1 bar)	10	0	0	3	0	10
Bomb Pop, Jr. (1 bar)	25	0	0	7	0	10
Chocolate Fudge Lites (2 bars)	70	1	0	17	0	120
Citrus Lites (1 bar)	20	0	0	5	0	10
FROZEN YOGURTS						
Ben & Jerry's Low-Fat Frozen Yogurt, Apple Pie or Cherry Garcia (1/2 cup)	170	3	2	31	0	70-85
Banana Strawberry (1/2 cup)	160	2	1	32	1	60
Blueberry (1/2 cup)	160	2	1	33	1	60
Blueberry Cheesecake (1/2 cup)	150	2	2	29	0	90
Chocolate Raspberry Swirl (1/2 cup)	200	3	2	40	1	75
Blue Bell Lowfat Frozen Yogurt, Cookies N Cream or Double Chocolate Chunk (1/2 cup)	130	3	2	23	0	75-80
Pecan Pralines N Cream (1/2 cup)	140	2	1	26	0	80
Strawberry Cheesecake (1/2 cup)	120	2	1	24	0	135

	Calories	Fat g	Saturated Fat g	Carbohydrate g	Fiber g	Sodium mg
Blue Bell *(continued)*						
Vanilla Chocolate Twist or Vanilla (1/2 cup)	120	2	1	22	0	65-70
Nonfat Frozen Yogurt, Banana Split (1/2 cup)	110	0	0	25	0	55
Burgundy Cherry (1/2 cup)	120	0	0	26	0	65
Chocolate (1/2 cup)	110	0	0	24	0	65
Fruit Cocktail (1/2 cup)	110	0	0	24	0	60
Strawberry (1/2 cup)	110	0	0	23	0	55
Colombo Shoppe Style Low Fat Frozen Yogurt, Banana Split (1/2 cup)	140	2	1	25	0	60
Caramel Fudge Sundae (1/2 cup)	140	2	1	27	0	80
Chocolate Peanut Butter Twist (1/2 cup)	140	3	1	23	1	65
Old World Chocolate (1/2 cup)	130	2	1	23	0	75
Raspberry Peach Melba (1/2 cup)	130	2	1	24	0	60
Simply Vanilla (1/2 cup)	120	2	1	22	0	65
Strawberries 'N Cream (1/2 cup)	130	2	1	23	0	65
Vanilla Chocolate Twist (1/2 cup)	120	2	1	23	0	70
Slender Scoops Frozen Yogurt, Black Cherry Chill or Cappuccino (1/2 cup)	80	0	0	17	0	65-75
Chocolate Bliss (1/2 cup)	80	0	0	17	1	70
Double Fudge Paradise (1/2 cup)	90	0	0	18	1	80
Vanilla Fudge Heaven (1/2 cup)	90	0	0	19	<1	80
Vanilla Silk (1/2 cup)	80	0	0	16	0	70
Dannon Light Nonfat Hard Frozen Yogurt w/Aspartame, Cappuccino (1/2 cup)	80	0	0	19	0	70
Cherry Vanilla Swirl (1/2 cup)	90	0	0	21	0	65
Chocolate (1/2 cup)	80	0	0	21	1	60
Lemon Chiffon (1/2 cup)	90	0	0	22	0	65
Peach (1/2 cup)	80	0	0	20	0	60
Strawberry (1/2 cup)	80	0	0	19	1	65
Vanilla (1/2 cup)	80	0	0	21	0	65
Light Nonfat Soft Frozen Yogurt w/Aspartame, Chocolate (1/2 cup)	70	0	0	13	1	60
Mixed Berry or Vanilla (1/2 cup)	70	0	0	13	0	60

	Calories	Fat g	Saturated Fat g	Carbohydrate g	Fiber g	Sodium mg
Pure Indulgence Hard Frozen Yogurt w/Aspartame, Cherry Chocolate Cherry (1/2 cup)	150	3	1	26	0	85
Vanilla (1/2 cup)	130	2	1	22	0	85
Dreyer's Fat Free Frozen Yogurt, Banana Strawberry or Raspberry (1/2 cup)	80	0	0	18	NA	50
Black Cherry Vanilla Swirl (1/2 cup)	90	0	0	19	NA	65
Chocolate Fudge (1/2 cup)	100	0	0	21	NA	75
Chocolate, Pine-Orange Paradise or Strawberry (1/2 cup)	90	0	0	18	NA	55-60
Vanilla Chocolate Swirl or Vanilla (1/2 cup)	90	0	0	18	NA	65
Frozen Yogurt, Boysenberry Vanilla Swirl, Orange Vanilla Swirl, Raspberry Vanilla Swirl or Vanilla (1/2 cup)	100	3	2	17	NA	30
Chocolate (1/2 cup)	100	3	2	17	NA	30
Citrus Heights (1/2 cup)	80	3	2	18	NA	25
Marble Fudge (1/2 cup)	110	3	2	19	NA	35
Perfectly Peach or Raspberry (1/2 cup)	100	3	2	17	NA	25
Edy's Fat Free Frozen Yogurt, Black Cherry Vanilla Swirl (1/2 cup)	90	0	0	19	NA	65
Chocolate Fudge (1/2 cup)	100	0	0	21	NA	75
Chocolate, Pine-Orange Paradise or Strawberry (1/2 cup)	90	0	0	18	NA	55-60
Raspberry (1/2 cup)	80	0	0	18	NA	50
Vanilla Chocolate Swirl or Vanilla (1/2 cup)	90	0	0	18	NA	65
Frozen Yogurt, Chocolate (1/2 cup)	100	3	2	17	NA	30
Citrus Heights (1/2 cup)	80	3	2	18	NA	25
Marble Fudge (1/2 cup)	110	3	2	19	NA	35
Orange Vanilla Swirl, Raspberry Vanilla Swirl or Vanilla (1/2 cup)	100	3	2	17	NA	30
Perfectly Peach, Raspberry or Strawberry (1/2 cup)	100	3	2	17	NA	25
Häagen-Dazs Frozen Yogurt, Orange Tango (1/2 cup)	130	1	1	26	0	25
Pina Colada (1/2 cup)	130	2	1	26	0	25

	Calories	Fat g	Saturated Fat g	Carbohydrate g	Fiber g	Sodium mg
Frozen Yogurts (continued)						
Häagen-Dazs (continued)						
Raspberry Rendezvous (½ cup)	130	2	1	26	1	25
Strawberry Duet (½ cup)	130	2	1	26	<1	25
"TCBY" Frozen Yogurt, Classic Vanilla (½ cup)	110	2	1	21	0	50
Cookies 'N Cream or Pecan Praline Crisp (½ cup)	120	3	1	23	0	70-80
Dutch Chocolate (½ cup)	100	2	1	20	<1	40
Homestyle Banana Pudding (½ cup)	120	2	1	22	0	55
Peach (½ cup)	110	1	1	21	0	45
Peanut Butter Fudge Sundae (½ cup)	110	2	1	23	<1	50
Summertime Strawberry (½ cup)	100	1	1	20	0	40
Gourmet Collection Frozen Yogurt, Blueberry Cheesecake (½ cup)	140	2	2	27	0	55
Brazil & Cashew Nut Crunch (½ cup)	160	3	2	30	0	85
Honey Almond Vanilla (½ cup)	150	3	2	27	0	75
Strawberry White Chocolate Almond Crunch (½ cup)	130	2	2	26	0	55
Triple Chocolate Brownie (½ cup)	150	3	2	29	1	55
Wells' Blue Bunny Nonfat Frozen Yogurt, Burgundy Cherry (½ cup)	100	0	0	22	0	55
Cookies N Cream (½ cup)	100	0	0	21	0	80
Neapolitan (½ cup)	90	0	0	20	0	65
Peach or Vanilla (½ cup)	90	0	0	19	0	60-65
Strawberry (½ cup)	90	0	0	20	0	55
Strawberry Cheesecake (½ cup)	100	0	0	23	0	60
Sweet Freedom (No Added Sugar) Lowfat Frozen Yogurt, Burgundy Cherry (½ cup)	70	2	1	16	0	50
Chocolate (½ cup)	80	2	1	16	0	65
Peach or Strawberry (½ cup)	70	2	1	15	0	50
Vanilla (½ cup)	70	2	1	15	0	60
Yarnell's Guilt Free Nonfat Frozen Yogurt, Black Cherry (½ cup)	80	0	0	17	0	80
Chocolate Fudge (½ cup)	80	0	0	19	0	80
Peach (½ cup)	70	0	0	17	0	60
Strawberry Swirl (½ cup)	80	0	0	17	0	60
Vanilla (½ cup)	80	0	0	16	0	60

	Calories	Fat g	Saturated Fat g	Carbohydrate g	Fiber g	Sodium mg
ICE CREAM CONES						
Delicious Jumbo Cake Cup Cone (1 cone)	25	0	0	6	0	25
Rainbow Color Cup Cone (1 cone)	20	0	0	4	0	20
Sugar Cones (1 cone)	45	0	0	9	0	5
Vanilla Cake Cup Cone (1 cone)	20	0	0	4	0	20
Keebler Assorted Color Cups or Ice Creme Cups (1 cup)	15	0	0	4	0	20
Sugar Cones (1 cone)	50	1	0	11	0	35
Waffle Bowls (1 bowl)	50	1	0	10	0	25
Waffle Cones (1 cone)	50	1	0	10	0	25
Nabisco Comet Cups (1 cone)	20	0	0	4	0	20
Comet Sugar Cones (1 cone)	50	0	0	11	<1	40
Comet Waffle Cones (1 cone)	70	1	0	14	1	30
Oreo Chocolate Cones (1 cone)	50	1	0	10	<1	110
Teddy Grahams Cinnamon Cones (1 cone)	60	1	0	13	<1	55
ICE CREAMS AND ICE MILKS						
Higher-Fat						
Ice Cream, Chocolate, Rich (16% fat) (½ cup)	257	17	11	24	0	60
Ice Cream, Chocolate, Regular (11% fat) (½ cup)	143	7	4	19	0	50
Lower-Fat						
Most Brands, Ice Milk, Chocolate (½ cup)	92	3	2	15	0	56
Blue Bell Diet Ice Cream, Banana Berry (½ cup)	100	0	0	21	1	60
Chocolate (½ cup)	100	0	0	21	0	70
Neapolitan (½ cup)	100	0	0	24	0	75
Orange Pineapple (½ cup)	100	0	0	20	0	85
Strawberry (½ cup)	100	0	0	21	1	80
Vanilla Bean (½ cup)	100	0	0	21	0	85
Borden Fat Free Ice Cream, Black Cherry, Chocolate or Peach (½ cup)	90	0	0	19	0	45
Strawberry or Vanilla (½ cup)	80	0	0	18	0	45
Light Ice Cream, Chocolate Flavored (½ cup)	110	3	2	18	0	60
Chocolate Revel (½ cup)	100	2	1	18	0	55
Neapolitan Flavored or						

Ice Creams and Ice Milks (continued)	Calories	Fat g	Saturated Fat g	Carbohydrate g	Fiber g	Sodium mg
Borden (continued)						
Strawberry Revel (1/2 cup)	90	2	2	16	0	55
Orange Pineapple (1/2 cup)	90	2	1	17	0	55
Strawberry Flavored or Vanilla (1/2 cup)	80	2	1	15	0	50
Low Fat Ice Cream, Cherry Vanilla or Neapolitan (1/2 cup)	110	2	1	20	0	40
Chocolate (1/2 cup)	110	2	1	21	0	50
Chocolate Chip Cookie Dough (1/2 cup)	120	3	2	23	0	60
Chocolate Marshmallow Swirl (1/2 cup)	110	2	2	21	0	50
Chocolate Swirl or Cookies 'N Cream (1/2 cup)	110	2	1	20	0	45-55
Orange Sherbet N' Cream or Strawberry (1/2 cup)	100	2	1	19	0	35
Vanilla (1/2 cup)	100	2	1	18	0	35
Dreyer's Grand Fat Free Ice Cream, Black Cherry Vanilla (1/2 cup)	100	0	0	21	NA	70
Chocolate Fudge or Marble Fudge (1/2 cup)	100	0	0	23	NA	75
Mint Fudge (1/2 cup)	100	0	0	22	NA	75
Raspberry Vanilla Swirl (1/2 cup)	70	0	0	18	NA	35
Strawberry (1/2 cup)	90	0	0	20	NA	55
Vanilla (1/2 cup)	90	0	0	20	NA	65
Vanilla Chocolate Swirl (1/2 cup)	80	0	0	20	NA	45
Edy's Grand Fat Free Ice Cream, Black Cherry Vanilla (1/2 cup)	100	0	0	21	NA	70
Chocolate Fudge or Marble Fudge (1/2 cup)	100	0	0	23	NA	75
Mint Fudge (1/2 cup)	100	0	0	22	NA	75
Raspberry Vanilla Swirl (1/2 cup)	70	0	0	18	NA	35
Strawberry (1/2 cup)	90	0	0	20	NA	55
Vanilla (1/2 cup)	90	0	0	20	NA	65
Vanilla Chocolate Swirl (1/2 cup)	80	0	0	20	NA	45
Gisé Crème Glacé (4 fl oz)	33	0	0	7	1	0
Healthy Choice Ice Cream, Black Forest (1/2 cup)	120	2	1	23	1	50
Bordeaux Cherry Chocolate Chip (1/2 cup)	110	2	2	19	<1	55

	Calories	Fat g	Saturated Fat g	Carbohydrate g	Fiber g	Sodium mg
Butter Pecan Crunch, Cappuccino Chocolate Chunk or Malt Caramel Cone (1/2 cup)	120	2	1	22	1	60
Cookies 'N Cream (1/2 cup)	120	2	2	21	<1	90
Double Fudge Swirl (1/2 cup)	120	2	2	21	1	50
Fudge Brownie (1/2 cup)	120	2	1	22	2	55
Mint Chocolate Chip (1/2 cup)	120	2	1	21	<1	50
Peanut Butter Cookie Dough 'N Fudge (1/2 cup)	120	2	1	22	<1	60
Praline & Caramel (1/2 cup)	130	2	1	25	<1	70
Rocky Road (1/2 cup)	140	2	1	28	2	60
Vanilla (1/2 cup)	100	2	2	18	1	50
Milky Way Low Fat Chocolate Malt, Milk Shake (1 cup)	220	3	2	44	2	135
Wells' Blue Bunny Health Smart Nonfat No Sugar Added Ice Cream, Burgundy Cherry, Chocolate, Peach, Raspberry or Strawberry (1/2 cup)	70	0	0	17	0	70
Vanilla Flavored (1/2 cup)	80	0	0	18	0	75
Nonfat Ice Cream, Burgundy Cherry (1/2 cup)	110	0	0	25	0	60
Chocolate (1/2 cup)	110	0	0	22	0	75
Cookies & Cream (1/2 cup)	120	0	0	27	0	80
Neapolitan (1/2 cup)	70	0	0	24	0	65
Peach (1/2 cup)	100	0	0	22	0	55
Strawberry (1/2 cup)	110	0	0	24	0	55
Vanilla Flavored (1/2 cup)	120	0	0	26	0	65
Yarnell's Guilt Free Nonfat Ice Cream, Banana Nut Crunch (1/2 cup)	80	0	0	20	0	85
Blueberry Swirl, Mint Fudge, Strawberry, Vanilla Brownie or Vanilla Fudge (1/2 cup)	80	0	0	19	0	80
Chocolate (1/2 cup)	80	0	0	20	0	80
Praline Pecan Crunch (1/2 cup)	80	0	0	21	0	85
Triple Chocolate (1/2 cup)	80	0	0	19	0	90
Vanilla (1/2 cup)	80	0	0	19	0	70

	Calories	Fat g	Saturated Fat g	Carbohydrate g	Fiber g	Sodium mg
ICES, SHERBETS, AND SORBETS						
Blue Bell Sherbet, Lime, Orange or Rainbow (½ cup)	130	1	1	28	0	30
Pineapple (½ cup)	120	1	1	27	0	30
Strawberry (½ cup)	120	1	1	27	0	25
Tropical Fruit (½ cup)	120	1	1	28	0	25
Häagen-Dazs Sorbet, Mango (½ cup)	120	0	0	30	<1	0
Raspberry (½ cup)	120	0	0	30	3	0
Strawberry (½ cup)	130	0	0	33	1	0
Zesty Lemon (½ cup)	120	0	0	31	<1	5
Mama Tish's No Sugar Added Italian Ices, Lemon (4 fl oz)	50	0	0	12	0	5
Strawberry (4 fl oz)	40	0	0	10	0	10
Original Italian Ices, Cherry (4 fl oz)	100	0	0	24	0	0
Chocolate (4 fl oz)	100	0	0	24	1	125
Lemon (4 fl oz)	100	0	0	24	0	5
Lemon-Lime or Pineapple-Banana-Orange (4 fl oz)	90	0	0	23	0	0
Pineapple-Coconut or Tropical (4 fl oz)	90	0	0	22	0	0
Raspberry (4 fl oz)	100	0	0	25	0	5
Strawberry (4 fl oz)	80	0	0	21	0	5
Mazzone's Italian Ice, Cherry (3.5 fl oz)	70	0	0	16	0	0
Lemon, Orange or Watermelon (3.5 fl oz)	60	0	0	15	0	0
Lime (3.5 fl oz)	60	0	0	14	0	0
Rainbow (3.5 fl oz)	60	0	0	16	0	0
Sorbetto Molle Soft Italian Sorbet, Lemon (4 fl oz)	113	0	0	27	0	10
Passion Fruit (4 fl oz)	101	0	0	24	0	5
Raspberry (4 fl oz)	83	0	0	19	0	5
Strawberry (4 fl oz)	116	0	0	28	0	15
Wells' Blue Bunny Ol' Fashion Premium Sherbet, Orange or Raspberry (½ cup)	110	1	1	26	0	35
Sherbet, Fuzzy Navel (½ cup)	130	1	1	30	0	35
Lime or Rainbow (½ cup)	110	1	1	27	0	35
Orange, Raspberry or Strawberry (½ cup)	110	1	1	26	0	35

Ices, Sherbets, and Sorbets (continued)	Calories	Fat g	Saturated Fat g	Carbohydrate g	Fiber g	Sodium mg
Pina Colada (1/2 cup)	120	2	1	28	0	35
Pineapple (1/2 cup)	110	1	1	25	0	35
Strawberry Colada (1/2 cup)	130	1	1	31	0	35
Strawberry Margarita (1/2 cup)	130	1	1	32	0	35
Tropical Neapolitan Cooler (1/2 cup)	120	1	1	29	0	35
Wildberry Crumble (1/2 cup)	140	2	1	31	0	50

NON-DAIRY FROZEN DESSERTS

	Calories	Fat g	Saturated Fat g	Carbohydrate g	Fiber g	Sodium mg
Sweet Nothings Nonfat Non-Dairy Frozen Desserts, Black Leopard, Chocolate Mandarin, Chocolate, Mango Raspberry, Raspberry Swirl or Very Berry Blueberry (1/2 cup)	100	0	0	23	0	5
Espresso Fudge, Tiger Stripes or Vanilla (1/2 cup)	110	0	0	25	0	5

FRUITS

Most fruits naturally contain little or no fat and are low in sodium. Avocado and olives are exceptions since they do contain fat; they are listed in the Fats section beginning on page 141. Fruit snacks are found in the Snacks section beginning on page 219. The foods in this section contain a maximum of 3 grams of fat and 1 gram of saturated fat per serving.

Canned Fruits

	Calories	Fat g	Saturated Fat g	Carbohydrate g	Fiber g	Sodium mg
CANNED FRUITS						
APPLESAUCE, CANNED						
Most Brands, Applesauce, Sweetened (¹/₂ cup)	97	0	0	25	2	4
Unsweetened (¹/₂ cup)	52	0	0	14	2	2
America's Choice Apple Sauce, Old Fashioned Unsweetened (¹/₂ cup)	50	0	0	15	2	30
Original (¹/₂ cup)	90	0	0	23	2	30
APRICOTS, CANNED						
Most Brands, Apricot Halves, in heavy syrup (¹/₂ cup)	107	0	0	28	2	5
In juice or in water (¹/₂ cup)	35	0	0	8	2	1
In light syrup (¹/₂ cup)	105	0	0	27	2	5
America's Choice Unpeeled Apricot Halves in Pear Juice Concentrate & Water (¹/₂ cup)	40	0	0	12	1	10
Del Monte Apricots in water (¹/₂ cup halves)	40	0	0	10	1	10
Lite Apricot Halves in Extra Lite Syrup (¹/₂ cup)	60	0	0	16	1	10

	Calories	Fat g	Saturated Fat g	Carbohydrate g	Fiber g	Sodium mg

Canned Fruits *(continued)*

BLACKBERRIES, CANNED

	Calories	Fat g	Saturated Fat g	Carbohydrate g	Fiber g	Sodium mg
Blackberries in syrup (½ cup)	116	0	0	30	3	0

BLUEBERRIES, CANNED

Blueberries in syrup (½ cup)	110	0	0	28	1	5

BOYSENBERRIES, CANNED

Boysenberries in syrup (½ cup)	114	0	0	29	3	0

CHERRIES, CANNED

Most Brands, Cherries, in heavy syrup (½ cup)	105	0	0	27	2	4
In juice or in water (½ cup)	57	1	0	13	1	2
In light syrup (½ cup)	83	0	0	21	2	3
America's Choice Maraschino Cherries or Maraschino Cherries w/Stems (1 cherry)	10	0	0	2	0	0
Del Monte Dark Sweet Cherries, pitted or whole (½ cup)	100	0	0	24	<1	10

CRANBERRY SAUCES, CANNED

Most Brands, Cranberry Sauce, Sweetened (½ cup)	216	0	0	53	2	35
Ocean Spray Cranberries, Jellied (2 ¾ oz)	110	0	0	27	<1	5
Whole Berry (2 ¾ oz)	112	0	0	28	1	8

FIGS, CANNED

Figs, in heavy syrup (½ cup)	114	0	0	30	2	2
In light syrup (½ cup)	111	0	0	29	2	1
In water (½ cup)	56	0	0	15	2	1

GRAPEFRUIT, CANNED

Grapefruit, in juice or in water (½ cup)	31	0	0	8	1	0
In light syrup (½ cup)	76	0	0	20	1	3

LYCHEES, CANNED

Ka-me Lychees in Syrup, whole pitted (15 pieces)	130	0	0	32	0	26

MANGO, CANNED

Ka-me Mango (4 pieces)	102	0	0	25	0	10

MIXED FRUIT, CANNED

Most Brands, Fruit Cocktail, in heavy syrup (½ cup)	93	0	0	24	2	8

	Calories	Fat g	Saturated Fat g	Carbohydrate g	Fiber g	Sodium mg
Most Brands, Fruit Cocktail *(continued)*						
In juice (1/2 cup)	55	0	0	14	2	5
In light syrup (1/2 cup)	88	0	0	23	2	7
In water (1/2 cup)	56	0	0	15	2	5
America's Choice Chunky Mixed Fruit, in Light Syrup (1/2 cup)	70	0	0	18	1	15
In Water (1/2 cup)	40	0	0	10	1	10
Fruit Cocktail in Pear Juice from Concentrate (1/2 cup)	60	0	0	10	1	10
Fruit Mix, in Light Syrup (1/2 cup)	80	0	0	18	1	5
In Pear Juice from Concentrate (1/2 cup)	60	0	0	13	1	5
Mixed Fruit in Heavy Syrup (1 fruit cup)	100	0	0	24	1	10
Del Monte Tropical Fruit Salad in Light Syrup w/Passion Fruit Juice (1/2 cup)	80	0	0	21	1	10
Fruit Naturals, Chunky Mixed Fruit in Fruit Juices from Concentrate (1/2 cup)	60	0	0	15	1	10
Fruit Cocktail in Fruit Juices from Concentrate (1/2 cup)	60	0	0	15	1	10
Mixed Fruits in Juice (4.5 oz can)	60	0	0	16	1	10
Lite, Chunky Mixed Fruit in Extra Light Syrup (1/2 cup)	60	0	0	15	1	10
Fruit Cocktail in Extra Light Syrup (1/2 cup)	60	0	0	15	1	10
Mixed Fruits in Extra Light Syrup (4.5 oz can)	80	0	0	15	1	10
ORANGES, CANNED						
Del Monte Mandarin Oranges in Light Syrup (1/2 cup)	80	0	0	19	<1	10
PAPAYA, CANNED						
Ka-me Papaya (3/4 cup)	120	0	0	29	1	15
PEACHES, CANNED						
Most Brands, Peaches, in heavy syrup (1/2 cup)	95	0	0	26	2	8
In juice (1/2 cup)	32	0	0	8	1	0
In light syrup (1/2 cup)	93	0	0	25	2	8
In water (1/2 cup)	31	0	0	7	1	0
Spiced (1/2 cup)	92	0	0	25	2	7

	Calories	Fat g	Saturated Fat g	Carbohydrate g	Fiber g	Sodium mg
America's Choice Sliced Peaches in Pear Juice Concentrate & Water (1/2 cup)	60	0	0	14	1	10
Del Monte Spiced Peaches, whole (1/2 cup)	100	0	0	24	<1	10
Naturals, Diced Peaches in Peach Juice (4.5 oz can)	60	0	0	16	1	10
Sliced Yellow Cling Peaches in Peach Juice from Concentrate (1/2 cup)	60	0	0	15	1	10
Lite, Diced Yellow Cling Peaches in Extra Light Syrup (4.5 oz can)	60	0	0	16	1	10
Sliced Freestone Peaches in Extra Light Syrup (1/2 cup)	60	0	0	14	1	10
Yellow Cling Peaches in Extra Light Syrup (1/2 cup)	60	0	0	15	1	10
PEARS, CANNED						
Most Brands, Pears, in heavy syrup (1/2 cup halves)	94	0	0	24	4	6
In juice or in water (1/2 cup halves)	36	0	0	9	2	0
In light syrup (1/2 cup halves)	92	0	0	24	4	6
America's Choice Pears in Pear Juice Concentrate (1/2 cup)	60	0	0	14	1	10
Del Monte Fruit Naturals Pears in Pear Juice from Concentrate or Lite Pears in Extra Light Syrup (1/2 cup)	60	0	0	15	1	10
PINEAPPLE, CANNED						
Most Brands, Pineapple Chunks, in juice (1/2 cup)	75	0	0	20	2	1
In light syrup (1/2 cup)	66	0	0	17	2	1
In water (1/2 cup)	74	0	0	19	2	1
Dole Pineapple, Chunks or Tidbits (1/2 cup)	60	0	0	15	1	10
Crushed (1/2 cup)	70	0	0	17	1	10
Slices (2 slices)	60	0	0	15	1	10
PLUMS, CANNED						
Plums, in heavy syrup (1/2 cup)	115	0	0	30	3	25
In juice (1/2 cup)	52	1	0	12	2	0
In light syrup (1/2 cup)	112	0	0	29	3	24
In water (1/2 cup)	51	1	0	12	2	0

	Calories	Fat g	Saturated Fat g	Carbohydrate g	Fiber g	Sodium mg
PRUNES, CANNED						
Prunes in syrup (1/2 cup)	143	0	0	37	3	2
RASPBERRIES, CANNED						
Raspberries in syrup (1/2 cup)	129	0	0	33	4	1
STRAWBERRIES, CANNED						
Strawberries in syrup (1/2 cup)	122	0	0	33	2	4
TANGERINES, CANNED						
Tangerines, in juice (1/2 cup)	55	0	0	14	1	1
In light syrup (1/2 cup)	77	0	0	21	1	8
DRIED FRUITS						
APPLES, DRIED						
Apples, uncooked (1/2 cup)	104	0	0	28	4	37
APRICOTS, DRIED						
Apricots, uncooked (10 halves)	83	0	0	22	3	3
CURRANTS, DRIED						
Currants (1/4 cup)	108	0	0	28	1	4
DATES, DRIED						
Most Brands, Dates (5)	114	0	0	31	2	1
Dole Pitted Dates (1/4 cup)	120	0	0	31	3	10
FIGS, DRIED						
Most Brands, Figs, uncooked (2)	95	0	0	24	3	4
MIXED FRUIT, DRIED						
Del Monte Mixed Dried Fruit (1/3 cup)	110	0	0	30	5	50
PEACHES, DRIED						
Peaches, uncooked (1/4 cup halves)	96	0	0	24	3	3
PEARS, DRIED						
Pears, uncooked (1/4 cup halves)	118	0	0	31	5	3
PINEAPPLE, DRIED						
Fisher Dried Pineapple (30 pieces)	140	0	0	35	1	20
PRUNES, DRIED						
Most Brands, Prunes, uncooked (5)	100	0	0	26	3	2
Dole Pitted Prunes (1/4 cup)	110	0	0	26	2	5

	Calories	Fat g	Saturated Fat g	Carbohydrate g	Fiber g	Sodium mg
RAISINS, DRIED						
Most Brands, Raisins (1/4 cup)	116	0	0	31	1	5
Del Monte Golden Raisins (1/4 cup)	130	0	0	31	2	10
Dole Raisins (1/4 cup)	130	0	0	31	2	10
FRESH FRUITS						
Apple (2 ¾" diam)	81	1	0	21	3	0
Apricots (2)	34	0	0	8	2	1
Banana (8 ¾" long)	105	1	0	27	2	1
Blackberries (1 cup)	75	1	0	18	5	0
Blueberries (1 cup)	81	1	0	20	2	9
Boysenberries (1 cup)	74	1	0	18	5	0
Cantaloupe (1 cup cubes)	56	1	0	13	1	14
Casaba Melon (1 cup cubes)	60	0	0	16	1	17
Cherries (1 cup)	104	1	0	24	2	0
Cranberries, chopped (½ cup)	27	0	0	7	2	1
Figs (2 large)	95	0	0	25	4	1
Gooseberries (1 cup)	66	1	0	15	4	1
Grapefruit (½ of a 4" diam)	47	0	0	12	2	0
Grapes (1 cup)	114	1	0	28	1	3
Guava (1)	46	1	0	11	5	3
Honeydew Melon (1 cup cubes)	60	0	0	16	1	17
Kiwifruit (1 med)	46	0	0	11	1	4
Kumquat (1)	12	0	0	3	1	1
Lemon (1 med)	17	0	0	5	1	1
Lime (1)	19	0	0	6	1	1
Loganberries (1 cup)	81	1	0	19	5	1
Mango (½)	67	0	0	18	3	2
Mulberries (1 cup)	78	1	0	20	2	8
Nectarine (2½" diam)	67	1	0	16	2	0
Orange (2 ⅝" diam)	62	0	0	15	3	0
Papaya (1 cup cubes)	55	0	0	14	4	4
Passion Fruit (1)	11	0	0	3	1	1
Peach (2½" diam)	37	0	0	5	1	0
Pear (2½" diam)	98	1	0	13	6	0
Persimmon (1)	118	0	0	31	3	2
Pineapple (1 cup diced)	76	1	0	19	2	2

	Calories	Fat g	Saturated Fat g	Carbohydrate g	Fiber g	Sodium mg
Fresh Fruits *(continued)*						
Plantain, raw (1)	278	0	0	75	3	12
Plum (2 1/8" diam)	36	0	0	9	1	0
Pomegranate (3 3/8" diam)	105	1	0	26	6	5
Raspberries (1 cup)	60	1	0	14	3	0
Rhubarb (1 cup diced)	9	0	0	3	2	1
Strawberries (1 cup)	45	1	0	10	2	1
Tangerine (2 3/8" diam)	37	0	0	9	1	1
Watermelon (2 cups diced)	102	1	0	23	1	6
FROZEN FRUITS						
Most Brands, Blackberries, unsweetened (1 cup)	74	1	0	18	5	2
Blueberries, unsweetened (1 cup)	129	1	0	33	3	14
Boysenberries, unsweetened (1 cup)	74	1	0	18	5	0
Cantaloupe (1 cup cubes)	56	1	0	13	1	14
Grapefruit Sections (1/2 cup)	31	0	0	8	1	0
Loganberries (1 cup)	81	1	0	6	5	1
Melon Balls (1 cup)	64	1	0	16	1	14
Peaches, sweetened (1/2 cup slices)	92	0	0	25	2	7
Pineapple Chunks, sweetened (1/2 cup)	105	0	0	27	2	1
Raspberries, sweetened (1/2 cup)	129	0	0	33	4	1
Rhubarb, unsweetened, uncooked (1 cup)	10	0	0	3	2	1
Strawberries, sweetened (1/2 cup)	122	0	0	33	2	4
Strawberries, unsweetened (1/2 cup)	33	0	0	8	2	1
Campbell's Kitchen Homestyle, Cinnamon Scalloped Apples (1/2 cup)	110	2	1	24	NA	80

JUICES

Fruit and vegetable juices contain little or no fat and saturated fat. Values for many of the foods in this section are given for "most brands." Foods in this section of the Guide do not exceed the cutoff points of 3 grams of fat and 1 gram of saturated fat per serving. Most vegetable juices are high in sodium. Individuals needing to limit their intake of sodium (or salt) may wish to try low-sodium vegetable juices.

Fruit Juices	Calories	Fat g	Saturated Fat g	Carbohydrate g	Fiber g	Sodium mg
FRUIT JUICES						
APPLE JUICES						
Most Brands, Apple Juice, unsweetened, ready-to-serve (8 fl oz)	117	0	0	29	0	7
Betty Crocker Squeezit 100, Acrobat Apple (6 2/3 fl oz bottle)	110	0	0	27	0	20
Dole 100% Juice, Apple Juice, ready-to-serve (10 fl oz)	160	0	0	39	0	25
Hansen's Natural Apple Juice, ready-to-serve (8 fl oz)	100	0	0	25	0	15
Just Pik't 100% Pure Frozen Apple Juice, Fresh Pressed, ready-to-serve (8 fl oz)	120	0	0	30	0	60
Ocean Spray Apple Juice, from frozen (8 fl oz)	110	0	0	28	0	35
APRICOT NECTAR						
Apricot Nectar, sweetened, ready-to-serve (8 fl oz)	141	0	0	36	2	8

	Calories	Fat g	Saturated Fat g	Carbohydrate g	Fiber g	Sodium mg
BERRY JUICES						
Betty Crocker Squeezit 100, Berry (6 2/3 fl oz bottle)	100	0	0	24	0	20
Dole 100% Juice, Country Raspberry, ready-to-serve or from frozen (8 fl oz)	140	0	0	34	0	30
Smucker's Naturally 100% Fruit Juice, Boysenberry, ready-to-drink (8 fl oz)	120	0	0	30	NA	10
Red Raspberry, ready-to-drink (8 fl oz)	120	0	0	30	NA	10
CHERRY JUICES						
Dole 100% Juice, Mountain Cherry, ready-to-serve or from frozen (8 fl oz)	120	0	0	30	0	30
Smucker's Naturally 100% Fruit Juice, Black Cherry, ready-to-drink (8 fl oz)	130	0	0	31	NA	10
GRAPE JUICES						
Most Brands, Grape Juice, sweetened, ready-to-serve (8 fl oz)	154	0	0	38	1	8
Betty Crocker Squeezit 100, Caped Grape (6 2/3 fl oz bottle)	110	0	0	24	0	20
GRAPEFRUIT JUICES						
Most Brands, Grapefruit Juice, sweetened, ready-to-serve (8 fl oz)	115	0	0	28	0	5
Unsweetened, ready-to-serve (8 fl oz)	94	0	0	22	0	2
Dole 100% Juice, Sun Ripe Grapefruit, ready-to-serve (10 fl oz)	160	0	0	39	0	45
Florida's Natural Juice, Ruby Red Premium Grapefruit, ready-to-serve (8 fl oz)	100	0	0	24	0	0
Just Pik't Fresh Squeezed Grapefruit, ready-to-serve (8 fl oz)	100	0	0	24	0	0
Ocean Spray Grapefruit Juice, ready-to-drink (8 fl oz)	100	0	0	24	<1	35
LEMON JUICE						
Lemon Juice (1 tsp)	1	0	0	0	0	1
LIME JUICE						
Lime Juice (1 tsp)	1	0	0	0	0	1
MIXED FRUIT JUICES						
Most Brands, Orange & Grapefruit Juice, unsweetened, ready-to-drink (8 fl oz)	103	0	0	25	0	2

	Calories	Fat g	Saturated Fat g	Carbohydrate g	Fiber g	Sodium mg
Pineapple-Grapefruit Juice, unsweetened, ready-to-drink (8 fl oz)	117	0	0	28	1	2
Betty Crocker Squeezit 100, Pilot Punch (6 2/3 fl oz bottle)	110	0	0	24	0	20
Dole 100% Juice, Pine-Orange Banana, ready-to-serve (8 fl oz)	130	0	0	29	0	20
Pine-Passion Banana, ready-to-serve or from frozen (8 fl oz)	120	0	0	29	0	20
Pineapple Orange, from frozen (8 fl oz)	120	0	0	29	0	20
Ready-to-serve (8 fl oz)	120	0	0	27	0	20
Tropical Fruit, from frozen (8 fl oz)	140	0	0	34	0	30
Ready-to-serve (8 fl oz)	140	0	0	35	0	30
Florida's Natural Juice Premium, Orange Pineapple, ready-to-serve (8 fl oz)	130	0	0	31	0	0
Minute Maid Orange Blend, ready-to-serve (10 oz)	150	0	0	37	0	0
Smucker's Naturally 100% Fruit Juice, Apple-Cranberry, ready-to-drink (8 fl oz)	120	0	0	32	NA	10
ORANGE JUICES						
Most Brands, Orange Juice, unsweetened, ready-to-drink or from frozen (8 fl oz)	112	0	0	25	1	2
Florida's Natural Premium Orange Juice, Home Squeezed Style or Regular, ready-to-serve (8 fl oz)	120	0	0	29	0	0
Just Pik't Fresh Squeezed Orange Juice, ready-to-serve (8 fl oz)	120	0	0	29	0	0
Ocean Spray Orange Juice, from frozen (8 fl oz)	120	0	0	31	0	35
PAPAYA NECTAR						
Papaya Nectar, sweetened, ready-to-drink (8 fl oz)	149	0	0	36	1	12
PASSION FRUIT JUICE						
Passion Fruit Juice, ready-to-drink (8 fl oz)	139	0	0	34	1	3
PEACH JUICES						
Most Brands, Peach Nectar, sweetened, ready-to-drink (8 fl oz)	134	0	0	35	2	17
Dole 100% Juice, Orchard Peach, ready-to-serve or from frozen (8 fl oz)	140	0	0	34	0	30

	Calories	Fat g	Saturated Fat g	Carbohydrate g	Fiber g	Sodium mg
Peach Juices *(continued)*						
Smucker's Naturally 100% Fruit Juice, Peach, ready-to-drink (8 fl oz)	120	0	0	30	NA	10
PEAR NECTAR						
Pear Nectar, sweetened, ready-to-drink (8 fl oz)	148	0	0	39	2	2
PINEAPPLE JUICES						
Most Brands, Pineapple Juice, unsweetened, ready-to-drink (8 fl oz)	139	0	0	34	1	2
Dole 100% Juice, Pineapple, from frozen (8 fl oz)	130	0	0	30	0	20
Ready-to-serve (8 fl oz)	130	0	0	29	0	20
Unsweetened, ready-to-serve (8 fl oz)	120	0	0	29	0	10
PRUNE JUICES						
Most Brands, Prune Juice, ready-to-drink (8 fl oz)	181	0	0	45	1	11
Del Monte Prune Juice, ready-to-serve (6 fl oz)	170	0	0	43	1	20
TANGERINE JUICES						
Dole 100% Juice, Mandarin Tangerine, ready-to-serve (8 fl oz)	140	0	0	35	0	30
Minute Maid Tangerine Juice, from frozen (8 fl oz)	120	0	0	29	0	0
VEGETABLE JUICES						
CARROT JUICES						
Most Brands, Carrot Juice (8 fl oz)	98	0	0	23	2	71
Just Pik't Carrot Juice (5.5 fl oz)	44	0	0	11	0	0
MIXED VEGETABLE JUICES						
Most Brands, Vegetable Juice Cocktail (8 fl oz)	46	0	0	11	1	887
No Salt Added, ready-to-serve (8 fl oz)	46	0	0	11	1	56
Del Monte Vegetable Cocktail (8 oz)	50	0	0	12	1	490
Smucker's Vegetable Juice, Hearty (8 fl oz)	58	0	0	13	NA	714
Hearty Hot & Spicy (8 fl oz)	58	0	0	13	NA	650
V8 Vegetable Juice (8 fl oz)	50	0	0	10	1	620
Light in Sodium & Tangy (1 cup)	60	0	0	11	1	340

	Calories	Fat g	Saturated Fat g	Carbohydrate g	Fiber g	Sodium mg
Vegetable Juices (continued)						
Low Sodium (8 fl oz)	60	0	0	11	2	140
Picante (8 fl oz)	50	0	0	9	1	690
Spicy Hot (8 fl oz)	50	0	0	10	1	780
SAUERKRAUT JUICE						
Bush's Sauerkraut Juice (8 fl oz)	14	1	0	1	0	1,670
TOMATO JUICES						
Most Brands, Tomato Juice (8 fl oz)	41	0	0	10	2	877
No Salt Added (8 fl oz)	41	0	0	10	2	24
America's Choice Tomato Juice (8 fl oz)	40	0	0	7	0	550
Campbell's Tomato Juice (8 fl oz)	50	0	0	9	1	860
Low Sodium Tomato Juice w/Enhanced Tomato Flavor (8 fl oz)	50	0	0	10	1	140
Tomato Del Mar (8 fl oz)	110	1	1	26	1	880
Del Monte Snap-E-Tom (8 fl oz)	50	0	0	11	2	670
OTHER JUICES						
Gorton's Clam Juice (10.6 oz can)	0	0	0	0	0	740

MAIN DISHES AND MEAL-TYPE PRODUCTS

Main dishes and meal-type products included in this section of the Guide are low in fat and saturated fat *as purchased* or when *prepared according to package directions*. The foods in this section can be used as a main dish (entrée, pizza, etc.) or as an entire breakfast, lunch, or dinner meal.

To be included in the Guide, a main dish or meal-type product may provide no more fat and saturated fat than the cutoff points indicated in the first table below. Since the cutoff points are applied to 100 grams (g), which is about 3½ ounces (oz), of these products, the actual cutoff points for each product will depend on its total weight. To help you evaluate main dishes and meal-type products not in the Guide, the second table below provides the cutoff points for fat and saturated fat for products of different weights. For example, a meal-type product weighing 12 oz and providing 9 g of fat and 2 g of saturated fat qualifies for inclusion in the Guide and is a good choice for a cholesterol-lowering eating pattern. Foods in this section of the Guide meet the FDA definitions of "low fat" and "low saturated fat."

CUTOFF POINTS FOR MAIN DISHES AND MEAL-TYPE PRODUCTS

Fat g	Saturated Fat g
3 g per 100g*	1 g per 100 g
and	and
30% of calories	10% of calories

*100 g = about 3½ oz.

CUTOFF POINTS AT VARIOUS WEIGHTS OF MAIN DISHES AND MEAL-TYPE PRODUCTS

Weight of Product oz	Fat g	Saturated Fat g
5	4	1
6	5	2
7	6	2
8	7	2
9	8	3
10	9	3
11	9	3
12	10	3
13	11	4

Canned and Shelf-Stable Entrées and Dinners	Calories	Fat g	Saturated Fat g	Carbohydrate g	Fiber g	Sodium mg
CANNED AND SHELF-STABLE ENTRÉES AND DINNERS						
Higher-Fat						
Beef Stew (7.5 oz)	237	15	6	11	2	1,142
Chili w/o Beans (7.4 oz)	260	16	6	13	3	599
Lower-Fat						
Aunt Patsy's Pantry Chicken Chili, prep w/onions, chicken & green chilies (1 cup)	440	5	1	57	6	1,488
Lentil Chili, prep w/onions & tomato sauce (1 cup)	220	1	0	39	8	1,104
Souper Black Bean Chili, prep w/onions, tomato sauce & green chilies (1 cup)	230	1	0	45	8	1,248
Buckeye Beans & Herbs						
Black Bean Chili, prep w/onions, tomato sauce & chilies (bag) (1 cup)	260	1	0	48	9	1,248
Black Bean Chili, prep w/onions, tomato sauce & chilies (box) (1 cup)	240	1	0	48	9	1,248
White Chicken Chili, prep w/onions, chicken & chilies (1 cup)	430	5	1	54	5	984
Bush's Spaghetti (1 cup)	180	3	1	30	2	1,450
Spaghetti Rings (1 cup)	170	3	1	30	2	1,500

	Calories	Fat g	Saturated Fat g	Carbohydrate g	Fiber g	Sodium mg
Canned and Shelf-Stable *Entrées and Dinners (continued)*						
Chef Boyardee Sir Chomps-a-lot, Bite Size Cheese Ravioli (7.5 oz bowl)	170	0	0	35	2	790
Bite Size Cheese Tortellini (9.1 oz)	130	1	0	46	5	770
Di Giorno Light Varieties Cheese & Garlic Ravioli (1 cup)	270	2	1	45	1	580
Franco-American Spaghetti Pasta in Tomato & Cheese Sauce (1 cup)	210	2	1	41	3	1,020
Spaghetti in Tomato Sauce w/Cheese (7 3/4 oz)	180	2	1	36	2	890
Spaghettios Garfield Pizzos (1 cup)	210	3	1	39	2	910
Spaghettios Pasta in Tomato & Cheese Sauce (1 cup)	190	2	1	36	2	990
Spaghettios Pasta in Tomato & Cheese Sauce 7.5 oz can)	160	2	1	31	2	840
Health Valley Fat-Free Chili, 3 Bean, Mild Black Bean or Spicy Black Bean (1/2 cup)	80	0	0	15	7	160
Vegetarian Chili w/Beans, Mild or Spicy (1/2 cup)	80	0	0	15	7	100
Mild or Spicy, No Salt (1/2 cup)	80	0	0	15	7	35
Vegetarian Chili w/Lentils, Mild (1/2 cup)	80	0	0	14	6	100
Mild, No Salt (1/2 cup)	80	0	0	14	6	50
Vegetarian Cuisine, Amaranth Garden Vegetable (1 cup)	160	0	0	31	9	290
Lentil Garden Vegetable (1 cup)	160	1	0	34	12	240
Tofu Baked Beans (1 cup)	170	1	0	27	16	270
Tofu Black Bean (1 cup)	170	1	0	28	15	290
Tofu Lentil (1 cup)	160	1	0	29	16	290
Western Black Bean (1 cup)	230	1	0	40	19	230
Hormel Roast Beef w/Gravy (2 oz)	60	2	1	1	0	280
Top Shelf Chicken Cacciatore Two Minute Entree (10 oz bowl)	210	3	1	26	3	850
La Choy Chow Mein Entrees, Beef (3/4 cup)	40	2	1	5	2	960
Meatless (3/4 cup)	25	<1	0	5	2	860
Libby's Diner Pasta Spirals & Chicken (7.75 oz)	130	4	1	16	4	980
Spaghetti & Meatballs (7.75 oz)	190	5	2	27	2	940
Roast Beef w/Gravy (2/3 cup)	140	3	2	2	0	800

	Calories	Fat g	Saturated Fat g	Carbohydrate g	Fiber g	Sodium mg
Lunch Bucket Elbows'n Tomato Sauce (7 1/2 oz container)	160	2	1	31	3	830
Nile Spice Chili'n Beans (1.5 oz dry pkg)	150	2	0	25	6	670
Pritikin Three Bean Chili (1/2 cup)	90	1	0	19	5	170
Progresso Cheese Ravioli (1 cup)	220	2	1	43	4	930
Weight Watchers Chunky Beef Stew (7.5 oz)	120	2	1	14	4	450

FROZEN ENTRÉES AND DINNERS

Higher-Fat

	Calories	Fat g	Saturated Fat g	Carbohydrate g	Fiber g	Sodium mg
Beef Stroganoff Dinner (10 oz)	320	14	6	25	3	1,078
Chicken Pot Pie (10 oz)	530	32	11	37	5	954
Lasagna (10 oz)	370	13	7	37	3	863
Fried Chicken Dinner (9 oz)	504	29	8	41	4	1,132

Lower-Fat

	Calories	Fat g	Saturated Fat g	Carbohydrate g	Fiber g	Sodium mg
Gorton's Stir Fry Kit Sweet & Sour (10 oz)	270	2	0	54	2	550
Teriyaki (10 oz)	290	2	0	56	1	1,470
Green Giant Garden Gourmet Right for Lunch, Asparagus Pilaf (9.5 oz)	190	4	2	37	3	610
Tortellini Provencale (9.5 oz)	260	6	2	44	3	840
Healthy Choice Classics, Beef Broccoli Beijing (12 oz)	330	3	1	55	5	500
Cacciatore Chicken (12.5 oz)	260	3	1	36	6	510
Chicken Francesca (12.5 oz)	360	5	2	51	5	500
Country Inn Roast Turkey (10 oz)	250	4	1	29	6	530
Ginger Chicken Hunan (12.6 oz)	350	3	1	59	5	430
Mesquite Beef Barbecue (11 oz)	310	4	2	45	6	490
Pasta Italiano (12 oz)	340	4	1	60	6	360
Pasta Shells Marinara (12 oz)	360	3	2	59	5	390
Salisbury Steak (11 oz)	260	6	3	32	5	500
Sesame Chicken Shanghai (12 oz)	310	5	1	42	5	460
Shrimp and Vegetables Maria (12.5 oz)	260	2	1	46	5	540
Turkey Fettuccine alla Crema (12.5 oz)	350	4	2	50	5	370
Dinners, Beef & Peppers Cantonese (11.5 oz)	270	5	3	40	5	560
Beef Enchiladas Rio Grande (13.4 oz)	410	8	3	70	9	480
Beef Tips w/BBQ Sauce (11 oz)	290	6	3	40	5	270
Chicken Broccoli Alfredo (12.1 oz)	370	8	3	53	6	470

Frozen Entrées and Dinners (continued)	Calories	Fat g	Saturated Fat g	Carbohydrate g	Fiber g	Sodium mg
Healthy Choice Dinners (continued)						
Chicken Cantonese (11.3 oz)	210	1	0	31	5	360
Chicken Dijon (11 oz)	280	4	2	41	9	410
Chicken Parmigiana (11.5 oz)	300	2	1	47	6	490
Chicken Picante (11.3 oz)	220	2	2	30	6	330
Chicken Teriyaki (12.25 oz)	270	2	1	42	5	420
Country Herb Chicken (11.5 oz)	270	4	2	40	6	340
Country Turkey and Pasta (12.6 oz)	300	4	2	42	6	450
Lemon Pepper Fish (10.7 oz)	290	5	1	47	7	360
Mesquite Chicken BBQ (10.5 oz)	320	2	1	55	6	290
Shrimp Marinara (10.5 oz)	220	1	0	44	5	220
Smoky Chicken Barbecue (12.75 oz)	380	5	2	57	7	450
Southwestern Glazed Chicken (12.5 oz)	300	3	1	48	6	430
Sweet & Sour Chicken (11.5 oz)	310	5	1	42	5	250
Traditional Beef Tips (11.25 oz)	260	5	2	32	6	390
Traditional Breast of Turkey (10.5 oz)	280	3	1	40	7	460
Traditional Salisbury Steak (11.5 oz)	320	6	3	48	7	470
Yankee Pot Roast (11 oz)	280	5	2	38	5	460
Entrées, Beef Macaroni Casserole (8.5 oz)	200	1	1	34	5	450
Beef Pepper Steak Oriental (9.5 oz)	250	4	2	34	3	470
Beef Tips Francais (9.5 oz)	280	5	2	40	4	520
Cheddar Broccoli Potatoes (10 oz)	310	5	2	53	8	550
Cheese Ravioli Parmigiana (9 oz)	250	4	2	44	6	290
Chicken & Vegetables Marsala (11.5 oz)	220	1	0	32	3	440
Chicken Bangkok (9.5 oz)	270	4	1	35	5	390
Chicken Enchilada Suiza (10 oz)	270	4	2	43	5	440
Chicken Fettuccine Alfredo (8.5 oz)	250	3	1	34	3	370
Chicken Imperial (9 oz)	230	4	1	31	3	470
Country Glazed Chicken (8.5 oz)	200	2	1	30	3	480
Country Roast Turkey w/Mushrooms (8.5 oz)	220	4	1	28	3	440
Fettuccine Alfredo (8 oz)	240	5	2	39	3	430
Fiesta Chicken Fajitas (7 oz)	260	4	1	36	5	410
French Bread Pizza, Cheese (1 pizza = 5.6 oz)	310	4	2	49	6	470
Garden Potato Casserole (9.25 oz)	200	4	2	30	6	520

	Calories	Fat g	Saturated Fat g	Carbohydrate g	Fiber g	Sodium mg
Homestyle Turkey w/Vegetables (9.5 oz)	260	2	1	34	3	490
Honey Mustard Chicken (9.5 oz)	260	2	0	40	4	550
Lasagna Roma (13.5 oz)	390	5	2	60	9	550
Macaroni & Cheese (9 oz)	290	5	2	45	4	580
Mandarin Chicken (10 oz)	280	3	0	44	4	520
Spaghetti Bolognese (10 oz)	260	3	1	43	5	470
Vegetable Pasta Italiano (10 oz)	220	1	0	44	6	340
Zucchini Lasagna (14 oz)	330	2	1	58	11	310
Lean Cuisine Angel Hair Pasta (10 oz)	210	4	1	35	4	420
Baked Chicken w/Whipped Potatoes & Stuffing (8 oz)	240	5	1	31	3	480
Beef Pot Roast w/Whipped Potatoes (9 oz)	210	7	2	21	3	570
Cafe Classics, Bow Tie Pasta & Chicken (9 1/2 oz)	270	6	2	34	5	550
Calypso Chicken (8 1/2 oz)	280	6	2	42	3	590
Cheese Lasagna w/Chicken Scaloppini (10 oz)	290	8	3	34	4	560
Chicken Carbonara (9 oz)	290	8	2	32	4	540
Chicken Mediterranean (10 1/8 oz)	250	4	1	35	4	570
Chicken Piccata (9 oz)	290	6	2	45	1	540
Grilled Chicken Salsa (8 7/8 oz)	240	6	2	32	4	550
Herb Roasted Chicken (8 oz)	210	5	1	25	4	430
Sirloin Beef Peppercorn (8 3/4 oz)	210	7	2	24	4	480
Cheddar Bake w/Pasta (9 oz)	220	6	2	29	3	560
Chicken a l'Orange (9 oz)	260	3	1	40	1	260
Chicken & Vegetables (10 1/2 oz)	240	5	1	30	5	520
Chicken Chow Mein w/Rice (9 oz)	210	5	1	28	2	510
Chicken Enchilada Suiza (9 oz)	290	5	2	48	5	530
Chicken Fettucini (9 oz)	270	6	3	33	2	580
Chicken in Honey Barbecue Sauce (8 3/4 oz)	250	5	1	35	6	560
Chicken in Peanut Sauce (9 oz)	280	6	1	33	3	590
Chicken Italiano (9 oz)	270	6	2	31	3	560
Chicken Marsala & Vegetables (8 1/8 oz)	180	4	1	13	5	470
Chicken Oriental (9 oz)	260	6	1	30	3	530

	Calories	Fat g	Saturated Fat g	Carbohydrate g	Fiber g	Sodium mg
Lean Cuisine *(continued)*						
Chicken Parmesan & Pasta (10⅞)	220	5	2	22	5	530
Classic Cheese Lasagna (11½ oz)	290	6	3	38	5	560
Fettucini Alfredo (9 oz)	270	7	3	38	2	590
Fettucini Primavera (10 oz)	260	8	3	33	4	580
Fiesta Chicken (8½ oz)	240	5	1	31	3	590
Fish Divan (10⅜ oz)	210	6	1	15	3	490
Glazed Chicken w/Vegetable Rice (8½ oz)	240	6	1	24	2	460
Homestyle Turkey (9⅜ oz)	230	6	2	26	3	590
Honey Mustard Chicken w/Vegetable Rice (7½ oz)	250	5	1	32	4	460
Lasagna w/Meat Sauce (10¼ oz)	270	6	3	34	5	560
Lunch Express, Broccoli & Cheddar Cheese Sauce over Baked Potato (10¼ oz)	250	9	4	28	6	490
Cheese Lasagna Casserole (9½ oz)	270	7	3	38	5	590
Chicken Fettucini w/Broccoli (10¼ oz)	290	8	4	38	3	570
Macaroni & Cheese & Broccoli (9¾ oz)	240	6	3	35	5	460
Mandarin Chicken (9¾ oz)	270	6	1	41	2	520
Mexican-Style Rice w/Chicken (9 oz)	270	8	2	39	3	590
Pasta & Chicken Marinara (9⅛ oz)	270	6	2	38	4	540
Pasta & Tuna Casserole (9¾ oz)	280	6	2	39	4	590
Pasta & Turkey Dijon (9⅞ oz)	270	6	2	37	6	570
Teriyaki Stir-Fry (9 oz)	260	5	1	39	4	550
Macaroni & Beef (10 oz)	280	8	2	40	3	550
Marinara Twist (10 oz)	240	3	1	42	4	440
Meatloaf & Whipped Potatoes (9⅜ oz)	250	7	2	25	5	570
Oriental Beef (9 oz)	250	8	3	30	4	480
Rigatoni (9 oz)	180	4	2	25	4	560
Roasted Turkey Breast (9¾ oz)	290	4	1	48	3	530
Spaghetti w/Meat Sauce (11½ oz)	290	6	2	45	4	550
Spaghetti w/Meatballs (9½ oz)	290	7	2	40	4	520
Stuffed Cabbage (9½ oz)	220	7	2	27	5	460
Swedish Meatballs w/Pasta (9½ oz)	290	8	3	32	3	590

	Calories	Fat g	Saturated Fat g	Carbohydrate g	Fiber g	Sodium mg
Sweet & Sour Chicken w/Vegetables & Rice (10 3/8 oz)	260	3	1	43	3	440
Three-Bean Chili w/Rice (9 oz)	210	6	2	32	7	460
Zucchini Lasagna (11 oz)	240	4	2	33	4	470
Stouffer's Entrees, Green Pepper Steak (10 1/2 oz)	330	9	3	45	3	650
Stuffed Pepper (10 oz pkg)	200	8	2	24	1	900
Lunch Express, Chicken Chow Mein w/Rice (10 5/8 oz)	260	4	1	43	3	940
Mexican-Style Chicken & Rice (9 1/8 oz)	280	8	1	40	4	540
Oriental Beef (9 5/8 oz)	260	8	2	34	4	1,220
Swanson Hungry Man, Turkey Dinner (Mostly White Meat) (11.5 oz pkg)	310	7	2	42	4	970
Yankee Pot Roast Dinner (16 oz pkg)	400	11	3	47	10	910
The Budget Gourmet Light & Healthy Dinners, Beef Sirloin Meatballs & Gravy (11 oz)	310	8	3	37	5	540
Beef Sirloin Salisbury Steak w/Red Skinned Potatoes (11 oz)	260	8	3	31	6	430
Chicken in Mesquite Barbecue Sauce (11 oz)	280	6	2	37	6	480
Herbed Chicken Breast w/Fettucini (11 oz)	300	8	3	34	5	620
Honey Mustard Chicken Breast (11 oz)	310	6	2	46	6	540
Roast Chicken Breast w/Herb Gravy (11 oz)	240	7	2	29	4	660
Shrimp Mariner (11 oz)	260	6	2	39	5	540
Sirloin of Beef in Wine Sauce (11 oz)	270	6	2	36	5	460
Special Recipe Sirloin of Beef (11 oz)	310	7	3	42	5	550
Stuffed Turkey Breast (11 oz)	260	6	2	29	7	660
Teriyaki Beef (10.75 oz)	310	6	2	46	7	600
Teriyaki Chicken Breast w/Oriental Style Vegetables (11 oz)	290	6	1	42	3	800
Yankee Pot Roast (10.5 oz)	270	7	3	32	8	430
Light & Healthy Entrees, Beef Sirloin Salisbury Steak (9 oz)	240	5	2	28	2	550
Chicken Oriental (9 oz)	300	6	2	44	6	700
Glazed Turkey (9 oz)	250	4	2	38	2	730
Mandarin Chicken (10 oz)	250	5	1	37	4	850

Frozen Entrées and Dinners (continued)	Calories	Fat g	Saturated Fat g	Carbohydrate g	Fiber g	Sodium mg
The Budget Gourmet						
Light & Healthy Entrees (continued)						
Orange Glazed Chicken Breast (9 oz)	300	2	1	56	1	920
Light & Healthy Special Selections, Chinese Style Vegetables & Chicken (10 oz)	290	9	2	42	4	720
Italian Style Vegetables & Chicken (10 oz)	280	7	2	44	3	660
Penne Pasta w/Chunky Tomato Sauce & Italian Sausage (10 oz)	330	8	3	49	6	530
Rigatoni in Cream Sauce w/Broccoli & Chicken (10.8 oz)	310	6	3	15	5	670
Spaghetti w/Chunky Tomato & Meat Sauce (10 oz)	320	7	3	49	4	470
Original Entrees, Sweet & Sour Chicken (10 oz)	330	5	1	55	4	700
Tyson Chicken Marsala (9 oz meal)	180	4	1	16	5	500
Chicken Mesquite (9 oz meal)	310	8	3	37	6	590
Chicken Piccata (9 oz meal)	190	3	1	18	2	530
Glazed Chicken w/Sauce (9.2 oz meal)	270	6	1	29	5	710
Grilled Chicken (7.8 oz meal)	220	3	1	24	5	540
Grilled Italian Style Chicken (9 oz meal)	210	4	1	16	5	500
Healthy Portion, BBQ Chicken (12.3 oz meal)	370	8	2	47	6	670
Chicken Marinara (13.8 oz meal)	420	5	1	60	6	370
Herb Chicken (13.8 oz meal)	450	3	1	65	5	370
Honey Mustard Chicken (13.8 oz meal)	400	3	1	60	6	510
Italian Style Chicken (13.8 oz meal)	390	4	2	54	5	430
Honey Roasted Chicken (9 oz meal)	220	4	1	37	6	590
Weight Watchers,						
Baked Cheese Ravioli (9 oz)	280	6	2	39	5	560
Barbecue Glazed Chicken (7.4 oz)	190	4	1	22	1	340
Broccoli & Cheese Baked Potato (10 oz)	230	7	2	34	6	510
Cheese Tortellini w/Tomato Sauce (9 oz)	290	4	2	51	3	510
Chicken Cordon Bleu (9 oz)	220	6	2	27	3	500
Chicken Enchiladas Suiza (9 oz)	230	7	2	25	8	530
Garden Lasagna (11 oz)	230	5	1	30	6	460
Grilled Chicken Suiza (8.6 oz)	240	6	2	25	3	590

	Calories	Fat g	Saturated Fat g	Carbohydrate g	Fiber g	Sodium mg
Italian Cheese Lasagna (11 oz)	300	8	3	28	7	560
Lasagna w/Meat Sauce (10.3 oz)	270	6	2	29	8	510
Macaroni & Beef (9.5 oz)	230	5	2	32	2	540
Macaroni & Cheese (9 oz)	260	6	2	43	7	550
Nacho Cheese Enchiladas (8.9 oz)	250	6	3	38	5	520
Roast Glazed Chicken (8.9 oz)	200	5	3	25	4	510
Smart Ones, Angel Hair Pasta (8.55 oz)	150	1	0	27	5	320
Chicken A L'Orange (8 oz)	200	1	0	35	2	320
Chicken Chow Mein (9 oz)	200	1	0	34	6	480
Chicken Francais (8.5 oz)	150	1	0	21	4	390
Chicken Marsala (8 oz)	110	1	0	15	1	340
Chicken Mirabella (9.2 oz)	160	1	0	25	5	480
Fiesta Chicken (8 oz)	200	1	1	34	3	460
Grilled Glazed Chicken (8 oz)	130	1	0	20	3	460
Honey Mustard Chicken (7.5 oz)	140	1	1	20	3	340
Lasagna Florentine (10 oz)	190	1	1	35	5	420
Lemon Herb Chicken Piccata (7.5 oz)	170	1	0	28	3	520
Pasta Portafino (9.5 oz)	150	1	0	29	4	270
Ravioli Florentine (8.5 oz)	170	1	0	29	6	530
Roast Turkey Medallions (8.5 oz)	190	1	0	34	4	490
Shrimp Marinara (8 oz)	150	1	0	28	3	400
Spaghetti w/Meat Sauce (10 oz)	240	7	2	28	8	490
Spring Vegetables w/Teriyaki Chicken (9 oz)	150	2	1	17	4	440
Tex-Mex Chicken (8.3 oz)	260	4	2	35	1	430
Tuna Noodle Casserole (9.5 oz)	240	7	3	30	5	580

MEAT, POULTRY, FISH, AND MEAT SUBSTITUTES

It is important to choose cuts of meat and poultry that are low in fat to help decrease fat, saturated fat, and cholesterol in your diet (see page 21 for information on cholesterol in food). Most fish (finfish and shellfish) are low in fat and saturated fat. According to food labeling guidelines for meat and poultry, these products may be labeled as "lean" or "extra lean" if they meet the cutoff points shown below. All the "meats" listed in this section can be classified as lean and many of them as extra lean.

Meat substitutes, many of which are made of soybean, are good sources of protein. The cutoff points for lean meat have been used to evaluate meat substitutes, which contain some fat; however, these products are much lower in saturated fat and usually contain no cholesterol.

Since fresh-cut meat usually does not carry a brand name, the values for many of the foods in this section are based on information from USDA handbooks and the Nutrition Data System, a software program.

CUTOFF POINTS FOR MEAT, POULTRY, FISH, AND MEAT SUBSTITUTES

	Fat g	Saturated Fat g
Lean cooked meat, poultry, and fish (3 oz)	9	3
Lean cooked meat, poultry, and fish (1 oz)	3	1
Extra-lean cooked meat, poultry, and fish (3 oz)	4	2
Extra-lean cooked meat, poultry, and fish (1 oz)	1	<1
Luncheon meats (2 oz)	6	2
Meat substitutes (3 oz)	9	3

	Calories	Fat g	Saturated Fat g	Carbohydrate g	Fiber g	Sodium mg
BEEF, CANNED AND SHELF-STABLE BEEF						
Higher-Fat						
Corned Beef (3 oz)	213	13	5	0	0	856
Lower-Fat						
Armour Star Sliced Dried Beef (7 slices)	60	2	1	2	0	1,370
Hormel Sliced Dried Beef (10 slices)	50	2	1	1	0	1,240
Tombstone Beef Jerky (1 stick)	35	0	0	<1	0	310
BEEF, FRESH						
Higher-Fat						
Brisket, untrimmed (3 oz)	286	22	9	0	0	53
Hamburger patty, grilled, prep w/salt (3 oz)	260	19	8	0	0	455
Prime Rib, untrimmed (3 oz)	310	25	10	0	0	54
Spare Ribs, untrimmed (3 oz)	401	36	15	0	0	43
Lower-Fat (prep w/o salt unless otherwise indicated)						
Bottom Round, *Choice,* lean only, braised (3 oz)	181	7	2	0	0	43
Roasted (3 oz)	164	7	2	0	0	56
Bottom Round, *Select,* lean only, braised (3 oz)	163	5	2	0	0	43
Roasted (3 oz)	146	5	2	0	0	56
Brisket, Flat Half, lean only, braised (3 oz)	162	5	2	0	0	54
Eye of Round, *Choice,* lean only, roasted (3 oz)	149	5	2	0	0	53
Select, roasted (3 oz)	132	3	1	0	0	53
Ground Beef, 4% fat, broiled (3 oz)	122	3	1	0	0	42
7% fat, broiled (3 oz)	165	6	2	0	0	55
10% fat, broiled (3 oz)	176	8	3	0	0	58
Prep w/salt (3 oz)	176	8	3	0	0	476
Rib, Small End, *Select,* lean only, broiled (3 oz)	168	7	3	0	0	59
Tenderloin, *Select,* lean only, broiled (3 oz)	170	8	3	0	0	54
Tip Round, *Choice,* lean only, roasted (3 oz)	153	5	2	0	0	55
Select, roasted (3 oz)	145	5	2	0	0	55
Top Loin, *Choice,* lean only, broiled (3 oz)	177	8	3	0	0	58
Select, broiled (3 oz)	157	6	2	0	0	58

	Calories	Fat g	Saturated Fat g	Carbohydrate g	Fiber g	Sodium mg
Beef, Fresh (continued)						
Top Round, *Choice,* lean only, braised (3 oz)	176	5	2	0	0	38
Select, braised (3 oz)	162	3	1	0	0	38
Top Sirloin, *Choice,* lean only, broiled (3 oz)	170	7	3	0	0	56
Select, broiled (3 oz)	153	5	2	0	0	56
Tripe, raw (3 oz)	84	3	2	0	0	39

BEEF, PRESEASONED

	Calories	Fat g	Saturated Fat g	Carbohydrate g	Fiber g	Sodium mg
Menu Maker by Rymer Teriyaki Seasoned Boneless Beef Rib Eye Steaks (7 oz serving)	240	10	4	4	0	560

CHICKEN, CANNED

	Calories	Fat g	Saturated Fat g	Carbohydrate g	Fiber g	Sodium mg
Hormel Chunk Breast of Chicken (2 oz)	60	2	1	0	0	100
No Salt (2 oz)	60	2	1	0	0	20
Chunk Chicken (2 oz)	70	3	1	0	0	200
Swanson Chunk Chicken (¼ cup)	90	3	1	2	0	200
Premium Chunk Chicken in Water (¼ cup)	90	3	1	1	0	240
Premium Chunk White Chicken in Water (¼ cup)	80	1	1	1	0	240

CHICKEN, FRESH OR FROZEN

Higher-Fat

	Calories	Fat g	Saturated Fat g	Carbohydrate g	Fiber g	Sodium mg
Chicken Patty, commercially pre-breaded (3 oz)	276	16	4	13	1	574
Chicken, Breast, breaded & fried (3 oz)	388	22	6	19	1	827
Drumstick, breaded & fried (1 drumstick = 3.5 oz)	329	20	6	15	1	669
Thigh, breaded & fried (1 thigh = 3 oz)	412	25	7	19	1	837

Lower-Fat

Most Brands (prep w/o salt)

	Calories	Fat g	Saturated Fat g	Carbohydrate g	Fiber g	Sodium mg
Chicken Breast, meat & skin, roasted (3 oz)	167	7	2	0	0	60
Stewed (3 oz)	156	6	2	0	0	53
Chicken Breast, w/o skin, roasted (3 oz)	140	3	1	0	0	63
Stewed (3 oz)	128	3	1	0	0	54
Chicken Thigh, w/o skin, stewed (1 thigh = 2 oz)	110	6	2	0	0	42
Chicken Wing, w/o skin, roasted (1 wing = 3/4 oz)	43	2	1	0	0	19
Stewed (1 wing = 1 oz)	50	2	1	0	0	21

	Calories	Fat g	Saturated Fat g	Carbohydrate g	Fiber g	Sodium mg
Chicken, Fresh or Frozen *(continued)*						
Dark Meat, w/o skin, roasted (3 oz)	174	8	2	0	0	79
Stewed (3 oz)	163	8	2	0	0	63
Drumstick, w/o skin, roasted (1 drumstick = 1.6 oz)	76	3	1	0	0	42
Stewed (1 drumstick = 1.6 oz)	78	3	1	0	0	37
Light Meat, w/o skin, roasted (3 oz)	147	4	1	0	0	65
Stewed (3 oz)	135	3	1	0	0	55
Light Meat, w/skin, stewed (3 oz)	171	8	2	0	0	54
Tyson Boneless Skinless Cooked Diced Chicken Meat (3 oz)	130	3	1	0	0	40
CHICKEN, PRESEASONED						
Chicken By George						
Lemon Herb Chicken (1 breast)	120	3	1	3	0	800
Lemon Oregano Chicken (1 breast)	130	4	1	3	0	600
Mesquite Barbecue Flavored Chicken (1 breast)	130	3	1	5	0	700
Menu Maker by Rymer Boneless Skinless Chicken Breasts, Butter Seasoned (3.5 oz)	110	2	1	2	0	430
Lemon Herb (3.5 oz)	110	1	0	2	0	290
Southern Style Breaded (3.5 oz)	130	1	0	13	0	1,070
Teriyaki Seasoned (3.5 oz)	110	1	0	3	0	400
FISH, CANNED						
Most Brands, Clams, drained solids (3 oz)	126	2	0	4	0	95
Crab, Blue (3 oz)	84	1	0	0	0	283
Mackerel, drained solids (3 oz)	132	5	2	0	0	322
Oyster, Eastern (3 oz)	58	2	1	3	0	95
Salmon, Chum, drained solids w/bone (3 oz)	120	5	1	0	0	414
Pink, solids w/bone & liquid (3 oz)	118	5	1	0	0	471
Sockeye, drained, solids w/bone (3 oz)	130	6	1	0	0	458
Shrimp, drained solids (3 oz)	102	2	0	0	0	143
Tuna, light in oil, drained solids (3 oz)	169	7	1	0	0	301
Light in water, drained solids (3 oz)	99	1	0	0	0	287
White in oil, drained solids (3 oz)	158	7	1	0	0	336
White in water, drained solids (3 oz)	108	3	1	0	0	320

	Calories	Fat g	Saturated Fat g	Carbohydrate g	Fiber g	Sodium mg
Crown-Prince Abalone Type Shellfish, Tidbits (¼ can = 1.8 oz)	45	0	0	0	0	270
Whole (¼ can = 1.7 oz)	50	0	0	0	0	250
Clams, Minced (½ can = 2.2 oz)	45	0	0	<1	0	310
Pacific (8 clams)	60	1	1	1	0	330
Whole Baby (¼ cup)	50	2	1	2	0	260
Crab Meat (½ can = 2.2 oz)	50	0	0	1	0	300
Fancy White (½ can = 2.2 oz)	50	0	0	0	0	340
Mackerel in water (¼ cup)	80	3	1	0	0	200
Sardines in Tomato Sauce (4.25 oz can)	90	2	1	3	1	480
Whole Oysters in Water (3 pieces)	70	3	2	4	0	150
Gorton's Cod Cakes (4 oz)	100	1	0	16	0	640
Ocean Chopped & Minced Clams, Undrained (¼ cup)	20	0	0	1	0	360
Ocean-Prince Sardines in Spring Water (4.25 oz can)	100	2	1	0	0	150
Progresso Minced Clams (¼ cup)	25	0	0	2	0	250

FISH, FRESH OR FROZEN

Higher-Fat

Fried Fish, breaded (3 oz)	310	15	4	19	1	857

Lower-Fat

Most Brands (prep w/o salt unless otherwise indicated)

Bass, Freshwater, cooked, dry heat (3 oz)	124	4	1	0	0	76
Bass, Striped, cooked, dry heat (3 oz)	105	3	1	0	0	75
Catfish, cooked, dry heat (3 oz)	129	7	2	0	0	68
Clams, cooked, moist heat (3 oz)	126	2	0	4	0	95
Cod, Atlantic, cooked, dry heat (3 oz)	89	1	0	0	0	66
Pacific, cooked, dry heat (3 oz)	70	1	0	0	0	60
Crab, Alaska King, cooked, moist heat (3 oz)	82	1	0	0	0	911
Blue, cooked, moist heat (3 oz)	87	2	0	0	0	237
Imitation, made from surimi (3 oz)	87	1	0	9	0	715
Crayfish, cooked, moist heat (3 oz)	74	1	0	0	0	83
Flounder, cooked, dry heat (3 oz)	99	1	0	0	0	89
Grouper, cooked, dry heat (3 oz)	100	1	0	0	0	45
Haddock, cooked, dry heat (3 oz)	95	1	0	0	0	74

Fish, Fresh or Frozen (continued)	Calories	Fat g	Saturated Fat g	Carbohydrate g	Fiber g	Sodium mg
Halibut, cooked, dry heat (3 oz)	119	3	0	0	0	59
Lobster, Northern, cooked, moist heat (3 oz)	83	1	0	1	0	323
Mussels, cooked, moist heat (3 oz)	147	4	1	6	0	313
Orange Roughy, cooked, dry heat (3 oz)	75	1	0	0	0	69
Oysters, cooked, dry heat (3 oz)	67	2	1	6	0	138
Raw (3 oz)	50	1	0	5	0	151
Perch, Fresh Water, cooked, dry heat (3 oz)	99	1	0	0	0	67
Ocean, cooked, dry heat (3 oz)	103	2	0	0	0	82
Pike, Northern, cooked, dry heat (3 oz)	96	1	0	0	0	42
Pollack, Walleye, cooked, dry heat (3 oz)	96	1	0	0	0	98
Redfish (see Ocean Perch)						
Rockfish, cooked, dry heat (3 oz)	103	2	0	0	0	65
Salmon, Atlantic, cooked, dry heat (3 oz)	155	7	1	0	0	48
Chinook, smoked (3 oz)	99	4	1	0	0	666
Chum, cooked, dry heat (3 oz)	131	4	1	0	0	54
Coho, cooked, moist heat (3 oz)	157	6	1	0	0	45
Pink, cooked, dry heat (3 oz)	127	4	1	0	0	73
Scallops, cooked in moist heat (3 oz)	98	1	0	3	0	225
Imitation, made from surimi (3 oz)	84	0	0	9	0	676
Scrod (see Cod, Atlantic)						
Shrimp, cooked, moist heat (3 oz)	84	1	0	0	0	190
Imitation, made from Surimi (3 oz)	86	1	0	8	0	599
Snapper, cooked, dry heat (3 oz)	109	2	0	0	0	48
Sole (see Flounder)						
Swordfish, cooked, dry heat (3 oz)	132	4	1	0	0	98
Trout, Rainbow, cooked, dry heat (3 oz)	128	5	1	0	0	48
Tuna, Bluefin, fresh, cooked, dry heat (3 oz)	157	5	1	0	0	43
Yellowfin, fresh, cooked, dry heat (3 oz)	118	1	0	0	0	40
Whitefish, smoked (3 oz)	92	1	0	0	0	866
Whiting, cooked, dry heat (3 oz)	98	1	0	0	0	112
Gorton's Seafood Stuffed Sole (1 portion = 5.4 oz)	150	2	1	17	0	500
Select Sole Country Herb (2 portions = 5.6 oz)	110	3	1	0	0	320
Mrs. Paul's Beach Haven Breaded Fish Sticks (4 sticks)	170	3	2	20	2	350
Fried Scallops (12 scallops)	210	8	2	22	1	420

	Calories	Fat g	Saturated Fat g	Carbohydrate g	Fiber g	Sodium mg
Mrs. Paul's *(continued)*						
Healthy Treasures,						
Breaded Fish Fillets (3 oz fillet)	130	3	1	16	1	220
Breaded Fish Fillets (4 oz fillet)	170	3	2	21	2	290
Breaded Fish Sticks (3 oz)	170	3	2	20	2	350
Kitchen Fillets in Sauce (4 oz fillet)	120	5	2	4	1	450
Premium Fillets, Cod (4.5 oz fillet)	250	11	3	24	2	510
Flounder (4.5 oz fillet)	250	13	4	22	2	510
Haddock (4.5 oz fillet)	230	11	3	18	2	450
Sole (4.5 oz fillet)	250	13	4	22	2	510
Van de Kamp's Breaded Whole Shrimp (7 shrimp)	240	10	2	26	2	520
Crisp & Healthy Breaded Fish,						
Fillets (2 fillets = 3.5 oz)	150	3	1	20	0	380
Sticks (6 sticks = 4 oz)	180	3	1	26	0	440
Lightly Breaded Fillets, Cod (4 oz fillet)	220	10	2	19	0	410
Flounder (4 oz fillet)	230	11	2	19	0	400
Haddock (4 oz fillet)	220	10	2	19	0	410
Sole (4 oz fillet)	220	11	2	17	0	410
Natural Fillets, Flounder (4 oz fillet)	110	2	0	0	0	105
Sole (4 oz fillet)	110	2	0	0	0	125
GAME (prep w/o salt)						
Beefalo, cooked, roasted (3 oz)	160	5	2	0	0	70
Elk, cooked, roasted (3 oz)	124	2	1	0	0	52
Goat, cooked, roasted (3 oz)	122	3	1	0	0	73
Horse, cooked, roasted (3 oz)	149	5	2	0	0	47
Moose, cooked, roasted (3 oz)	114	1	0	0	0	58
Rabbit, Domesticated, roasted (3 oz)	167	7	2	0	0	40
Squirrel, cooked, roasted (3 oz)	116	3	0	0	0	80
Waterbuffalo, cooked, roasted (3 oz)	111	2	1	0	0	48
LAMB, FRESH						
Higher-Fat						
Ground Lamb (3 oz)	235	17	7	0	0	56
Lower-Fat (prep w/o salt)						
Cubes for Stew or Kabob (Leg & Shoulder), lean only, broiled (3 oz)	158	6	2	0	0	65

	Calories	Fat g	Saturated Fat g	Carbohydrate g	Fiber g	Sodium mg
Leg, Shank Half, *Choice,* lean only, roasted (3 oz)	153	6	2	0	0	56
Loin Chops, lean only, broiled (3 oz)	183	8	3	0	0	71
Loin, *Choice,* lean only, broiled (3 oz)	183	8	3	0	0	71
Roasted (3 oz)	171	8	3	0	0	56
Shoulder, Arm, *Choice,* lean only, broiled (3 oz)	170	8	3	0	0	70
Roasted (3 oz)	163	8	3	0	0	57

LUNCHEON MEAT

Higher-Fat

	Calories	Fat g	Saturated Fat g	Carbohydrate g	Fiber g	Sodium mg
Bologna, beef & pork (2 oz)	179	16	6	2	0	578
Hot Dog (2 oz jumbo)	182	17	6	1	0	638
Liverwurst (2 oz)	185	16	6	1	0	488
Pastrami, beef (2 oz)	198	17	6	2	0	696
Pepperoni (1 oz)	141	12	5	1	0	579
Salami, Genoa (2 oz)	237	20	7	1	0	1,055

Lower-Fat

	Calories	Fat g	Saturated Fat g	Carbohydrate g	Fiber g	Sodium mg
Most Brands, Chicken Roll (2 oz)	84	4	1	1	0	332
Dried Beef (1 oz)	47	1	1	1	0	984
Turkey Ham (2 oz)	73	3	1	0	0	565
Turkey Pastrami (2 oz)	80	4	1	1	0	593
Boar's Head Brand Baby Pastrami Seasoned Turkey Breast (3 oz)	90	1	0	0	0	590
Black Forest Ham (2 oz)	60	1	0	2	0	580
Branded or Smoked Deluxe Ham (2 oz)	60	1	0	2	0	560
Cajun Roast Beef (2 oz)	80	3	2	0	0	200
Chicken Breast (2 oz)	50	1	0	<1	0	420
Corned Beef Round (2 oz)	80	3	1	0	0	510
Corned Beef, First Cut Brisket (2 oz)	80	3	2	0	0	460
Cracked Pepper Mill Smoked Turkey Breast (2 oz)	60	1	0	<1	0	460
Deluxe Top Round, Low Sodium (2 oz)	90	3	2	0	0	80
Golden Turkey Breast, skin on (2 oz)	60	2	1	0	0	340
Skinless, (2 oz)	60	1	0	<1	0	350
Hickory Smoked Turkey Breast (2 oz)	70	2	1	<1	0	340
Maple Glazed Honey Coat Ham (2 oz)	60	1	0	3	0	570

	Calories	Fat g	Saturated Fat g	Carbohydrate g	Fiber g	Sodium mg
Boar's Head Brand *(continued)*						
Maple Glazed Honey Coat Turkey Breast (2 oz)	70	1	0	2	0	440
Oven Roasted Top Round, No Salt Added (2 oz)	90	3	2	0	0	40
Ovengold Roast Breast of Turkey (2 oz)	60	1	0	0	0	350
Pastrami Round (2 oz)	70	3	1	<1	0	530
Pastrami Seasoned Turkey Breast (2 oz)	60	1	0	0	0	390
Pastrami, First Cut Brisket (2 oz)	90	4	2	2	0	620
Premium Turkey Breast, 25% Lower Sodium, skin on (2 oz)	60	2	1	<1	0	310
Skinless (2 oz)	60	1	0	<1	0	340
Seasoned Fresh Roasted Ham (2 oz)	80	3	2	1	0	310
Sweet Slice Boneless Smoked Ham (3 oz)	110	5	2	<1	0	780
Virginia Brand Ham (2 oz)	60	1	0	3	0	560
Butterball Skinless Turkey Breast, Honey Roasted & Smoked (2 oz)	60	0	0	2	0	490
Oven Roasted or Smoked (2 oz)	50	0	0	1	0	430-440
Oven Roasted, Low Sodium (2 oz)	50	0	0	1	0	310
Carl Buddig Beef (1.9 oz = 10 slices)	75	4	2	<1	0	790
Chicken (2½ oz pkg)	110	7	2	<1	0	680
Corned Beef (2½ oz pkg)	100	5	2	<1	0	950
Ham (2½ oz pkg)	120	7	3	<1	0	980
Honey Ham (2½ oz pkg)	120	7	3	3	0	760
Honey Roasted Turkey (2½ oz pkg)	110	6	2	3	0	780
Pastrami (2½ oz pkg)	100	5	2	<1	0	750
Turkey (2½ oz pkg)	110	7	3	<1	0	710
Continental Lean & Low 95% Fat Free Turkey Ham (1.2 oz slice)	30	1	0	1	0	380
96% Fat Free Cooked Ham (1.2 oz slice)	30	1	0	0	0	380
97% Fat Free, Ham (1 oz slice)	30	1	0	0	0	380
Turkey Breast (1.2 oz slice)	25	1	0	1	0	380
98% Fat Free Ham (1 oz slice)	25	1	0	0	0	380
Hafnia Lean & Low 95% Fat Free, Chopped Ham w/Natural Juices (1 oz slice)	35	1	0	1	0	380
Turkey Ham (1.2 oz slice)	30	1	0	1	0	380
97% Fat Free, Danish Ham (2 oz)	60	2	1	0	0	760

	Calories	Fat g	Saturated Fat g	Carbohydrate g	Fiber g	Sodium mg
Ham (1 oz slice)	30	1	0	0	0	380
Ham w/Natural Juices (1.2 oz slices)	30	1	0	0	0	380
98% Fat Free, Baked Cooked Ham w/Natural Juices (1 oz slice)	30	1	0	1	0	380
Danish Ham w/Natural Juices (2 oz)	50	1	0	0	0	760
Sliced (1 oz)	25	1	0	0	0	380
Thin Sliced (1.7 oz = 2 slices)	50	1	0	0	0	760
Ham or Ham w/Natural Juices (1 oz slice)	25	1	0	0	0	380
Ham w/Natural Juices, Lower Sodium (2 oz)	50	1	0	0	0	480
Sliced (1 oz)	25	1	0	1	0	240
Honey Ham w/Natural Juices (2 oz)	50	1	0	2	0	760
Turkey Breast (1 oz slice)	25	1	0	0	0	380
Healthy Choice 97% Fat Free Ham, Cooked (2 oz)	60	2	1	1	0	460
Honey (2 oz)	60	2	1	2	0	580
Smoked (2 oz)	60	2	1	1	0	390
Virginia Brand (2 oz)	60	2	1	1	0	510
Browned 99% Fat Free Turkey Breast (2 oz)	50	1	0	0	0	420
Corned Beef 97% Fat Free (2 oz)	60	2	1	0	0	460
Fat Free Turkey Breast, Honey Roasted & Smoked (2 oz)	60	0	0	2	0	410
Skinless (2 oz)	45	0	0	1	0	380
Smoked (2 oz)	50	0	0	2	0	410
Medium Roast Beef 97% Fat Free (2 oz)	60	2	1	1	0	450
Pastrami 97% Fat Free (2 oz)	60	2	1	1	0	500
Skinless Fat Free Chicken Breast (2 oz)	45	0	0	0	0	460
Structured Roast Beef 98% Fat Free (2 oz)	50	1	1	0	0	480
Louis Rich Carving Board Meats, Baked Ham w/Natural Juices (1.6 oz = 2 slices)	45	1	0	1	0	510
Honey Ham w/Natural Juices, Thin Carved (2.1 oz = 6 slices)	70	2	1	2	0	760
Honey Ham w/Natural Juices, Traditional Carved (1.6 oz = 2 slices)	50	2	1	1	0	530
Oven Roasted Turkey Breast, Thin Carved (2.1 oz = 6 slices)	60	1	0	0	0	740

	Calories	Fat g	Saturated Fat g	Carbohydrate g	Fiber g	Sodium mg
Louis Rich Carving Board Meats *(continued)*						
Oven Roasted Turkey Breast, Traditional Carved (1.6 oz = 2 slices)	40	1	0	0	0	560
Smoked Ham Cooked w/Natural Juices (1.6 oz=2 slices)	50	2	1	0	0	560
Smoked Turkey Breast (1.6 oz = 2 slices)	40	1	0	0	0	560
Chopped Turkey Ham, 10% water added (1 oz slice)	40	3	1	0	0	290
Deli-Thin, Fat Free Oven Roasted Turkey Breast (1.8 oz = 4 slices)	40	0	0	2	0	610
Oven Roasted Chicken Breast (1.8 oz = 4 slices)	60	2	1	1	0	620
Oven Roasted Turkey Breast (1.8 oz = 4 slices)	50	1	0	2	0	580
Smoked Turkey Breast (1.8 oz = 4 slices)	50	1	0	1	0	490
Turkey Ham, 10% water added (1.8 oz = 4 slices)	60	2	1	0	0	580
Deluxe Oven Roasted Chicken Breast (1 oz slice)	30	1	0	1	0	330
Fat Free Hickory Smoked or Oven Roasted Turkey Breast (1 oz slice)	25	0	0	1	0	300-310
Hickory Smoked Chicken Breast (1 oz slice)	30	1	0	1	0	360
Honey Cured Turkey Ham, 10% water added (2.2 oz = 3 slices)	15	2	1	2	0	660
Honey Roasted Turkey Breast (1 oz slice)	30	1	0	1	0	320
Oven Roasted Turkey Breast (1 oz slice)	30	1	0	1	0	310
Oven Roasted White Chicken (1 oz slice)	40	3	1	1	0	350
Sausage, Ground Turkey (2.5 oz)	110	6	3	3	0	580
Turkey & Cheddar Smoked (2 oz)	90	5	2	2	0	550
Turkey Links (2 oz = 2 links)	90	6	2	0	0	470
Turkey Polska Kielbasa (2 oz)	80	5	2	1	0	510
Turkey Smoked (2 oz)	90	5	2	2	0	510
Smoked Turkey Breast (1 oz slice)	25	1	0	0	0	260
Smoked White Turkey (1 oz slice)	30	1	0	0	0	290
Turkey Cotto Salami (1 oz slice)	40	3	1	0	0	290
Turkey Ham (2 oz)	60	2	1	1	0	640

	Calories	Fat g	Saturated Fat g	Carbohydrate g	Fiber g	Sodium mg
Turkey Ham, 10% water added (1 oz round slice)	35	1	1	0	0	300
Turkey Ham, 10% water added (2.2 oz = 3 square slices)	70	3	1	1	0	710
Turkey Ham, 15% water added (2 oz)	70	3	1	1	0	640
Turkey Pastrami (1.6 oz = 2 square slices)	45	2	0	0	0	520
Turkey Pastrami (2 oz)	70	2	1	1	0	590
Turkey Salami (1 oz slice)	45	3	1	0	0	290
Oscar Mayer Baked Ham (2.2 oz = 3 slices)	60	1	1	2	0	720
Boiled Ham (2.2 oz = 3 slices)	60	3	1	0	0	820
Canadian Style Bacon (1.6 oz = 2 slices)	50	2	1	0	0	600
Deli-Thin, Boiled Ham (1.8 oz = 4 slices)	50	2	1	0	0	680
Honey Glazed Chicken Breast (1.8 oz = 4 slices)	60	1	0	2	0	740
Honey Ham (1.8 oz = 4 slices)	60	2	1	2	0	630
Roast Beef (1.8 oz = 4 slices)	60	2	1	1	0	530
Roast Turkey (1.8 oz = 4 slices)	50	1	0	2	0	580
Smoked Cooked Ham (1.8 oz = 4 slices)	50	2	1	0	0	620
Smoked Honey Roasted Turkey (1.8 oz = 4 slices)	60	1	0	2	0	520
Ham, Lower Sodium (2.2 oz = 3 slices)	70	3	1	2	0	520
Healthy Favorites, Baked Ham (1.8 oz = 4 slices)	50	1	0	1	0	600
Bologna (1.6 oz = 2 slices)	45	1	0	2	0	510
Honey Ham (1.8 oz = 4 slices)	50	2	1	2	0	630
Hot Dogs made w/Turkey & Beef (2 oz = 1 link)	60	2	1	2	0	570
Oven Roasted Chicken Breast (1.8 oz = 4 slices)	40	0	0	1	0	620
Oven Roasted Turkey Breast (1.8 oz = 4 slices)	40	0	0	2	0	610
Smoked Cooked Ham (1.8 oz = 4 slices)	50	2	1	0	0	620
Smoked Turkey Breast (1.8 oz = 4 slices)	40	0	0	2	0	550
Honey Ham (2.2 oz=3 slices)	70	3	1	2	0	760
Honey Loaf (1 oz slice)	35	1	0	1	0	380
New England Brand Sausage (1.6 oz = 2 slices)	60	3	1	1	0	570
Smoked Cooked Ham (2.2 oz = 3 slices)	60	3	1	0	0	750

	Calories	Fat g	Saturated Fat g	Carbohydrate g	Fiber g	Sodium mg
MEAT SUBSTITUTES						
Green Giant Breakfast Patties (2 patties)	100	4	1	5	3	280
Breakfast Links (3 links)	110	5	1	5	2	340
Harvest Burgers, Italian Style (1 burger)	140	5	2	8	5	370
Original Flavor (1 burger)	140	4	2	8	5	380
Southwestern Style (1 burger)	140	4	2	9	5	370
Lifestream Natural Foods Vegi-Patties (1 patty)	140	3	0	16	4	440
PORK, CANNED						
Most Brands, Boneless Extra Lean Ham, roasted (3 oz)	116	4	1	0	0	966
Hormel Chunk Ham (2 oz)	90	6	2	0	0	600
Pickled Pigs Feet (2 oz)	80	6	2	0	0	530
PORK, FRESH OR PROCESSED						
Higher-Fat						
Bacon, regular cut, cooked (.5 oz = about 2 slices)	86	7	3	0	0	239
Bone-in Ham, untrimmed, meat only (3 oz)	238	18	7	0	0	912
Sausage (4 links, each 4" long x ½ diam" = 2 oz)	209	18	6	1	0	732
Ribs, Country-Style, untrimmed, meat only (3 oz)	275	21	8	0	0	26
Lower-Fat						
Most Brands (prep w/o salt unless otherwise indicated)						
Canadian Bacon, grilled (3 oz)	157	7	2	1	0	1,314
Loin Chops, boneless, lean only, broiled (3 oz)	173	7	2	0	0	55
Loin Roasts, boneless, lean only, roasted (3 oz)	165	6	2	0	0	38
Sirloin Chops, boneless, lean & fat, broiled (3 oz)	177	7	3	0	0	47
Lean only, broiled (3 oz)	164	6	2	0	0	48
Alpine Lace Boneless Cooked Ham, Less Sodium (2 oz)	60	2	1	1	0	380
Boar's Head Brand Canadian Style Bacon (2 oz)	70	3	1	1	0	560

	Calories	Fat g	Saturated Fat g	Carbohydrate g	Fiber g	Sodium mg
Baby Ham, Black Forest Brand (3 oz)	90	2	0	3	0	900
Maple Glazed Honey Coat (3 oz)	90	2	0	4	0	870
Virginia Smoked Gourmet (3 oz)	90	1	0	4	0	900
Hafnia Lean & Low Dinner Ham Steak (1 slice)	100	2	1	0	0	1,520
Louis Rich Baked Cooked Ham Dinner Slices (1 slice)	80	2	1	1	0	1,150
Oscar Mayer Dinner Ham, Slice (3 oz)	90	3	1	0	0	1,030
Steak (1 steak)	60	2	1	0	0	750
TURKEY, CANNED						
Hormel Chunk, Turkey (2 oz)	70	3	1	0	0	340
Turkey Ham (2 oz)	70	4	2	0	0	600
White Turkey (2 oz)	60	1	1	0	0	320
Swanson Premium Chunk, Turkey in Water (¼ cup)	100	4	1	2	0	230
White Turkey in Water (¼ cup)	90	2	1	4	1	220
TURKEY, FRESH, FROZEN, OR PROCESSED						
Higher-Fat						
Turkey Bacon (½ oz or about 2 slices)	61	5	1	0	0	390
Lower-Fat						
Most Brands (prep w/o salt)						
Dark Meat, w/o skin, roasted (3 oz)	159	6	2	0	0	67
Light Meat, meat only, roasted (3 oz)	133	3	1	0	0	54
Young Tom, dark meat w/o skin, roasted (3 oz)	158	6	2	0	0	70
Light meat, meat only, roasted (3 oz)	129	3	1	0	0	58
Light meat w/skin, roasted (3 oz)	163	7	2	0	0	57
Louis Rich Breast of Turkey Dinner Slices, Hickory Smoked (2.8 oz = 1 slice)	80	1	0	2	0	1,060
Honey Roasted (2.8 oz = 1 slice)	80	1	1	3	0	940
Oven Roasted (2.8 oz slice)	70	1	0	1	0	910
Ground Turkey (3 oz)	140	9	3	0	0	105
Oven Roasted Turkey Breast (2 oz)	60	2	1	2	0	640
Skinless Breast of Turkey, Barbecued (2 oz)	60	1	0	2	0	680
Hickory Smoked (2 oz)	60	1	0	1	0	760

Turkey, Fresh, Frozen, or Processed (continued)	Calories	Fat g	Saturated Fat g	Carbohydrate g	Fiber g	Sodium mg
Louis Rich Skinless Breast of Turkey (continued)						
Honey Roasted (2 oz)	60	1	0	2	0	690
Oven Roasted (2 oz)	50	1	0	1	0	650

PASTA, RICE, AND OTHER GRAIN PRODUCTS

Pasta, rice, and other grain products provide very little or no fat and saturated fat when they are cooked without added ingredients. However, when pasta, rice, or grain dishes have oil, butter, margarine, bacon, bacon fat, cheese, and/or meat fat added to them, the levels of fat and saturated fat are increased.

Servings of the foods included in this section of the Guide do not exceed the cutoff points of 3 grams of fat and 1 gram of saturated fat. Some packaged products not listed may qualify for the Guide when ingredients containing less fat are substituted for ingredients that are higher in fat.

Pasta and Pasta Mixes	Calories	Fat g	Saturated Fat g	Carbohydrate g	Fiber g	Sodium mg
PASTA AND PASTA MIXES						
Higher-Fat						
Crisp Chow Mein Noodles (1/2 cup)	121	7	1	13	1	101
Lower-Fat						
Aunt Patsy's Pantry Rabbit Pasta (2 oz dry)	210	1	0	42	2	5
Buckeye Beans and Herbs Pasta, Baseball, Football or Sports Ball (2 oz dry)	210	1	0	43	2	5
All-American, Bicycle, California Redwood, Evergreen, Funny Bunny, Hearts for Two, Hearty, Playful Dolphin, Starry Starry, Sunsational, Tree-Mendous Christmas (2 oz dry)	210	1	0	42	2	5

	Calories	Fat g	Saturated Fat g	Carbohydrate g	Fiber g	Sodium mg
Creamette Acini de Pepe, Capellini, Ditalini, Fettuccini, Large Shells, Linguine, Macaroni Elbows, Medium Shells, Mostaccioli, Nuggets, Raditore, Rigatoni, Rotini, Spaghetti, Vermicelli or Ziti (2 oz dry)	210	1	0	42	2	0
Jumbo Stuffing Shells (7 pieces)	210	1	0	36	1	0
Manicotti (3 pieces)	180	1	0	36	1	0
Spinach Fettuccini (2 oz dry)	210	1	0	42	1	25
Tri-Colored Rotini or Tri-colored Shells (2 oz dry)	210	1	0	42	1	20
Tri-Colored Wheels (2 oz dry)	210	1	0	42	2	20
Delmonico Capellini, Cut Ziti, Elbow Macaroni, Elbow Spaghetti, Lasagna, Mostaccioli, Rigatoni, Rotini, Shells, Spaghetti, Spaghettini or Vermicelli (2 oz dry)	210	1	0	42	2	0
Di Giorno Angel's Hair (2 oz dry)	160	1	0	31	1	190
Fettuccine, Herb Linguine or Linguine (2.5 oz dry)	190	2	0	39	2	125
Spinach Fettuccine (2.5 oz dry)	190	2	0	38	2	140
Formägg Alternative, Macaroni & Cheese Sauce, Penne Pasta Alfredo, Penne Pasta Primavera or Vegetable Pasta & Caesar Italian Garden (²/₃ cup prep)	190	2	0	35	0	470
Ka-me Bean Thread (Sai Fun) (1 cup)	190	0	0	50	1	0
Noodles, Chinese Plain or Chinese Wide Lo Mein (2 oz dry)	200	0	0	45	1	1
Curly (Chuka Soba) (2 oz dry)	200	1	0	42	1	310
Japanese Buckwheat (Shin Shu Soba) (2 oz dry)	200	1	0	40	2	80
Japanese Thick (Udon) (2 oz dry)	190	1	0	41	1	670
Somen (Tomoshiraga) (2 oz dry)	190	1	0	41	1	670
Rice Sticks (Py Mai Fun) (2 oz)	193	0	0	48	0	100
Kraft Light Italian Pasta Salad, prep as directed on box (³/₄ cup)	190	2	1	5	2	660
Mueller's Capellini, Elbows, Fettuccini, Jumbo Shells, Lasagna, Linguini, Macaroni, Ruffles, Seashells, Spaghetti, Super Shapes, Tricolor Twists, Twists or Vermicelli (2 oz dry)	210	1	0	42	1	0

Pasta and Pasta Mixes (continued)	Calories	Fat g	Saturated Fat g	Carbohydrate g	Fiber g	Sodium mg
Cholesterol-Free Noodle Style Pasta (2 oz dry)	210	1	0	42	1	10
Capellini, Fettuccini, Linguini, Napolina, Spaghetti or Vermicelli (2 oz dry)	210	1	0	43	1	0
P & R Acini de Pepe, Alphabets, Capellini, Cut Fusilli, Cut Ziti, Ditalini, Elbow Macaroni, Fettuccini, Jumbo Lasagna, Jumbo Shells, Large Elbow, Large Shells, Linguini, Manicotti, Medium Shells, Perciatelli, Ribbed Angle Cuts, Rigatoni, Rings, Rosa Marini, Rotelle, Small Rigatoni, Small Shells, Spaghetti, Spirals, Thin Spaghetti, Tubettini or Vermicelli (2 oz dry)	210	1	0	42	2	0
Pritikin Spiral Pasta (²/₃ cup)	190	1	0	40	4	10
Whole Wheat Thin Spaghetti (¹/₈ box)	190	1	0	40	5	0
San Giorgio Acini de Pepe, Alphabets, Capellini, Cut Fusilli, Cut Ziti, Ditalini, Elbow Macaroni, Jumbo Shells, Large Shells, Linguini, Medium Shells, Mostaccioli, Orzo, Perciatelli, Rigatoni, Rippled Lasagna, Rotini, Small Shells, Spaghetti, Spaghettini, Tubettini or Vermicelli (2 oz dry)	210	1	0	42	2	0
Skinner Alphabets, Dumplings, Fideo Enrollacio, Jumbo Elbow Macaroni, Large Elbow, Lasagna, Linguini, Long Spaghetti, Manicotti, Mostaccioli, Ready Cut Spaghetti, Rigatoni, Ripplets, Salad Macaroni, Short Cut Elbow Macaroni, Sea Shell Macaroni, Shell Macaroni, Thin Italian Style Spaghetti, Thin Spaghetti, Twirls, Twisted Vermicelli or Vermicelli (2 oz dry)	210	1	0	42	2	0
Spice Islands Quick Meals, Garlic & Herb Pasta (1 cup)	160	1	0	32	1	660
Pasta Primavera (1 cup)	170	2	1	30	15	470

RICE AND RICE MIXES

Higher-Fat

	Calories	Fat g	Saturated Fat g	Carbohydrate g	Fiber g	Sodium mg
Seasoned Rice Mix, prep w/margarine (²/₃ cup)	227	7	2	34	1	978
Fried Rice, prep w/oil (⁷/₈ cup)	194	7	1	27	2	717

	Calories	Fat g	Saturated Fat g	Carbohydrate g	Fiber g	Sodium mg
Lower-Fat						
Most Brands, Wild Rice, prep w/o fat or salt (1 cup)	166	1	0	35	1	5
Canilla Dorado Long Grain Rice Enriched Parboiled (¼ cup dry)	170	0	0	37	0	0
Carolina Extra Long Grain Rice, Brown (¼ cup dry)	150	1	0	32	1	0
White (¼ cup dry)	150	1	0	35	1	0
La Choy Chinese Fried Rice (¾ cup)	190	1	0	41	<1	820
Mahatma Extra Long Grain Rice, Brown (¼ cup dry)	150	1	0	32	1	0
White (¼ cup dry)	150	0	0	35	0	0
Mixes, Black Beans & Rice (2 oz dry)	200	2	0	39	6	850
Broccoli & Cheese (2 oz dry)	200	2	1	41	2	620
Jambalaya (2 oz dry)	190	1	0	43	<1	700
Long Grain & Wild Rice (2 oz dry)	190	1	0	41	2	1,240
Pilaf Rice (2 oz dry)	190	0	0	43	<1	820
Red Beans & Rice (2 oz dry)	190	1	0	40	7	790
Sesame Chicken Rice (2 oz dry)	190	2	0	41	1	970
Spanish Rice (2 oz dry)	180	1	0	42	2	760
Yellow Rice (2 oz dry)	190	0	0	43	<1	970
Minute Rice Boil-in-Bag, prep w/o fat or salt (1 cup)	190	0	0	42	0	10
Instant Whole Grain Brown, prep w/o fat or salt (⅔ cup)	170	2	0	34	2	10
Long Grain & Wild Rice Mix, prep w/o fat (1 cup)	230	1	0	50	1	960
Original, prep w/o fat or salt (¾ cup)	170	0	0	37	0	10
Premium Long Grain, prep w/o fat or salt (1 cup)	170	0	0	36	0	10
Old El Paso Spanish Rice (1 cup)	130	1	<1	28	2	1,340
Pritikin Dinner Rice Mixes, Mexican (⅓ cup dry)	200	2	0	43	4	105
Oriental (⅓ cup dry)	190	2	0	43	4	260
Spice Islands Quick Meals, Chicken Rice Pilaf (1 cup)	180	2	0	34	1	710
Curry Rice (1 cup)	190	3	0	35	3	340
Oriental Rice & Vegetables (1 cup)	180	3	0	33	13	600

	Calories	Fat g	Saturated Fat g	Carbohydrate g	Fiber g	Sodium mg
Rice and Rice Mixes (continued)						
Rice & Spicy Black Beans (1 cup)	190	1	0	34	7	200
Rice & Spicy Red Beans (1 cup)	180	1	0	34	6	560
Wild Rice & Vegetables (1 cup)	160	0	0	32	10	360
Success Beef Oriental, prep w/o fat (½ cup)	190	1	0	43	2	920
Broccoli & Cheese, prep w/o fat (½ cup)	200	2	1	41	2	690
Brown & Wild Rice, prep w/o fat (½ cup)	190	1	0	40	3	830
Brown Rice, prep w/o fat or salt (½ cup)	345	2	0	77	5	17
Classic Chicken Rice, prep w/o fat (½ cup)	150	1	0	32	1	720
Long Grain & Wild Rice, prep w/o fat (½ cup)	190	0	0	42	1	890
Rice Pilaf, prep w/o fat (½ cup)	200	0	0	44	2	630
Spanish Rice, prep w/o fat (½ cup)	190	1	0	43	1	780
White Rice, prep w/o fat or salt (½ cup)	190	0	0	44	<1	5
Van Camp's Spanish Rice (1 cup)	180	3	1	37	3	1,290
Water Maid Long Grain Rice (¼ cup dry)	160	0	0	37	1	0

OTHER GRAIN PRODUCTS

	Calories	Fat g	Saturated Fat g	Carbohydrate g	Fiber g	Sodium mg
Most Brands, Couscous, prep w/o fat or salt (1 cup)	201	0	0	41	2	6
Arrowhead Mills Bulgar (¼ cup dry)	150	1	0	33	4	0

SALAD DRESSINGS AND SANDWICH SPREADS

The only cutoff point used for foods included in this section of the Guide is 2 grams of saturated fat per serving *as purchased* or when *prepared according to package directions*. Regular salad dressings containing oil are included in this section of the Guide as long as they do not provide more than 2 grams of saturated fat per serving. Limited amounts of foods that are high in fat but contain smaller amounts of saturated fat are appropriate for a cholesterol-lowering eating pattern. Other foods that are high in fat and contain limited amounts of saturated fat are found in the Fats section of the Guide.

Bacon and Tomato *Salad Dressings*	Calories	Fat g	Saturated Fat g	Carbohydrate g	Fiber g	Sodium mg
BACON AND TOMATO **SALAD DRESSINGS**						
Henri's Salad Dressings, Bacon & Tomato (2 tbsp)	140	12	2	8	NA	290
Kraft Deliciously Right Reduced Calorie Dressing, Bacon & Tomato (2 tbsp)	60	5	1	3	0	300
BLUE CHEESE **SALAD DRESSINGS**						
Higher-Saturated Fat						
Bleu Cheese (Roquefort) Dressing (2 tbsp)	151	16	3	2	0	328
Lower-Saturated Fat						
Healthy Sensation! Salad Dressing, Blue Cheese (2 tbsp)	35	0	0	7	0	300
Henri's Light Salad Dressing, Blue Cheese (2 tbsp)	60	2	1	9	NA	430

Blue Cheese Salad Dressings (continued)	Calories	Fat g	Saturated Fat g	Carbohydrate g	Fiber g	Sodium mg
Kraft Free Salad Dressing, Blue Cheese Flavor (2 tbsp)	50	0	0	12	0	340
Marie's Luscious Creamy Low Fat Dressing, Blue Cheese (2 tbsp)	45	2	0	7	<1	270
Reduced Calorie Dressing & Dips, Chunky Blue Cheese (1 pkt)	150	11	2	11	1	360
Chunky Blue Cheese (2 tbsp)	100	7	1	7	1	250
Walden Farms Fat Free Dressing, Bleu Cheese (2 tbsp)	25	0	0	4	0	240
Weight Watchers Dressing Mix, Blue Cheese (1 tbsp)	8	0	0	1	NA	110
CAESAR SALAD DRESSINGS						
Kraft Deliciously Right Reduced Calorie Dressing, Caesar (2 tbsp)	60	5	1	2	0	560
Medford Farms Fat Free Dressing, Caesar (2 tbsp)	15	0	0	4	0	200
Newman's Own Salad Dressing, Caesar (2 tbsp)	150	16	2	1	0	450
Seven Seas Viva Salad Dressing, Caesar (2 tbsp)	120	12	2	2	0	500
Walden Farms Fat Free Salad Dressing, Caesar (2 tbsp)	25	0	0	4	0	360
Weight Watchers Salad Celebrations, Three Cheese Caesar (2 tbsp)	40	2	0	5	0	190
Salad Celebrations Fat Free Dressings, Caesar (2 tbsp)	10	0	0	1	0	390
Caesar (single serving pkt)	5	0	0	1	0	290
CATALINA SALAD DRESSINGS						
Kraft Free Salad Dressing, Catalina (2 tbsp)	45	0	0	11	0	360
Kraft Salad Dressings, Catalina w/Honey (2 tbsp)	140	12	2	8	0	310
Deliciously Right Reduced Calorie Dressing, Catalina French (2 tbsp)	80	4	1	9	0	400
CUCUMBER SALAD DRESSINGS						
Henri's Light Salad Dressing, Creamy Cucumber (2 tbsp)	60	2	0	11	NA	430

Cucumber Salad Dressings (continued)	Calories	Fat g	Saturated Fat g	Carbohydrate g	Fiber g	Sodium mg
Herb Magic Dressing, Creamy Cucumber (2 tbsp)	15	0	0	4	0	270
Weight Watchers Salad Dressing, Creamy Cucumber (1 tbsp)	18	0	0	4	0	85

FRENCH SALAD DRESSINGS

	Calories	Fat g	Saturated Fat g	Carbohydrate g	Fiber g	Sodium mg
Henri's Fat Free Salad Dressing, French (2 tbsp)	45	0	0	11	NA	240
Hearty French (2 tbsp)	140	11	2	9	NA	190
Original French (2 tbsp)	120	11	2	6	NA	210
Light Salad Dressings, Hearty French (2 tbsp)	60	2	0	10	NA	200
Original French (2 tbsp)	70	2	0	13	NA	280
Kraft Free Salad Dressing, French (2 tbsp)	50	0	0	12	0	300
Kraft Salad Dressings, Catalina French (2 tbsp)	140	11	2	8	0	390
Deliciously Right Reduced Calorie Dressing, French (2 tbsp)	50	3	1	6	0	260
French (2 tbsp)	120	12	2	4	0	260
Marie's Dressing & Dip, Tangy French (2 tbsp)	130	11	2	8	0	260
Pritikin Salad Dressings, French Style (2 tbsp)	35	0	0	8	0	130
Honey French (2 tbsp)	40	0	0	11	0	135
Weight Watchers Dressing Mix, French Style (1 tbsp)	3	0	0	1	NA	150
Salad Celebrations Fat Free, French Style (2 tbsp)	40	0	0	9	0	200
Wish-Bone Lite Salad Dressing, French Style (2 tbsp)	45	1	0	9	0	280

HERB SALAD DRESSINGS

	Calories	Fat g	Saturated Fat g	Carbohydrate g	Fiber g	Sodium mg
Good Seasons Salad Dressing Mix, Garlic & Herbs, prep w/vinegar, water & oil (2 tbsp)	140	15	2	1	0	340
Salad Dressing Mix for Fat Free Dressing, Zesty Herb, prep w/vinegar & water (2 tbsp)	10	0	0	2	0	260
Henri's Salad Dressing, Italian Herb (2 tbsp)	110	11	2	2	NA	410

	Calories	Fat g	Saturated Fat g	Carbohydrate g	Fiber g	Sodium mg
Medford Farms Fat Free Dressing, Creamy Dill (2 tbsp)	20	0	0	5	0	260

HONEY DIJON AND HONEY MUSTARD SALAD DRESSINGS

	Calories	Fat g	Saturated Fat g	Carbohydrate g	Fiber g	Sodium mg
Good Seasons Salad Dressing Mix, Honey Mustard, prep w/vinegar, water & oil (2 tbsp)	150	15	2	3	0	240
Salad Dressing Mix for Fat Free Dressing, Honey Mustard, prep w/vinegar & water (2 tbsp)	20	0	0	5	0	280
Healthy Sensation! Salad Dressing, Honey Dijon (2 tbsp)	45	0	0	10	0	390
Henri's Fat Free Salad Dressing, Honey Mustard (2 tbsp)	50	0	0	12	NA	180
Honey Mustard (2 tbsp)	100	6	1	10	NA	230
Kraft Free Salad Dressing, Honey Dijon (2 tbsp)	50	0	0	11	0	330
Kraft Salad Dressing, Honey Dijon (2 tbsp)	150	15	2	4	0	200
Marie's Dressing & Dip, Honey Mustard (2 tbsp)	160	15	2	8	<1	160
Medford Farms Fat Free Dressing, Honey Mustard (2 tbsp)	30	0	0	7	0	200
Pritikin Salad Dressings, Dijon Balsamic Vinaigrette (2 tbsp)	30	0	0	6	0	125
Honey Dijon (2 tbsp)	45	0	0	11	1	130
Smart Temptations Salad Dressing, French Honey Dijon (2 tbsp)	20	0	0	4	0	250
Walden Farms Fat Free Salad Dressing, Honey Dijon Vinaigrette (2 tbsp)	25	0	0	6	0	240
Weight Watchers Salad Celebrations Fat Free, Honey Dijon (2 tbsp)	45	0	0	11	0	150

ITALIAN SALAD DRESSINGS

	Calories	Fat g	Saturated Fat g	Carbohydrate g	Fiber g	Sodium mg
Good Seasons Salad Dressing Mixes for Fat Free Dressings, Creamy Italian, prep w/skim milk, vinegar & water (2 tbsp)	20	0	0	3	0	280
Italian, prep w/vinegar & water (2 tbsp)	10	0	0	3	0	290

Italian Salad Dressings (continued)	Calories	Fat g	Saturated Fat g	Carbohydrate g	Fiber g	Sodium mg
Good Seasons Italian Salad Dressing Mixes *(continued)*						
Salad Dressing Mixes for Reduced Calorie Dressings, Italian, prep w/vinegar, water & oil (2 tbsp)	50	5	1	1	0	280
Zesty Italian, prep w/vinegar, water & oil (2 tbsp)	140	15	2	1	0	220
Salad Dressing Mixes, Italian, prep w/vinegar, water & oil (2 tbsp)	140	15	2	1	0	320
Zesty Italian, prep w/vinegar, water & oil (2 tbsp)	50	5	1	2	0	260
Healthy Sensation! Salad Dressing, Italian (2 tbsp)	15	0	0	2	0	280
Henri's Creamy Garlic Italian (2 tbsp)	110	9	2	6	NA	290
Fat Free Salad Dressing, Italian (2 tbsp)	15	0	0	2	NA	320
Light Salad Dressing, Creamy Italian (2 tbsp)	50	2	0	8	NA	420
Traditional Italian (2 tbsp)	110	11	2	3	NA	560
Herb Magic Dressing, Italian (2 tbsp)	10	0	0	2	0	400
Kraft Free Salad Dressing, Italian (2 tbsp)	10	0	0	2	0	290
Kraft Salad Dressings, Deliciously Right Reduced Calorie Salad Dressings, Creamy Italian (2 tbsp)	50	5	1	3	0	250
Italian (2 tbsp)	70	7	1	3	0	240
House Italian (2 tbsp)	120	12	2	3	0	240
Oil-Free Italian Fat Free (2 tbsp)	5	0	0	2	0	450
Zesty Italian (2 tbsp)	110	11	2	2	0	530
Marie's Luscious Low Fat Dressing, Creamy Italian Herb (2 tbsp)	40	2	0	6	0	290
Reduced Calorie Dressing & Dips, Creamy Italian Garlic (2 tbsp)	90	7	1	6	1	240
Creamy Italian Garlic (1 pkt)	130	10	1	9	1	360
Medford Farms Fat Free Dressings, Creamy Italian (2 tbsp)	15	0	0	4	0	230
Italian (2 tbsp)	10	0	0	1	0	65
Newman's Own Light Dressing, Italian (2 tbsp)	20	1	0	3	0	380
Pritikin Salad Dressing, Italian (2 tbsp)	20	0	0	5	0	115
Seven Seas Creamy Italian (2 tbsp)	110	12	2	2	0	510

	Calories	Fat g	Saturated Fat g	Carbohydrate g	Fiber g	Sodium mg
Free Fat Free Dressing, Italian (2 tbsp)	10	0	0	2	0	480
Reduced Calorie Dressings, Creamy Italian (2 tbsp)	60	5	1	2	0	490
Italian w/Olive Oil, Oil Blend (2 tbsp)	50	5	1	2	0	450
Viva Italian (2 tbsp)	45	4	1	2	0	390
Viva Salad Dressing, Italian (2 tbsp)	110	11	2	2	0	580
Walden Farms Fat Free Salad Dressings, Creamy Italian w/Parmesan (2 tbsp)	25	0	0	4	0	360
Italian (2 tbsp)	10	0	0	2	0	290
Sodium Free (2 tbsp)	10	0	0	2	0	0
Sugar Free (2 tbsp)	0	0	0	0	0	290
w/Sun Dried Tomato (2 tbsp)	15	0	0	3	0	290
Weight Watchers Italian (single serving pkt)	8	0	0	1	0	270
Dressing Mixes, Creamy Italian (1 tbsp)	3	0	0	1	NA	180
Italian (1 tbsp)	2	0	0	0	NA	140
Salad Celebrations Fat Free Dressings, Creamy Italian (2 tbsp)	30	0	0	7	0	360
Italian (2 tbsp)	10	0	0	2	0	360
Wish-Bone Lite Salad Dressings, Creamy Italian (2 tbsp)	45	1	0	10	0	290
Italian (2 tbsp)	15	1	0	2	0	480

MAYONNAISE AND MAYONNAISE-TYPE SALAD DRESSINGS

	Calories	Fat g	Saturated Fat g	Carbohydrate g	Fiber g	Sodium mg
Best Foods Mayonnaise (1 tbsp)	100	11	2	0	0	80
Light Reduced Calorie (1 tbsp)	50	5	1	1	0	115
Reduced Fat Cholesterol Free Dressing (1 tbsp)	40	3	1	3	0	120
Blue Plate Mayonnaise (1 tbsp)	100	11	2	0	0	80
Reduced Fat Cholesterol Free Mayonnaise Dressing (1 tbsp)	50	5	1	<1	0	90
Heart-Beat Foods Smart Beat Mayonnaises, Canola Light Reduced Fat or Super Light Reduced Fat (1 tbsp)	35	3	0	2	NA	110
Fat Free (1 tbsp)	10	0	0	3	0	135
Nonfat Dressing (1 tbsp)	64	0	0	3	NA	130
Hellmann's Mayonnaise (1 tbsp)	100	11	2	0	0	80
Light Reduced Calorie (1 tbsp)	50	5	1	1	0	115

Mayonnaise and Mayonnaise-Type Salad Dressings (continued)	Calories	Fat g	Saturated Fat g	Carbohydrate g	Fiber g	Sodium mg
Hellmann's *(continued)*						
Reduced Fat Cholesterol Free Dressing (1 tbsp)	40	3	1	3	0	120
Kraft Free Mayonnaise, Fat Free Dressing (1 tbsp)	10	0	0	2	0	105
Kraft Light Mayonnaise, Light Dressing (1 tbsp)	50	5	1	1	0	110
Mayonnaise (1 tbsp)	100	11	2	0	0	75
Miracle Whip Dressings, Free Nonfat (1 tbsp)	15	0	0	3	0	120
Light (1 tbsp)	40	3	0	3	0	120
Salad Dressing (1 tbsp)	70	7	1	2	0	85
Weight Watchers Dressing, Fat Free Whipped (1 tbsp)	15	0	0	3	0	95
Mayonnaise, Fat Free (1 tbsp)	10	0	0	3	0	105
Light (1 tbsp)	25	2	0	1	0	130
Low Sodium (1 tbsp)	25	2	0	1	0	40
RANCH AND BUTTERMILK SALAD DRESSINGS						
Good Seasons Salad Dressing Mix for Reduced Calorie Dressing, Ranch, prep w/whole milk & mayonnaise (2 tbsp)	60	5	1	3	0	240
Salad Dressing Mix, Buttermilk Farm Style, prep w/whole milk & mayonnaise (2 tbsp)	120	12	2	2	0	260
Ranch, prep w/whole milk, water & mayonnaise (2 tbsp)	120	12	2	2	0	220
Healthy Sensation! Salad Dressing, Ranch (2 tbsp)	40	0	0	9	0	270
Henri's Fat Free Salad Dressing, Ranch (2 tbsp)	40	0	0	9	NA	340
Light Salad Dressings, Parmesan Ranch (2 tbsp)	60	2	1	10	NA	310
Ranch (2 tbsp)	60	2	0	11	NA	290
Herb Magic Dressing, Ranch (2 tbsp)	15	0	0	4	0	270
Kraft Deliciously Right Reduced Calorie Dressings, Cucumber Ranch (2 tbsp)	60	5	1	2	0	450
Ranch (2 tbsp)	110	11	2	2	0	310
Salsa Ranch (2 tbsp)	130	13	2	1	0	320

Ranch and Buttermilk Salad Dressings (continued)	Calories	Fat g	Saturated Fat g	Carbohydrate g	Fiber g	Sodium mg
Kraft Free Salad Dressings, Peppercorn Ranch (2 tbsp)	50	0	0	11	0	360
Ranch (2 tbsp)	50	0	0	11	0	310
Marie's Dressing & Dip, Bacon Ranch (2 tbsp)	150	16	2	3	0	200
Luscious Zesty Low Fat Dressing, Ranch (2 tbsp)	45	2	0	7	0	330
Reduced Calorie Dressing & Dips, Creamy Ranch (1 pkt)	140	10	1	11	1	360
Creamy Ranch (2 tbsp)	100	7	1	7	0	240
Medford Farms Fat Free Dressing, Ranch (2 tbsp)	20	0	0	4	0	230
Seven Seas Free Fat Free Dressing, Ranch (2 tbsp)	50	0	0	12	1	330
Reduced Calorie Dressing, Ranch (2 tbsp)	100	9	2	5	0	320
Smart Temptations Salad Dressing, Buttermilk Ranch (2 tbsp)	20	0	0	4	0	230
Walden Farms Fat Free Salad Dressing, Ranch or Ranch w/Sun Dried Tomato (2 tbsp)	25	0	0	4	0	290
Weight Watchers Salad Celebrations Fat Free, Ranch (2 tbsp)	35	0	0	7	0	270
Ranch (single serving pkt)	25	0	0	7	0	200

RUSSIAN SALAD DRESSINGS

	Calories	Fat g	Saturated Fat g	Carbohydrate g	Fiber g	Sodium mg
Henri's Salad Dressing, Russian (2 tbsp)	120	10	2	9	NA	190
Kraft Salad Dressing, Russian (2 tbsp)	130	10	2	10	0	280
Walden Farms Fat Free Salad Dressing, Russian (2 tbsp)	30	0	0	6	0	240
Weight Watchers Dressing Mix, Russian (1 tbsp)	4	0	0	1	NA	120
Salad Celebrations Dressing, Russian (2 tbsp)	45	2	0	8	0	190

SANDWICH SPREADS

	Calories	Fat g	Saturated Fat g	Carbohydrate g	Fiber g	Sodium mg
Best Foods Sandwich Spred (1 tbsp)	50	5	1	3	0	170
Blue Plate Sandwich Spread (1 tbsp)	75	7	1	3	0	105
Hellmann's Sandwich Spred (1 tbsp)	50	5	1	3	0	170
Kraft Sandwich Spread & Burger Sauce (1 tbsp)	50	5	1	3	0	100

	Calories	Fat g	Saturated Fat g	Carbohydrate g	Fiber g	Sodium mg
THOUSAND ISLAND SALAD DRESSINGS						
Healthy Sensation! Salad Dressing, Thousand Island (2 tbsp)	40	0	0	9	1	300
Henri's Fat Free Salad Dressing, Thousand Island (2 tbsp)	40	0	0	9	NA	260
Thousand Island (2 tbsp)	100	9	2	5	NA	230
Herb Magic Dressing, Thousand Island (2 tbsp)	15	0	0	4	0	170
Kraft Deliciously Right Reduced Calorie Dressing, Thousand Island (2 tbsp)	70	4	1	8	0	320
Thousand Island (2 tbsp)	110	10	2	5	0	310
Thousand Island w/Bacon (2 tbsp)	120	12	2	5	0	190
Kraft Free Salad Dressing, Thousand Island (2 tbsp)	45	0	0	11	0	300
Walden Farms Fat Free Dressing, Thousand Island (2 tbsp)	35	0	0	7	0	240
Weight Watchers Dressing Mix, Thousand Island (1 tbsp)	4	0	0	1	NA	140
Salad Celebrations Dressing, Thousand Island (2 tbsp)	45	2	0	8	0	190
Wish-Bone Lite Salad Dressings, Thousand Island (2 tbsp)	45	1	0	9	0	290
VINAIGRETTE SALAD DRESSINGS						
Herb Magic Dressing, Vinaigrette (2 tbsp)	10	0	0	3	0	270
Kraft Free Fat Free Dressing, Red Wine Vinegar (2 tbsp)	15	0	0	3	0	400
Marie's Zesty Fat Free Dressings, Classic Herb Vinaigrette (2 tbsp)	30	0	0	7	0	250
Honey Dijon Vinaigrette (2 tbsp)	50	0	0	11	0	125
Italian Vinaigrette (2 tbsp)	35	0	0	8	0	280
Raspberry Vinaigrette (2 tbsp)	35	0	0	8	0	35
Red Wine or White Wine (2 tbsp)	40	0	0	10	0	300-310
Medford Farms Fat Free Dressings, Balsamic Vinaigrette (2 tbsp)	10	0	0	2	0	240
Pritikin Salad Dressing, Raspberry Vinaigrette (2 tbsp)	45	0	0	11	0	70

	Calories	Fat g	Saturated Fat g	Carbohydrate g	Fiber g	Sodium mg
Seven Seas Free Fat Free Dressing, Red Wine Vinegar (2 tbsp)	15	0	0	3	0	400
Seven Seas Reduced Calorie Dressing, Red Wine Vinegar & Oil (2 tbsp)	60	5	1	2	0	310
Walden Farms Fat Free Salad Dressing, Raspberry Vinaigrette (2 tbsp)	20	0	0	4	0	290

OTHER SALAD DRESSINGS

Higher-Saturated Fat

	Calories	Fat g	Saturated Fat g	Carbohydrate g	Fiber g	Sodium mg
Sour Cream-Based Salad Dressing (2 tbsp)	145	16	3	2	0	354

Lower-Saturated Fat

	Calories	Fat g	Saturated Fat g	Carbohydrate g	Fiber g	Sodium mg
Henri's Light Salad Dressing, Tas-Tee (2 tbsp)	60	2	0	11	NA	220
Salad Dressing, Tas-Tee (2 tbsp)	110	9	2	8	NA	200
Herb Magic Dressings, Sweet-Sour (2 tbsp)	35	0	0	9	0	240
Zesty Tomato (2 tbsp)	10	0	0	3	0	220
Kraft Dressing, Coleslaw (2 tbsp)	150	12	2	8	0	420
Salad Dressings, Creamy Garlic (2 tbsp)	110	11	2	2	0	350
Salsa Zesty Garden (2 tbsp)	70	6	1	3	<1	280
Marie's Dressing, Cole Slaw (2 tbsp)	150	13	2	6	0	210
Dressing & Dip, Poppyseed (2 tbsp)	150	12	2	8	0	200
Luscious Low Fat Dressing, Creamy Parmesan (2 tbsp)	45	2	0	7	0	270
Old Dutch Dressing, Sweet/Sour (2 tbsp)	50	0	0	13	0	480
Seven Seas Salad Dressings, Green Goddess (2 tbsp)	120	13	2	1	0	260
Herbs & Spices (2 tbsp)	120	12	2	1	0	320
Red Wine Vinegar & Oil (2 tbsp)	110	11	2	2	0	510
Two Cheese Italian (2 tbsp)	70	7	1	3	0	240
Smart Temptations Salad Dressings, Cilantro Lime or Cracked Coriander (2 tbsp)	20	0	0	4	0	220
Lemon Peppercorn (2 tbsp)	20	0	0	0	0	250
Sun-Dried Tomato (2 tbsp)	20	0	0	4	0	280
Weight Watchers Salad Dressings, Creamy Peppercorn (1 tbsp)	8	0	0	2	0	85

SAUCES AND GRAVIES

All the sauces and gravies in the Guide are low in fat and saturated fat *as purchased* or when *prepared as indicated in the Guide.* The values given in the Guide are for the sauce or gravy only and do not include any food with which these products may be combined. For example, if ground beef is added to a spaghetti sauce found in this section of the Guide, values for the meat must be added to the values listed for the sauce. One serving of the foods included in this section of the Guide does not exceed the cutoff points of 3 grams of fat and 1 gram of saturated fat.

Barbecue Sauces	Calories	Fat g	Saturated Fat g	Carbohydrate g	Fiber g	Sodium mg
BARBECUE SAUCES						
America's Choice Barbecue Sauces, Hickory Smoked, Hot or Original (2 tbsp)	45	0	0	11	0	380
House of Tsang Barbecue Sauce, Hong Kong (1 tsp)	10	0	0	2	0	150
Hunt's Barbecue Sauces, Country Style (1 tbsp)	20	<1	0	5	<1	140
Hickory or Original (1 tbsp)	20	<1	0	5	<1	160
Homestyle (1 tbsp)	20	<1	0	6	<1	170
Kansas City Style (1 tbsp)	20	<1	0	5	<1	85
New Orleans Style (1 tbsp)	20	<1	0	5	<1	150
Southern Style or Western Style (1 tbsp)	20	<1	0	5	<1	170
Texas Style (1 tbsp)	20	<1	0	6	<1	150
Kraft Barbecue Sauces, Char-Grill or Teriyaki (2 tbsp)	60	1	0	12	0	430-440
Extra Rich Original (2 tbsp)	50	0	0	12	0	360
Garlic, Mesquite Smoke or Salsa Style (2 tbsp)	40	0	0	9	0	410-420

	Calories	Fat g	Saturated Fat g	Carbohydrate g	Fiber g	Sodium mg
Hickory Smoke (2 tbsp)	40	0	0	10	0	440
Hickory Smoke Onion Bits (2 tbsp)	50	0	0	11	<1	340
Honey (2 tbsp)	50	0	0	13	0	320
Hot (2 tbsp)	40	0	0	9	0	540
Hot Hickory Smoke (2 tbsp)	40	0	0	9	0	360
Italian Seasonings (2 tbsp)	45	1	0	10	0	280
Kansas City Style (2 tbsp)	45	0	0	11	<1	280
Onion Bits (2 tbsp)	50	0	0	11	0	340
Original (2 tbsp)	40	0	0	10	0	460
Thick 'N Spicy Barbecue Sauces, Hickory Smoke, Mesquite or Original (2 tbsp)	50	0	0	12	0	440
Honey (2 tbsp)	60	0	0	13	0	350
Kansas City Style (2 tbsp)	60	0	0	13	<1	280
Lawry's Barbecue sauce, Dijon & Honey (1 tbsp)	60	1	0	12	0	750
Open Pit BBQ Sauces, Hickory Flavor or Hot (2 tbsp)	50	0	0	11	0	380
Mesquite (2 tbsp)	50	1	0	11	0	440
Onion Flavor or Original (2 tbsp)	50	0	0	11	0	480-490
Original Flavor (2 tbsp)	50	0	0	11	0	450
Sweet Flavor (2 tbsp)	50	0	0	12	0	300
Thick & Tangy BBQ Sauces, Hickory or Onion (2 tbsp)	50	0	0	12	0	380-390

COOKING SAUCES

Higher-Fat

	Calories	Fat g	Saturated Fat g	Carbohydrate g	Fiber g	Sodium mg
Cheese Sauce, prep w/whole milk (1/4 cup)	141	11	6	4	0	360
Mushroom Sauce, prep w/whole milk (1/4 cup)	102	9	3	4	0	462

Lower-Fat

	Calories	Fat g	Saturated Fat g	Carbohydrate g	Fiber g	Sodium mg
Betty Crocker Recipe Sauces, Cacciatore (1/2 cup)	50	0	0	10	0	620
Parmigiana (1/2 cup)	60	1	1	10	0	490
Campbell's Simmer Chef Cooking Sauces, Golden Honey Mustard (1/2 cup)	150	2	0	30	1	400
Hearty Onion & Mushroom (1/2 cup)	50	1	0	9	1	670
Oriental Sweet & Sour (1/2 cup)	110	1	0	23	0	280

	Calories	Fat g	Saturated Fat g	Carbohydrate g	Fiber g	Sodium mg
Campbell's Simmer Chef Cooking Sauces *(continued)*						
Zesty Tomato Mexicali (½ cup)	90	3	1	16	1	400
Chelten House, Ham Glaze (2 tbsp)	50	0	0	14	0	20
Hot Chicken Wing Sauce (2 tbsp)	20	0	0	4	<1	135
Raisin Sauce (2 tbsp)	60	0	0	15	0	15
Del Monte Sloppy Joe Sauces, Hickory Flavor (¼ cup)	70	0	0	18	0	700
Italian Recipe (¼ cup)	70	0	0	16	0	700
Original (¼ cup)	70	0	0	16	0	680
Franco-American Cheese Sauce (¼ cup)	40	2	1	4	0	390
Green Giant Sloppy Joe Sandwich Sauce (¼ cup)	50	0	0	11	2	420
Hormel Not-So-Sloppy-Joe Sauce (¼ cup)	70	0	0	15	1	720
Hunt's Manwich Sauces, Chili Fixin's (5.3 oz)	110	<1	0	20	5	900
Extra Thick & Chunky (2.5 oz)	60	<1	0	15	2	640
Mexican (2.5 oz)	35	1	0	9	1	460
Sloppy Joe (2.5 oz)	40	<1	0	10	1	390
Lawry's Fajitas Skillet Sauce (1 tbsp)	15	0	0	2	0	600
Libby's Sloppy Joe Sauce (⅓ cup)	45	0	0	10	1	430
Muir Glen Organic Chef Sauces, Creole (½ cup)	60	2	0	12	2	290
Mexican (½ cup)	45	0	0	12	3	290
Newman's Own Spicy Simmer Sauce (½ cup)	70	3	0	10	3	600
Ragú Beef Tonight Simmer Sauces, Barbecue (½ cup)	110	1	0	26	3	800
Skillet Lasagna (½ cup)	80	2	1	13	2	730
Chicken Tonight Light Simmer Sauces, Honey Mustard (½ cup)	60	1	0	13	3	440
Italian Primavera (½ cup)	50	1	0	8	2	630
Sweet & Spicy (½ cup)	60	1	0	12	3	330
Chicken Tonight Simmer Sauces, Chicken Cacciatore (½ cup)	80	2	0	14	2	530
Oriental (½ cup)	60	1	0	13	1	750
Salsa (½ cup)	50	0	0	10	3	750
Spanish (½ cup)	70	2	0	11	2	710
Sweet & Sour (½ cup)	120	0	0	30	1	320

	Calories	Fat g	Saturated Fat g	Carbohydrate g	Fiber g	Sodium mg
Tabasco brand 7 Spice Chili Recipe, Original (1/2 cup)	50	1	0	8	3	115
Spicy (1/2 cup)	60	1	0	10	2	115
Village Saucerie Sauce & Recipe Mixes, Country Homestyle (2 tbsp)	45	0	0	8	0	530
Garden Herb (2 tbsp)	45	0	0	10	0	360
Garlic & Herb (2 tbsp)	45	0	0	10	0	460
Southwest (2 tbsp)	45	0	0	9	0	390
Weight Watchers Sauce Mix, Lemon Butter (1 tbsp)	7	0	0	1	0	90
Wolf Brand Chili Hot Dog Sauce (1 tbsp)	15	1	0	2	0	90
ENCHILADA SAUCES						
Las Palmas Enchilada Sauces, Green Chile (1/4 cup)	25	1	0	3	0	260
Hot (1/4 cup)	20	1	0	3	1	330
Original (1/4 cup)	15	1	0	2	1	310
Old El Paso Enchilada Sauce Mix (2 tsp dry)	10	0	0	2	<1	540
GRAVIES						
Higher-Fat						
Mushroom Gravy, canned (1/4 cup)	102	9	3	4	0	462
Lower-Fat						
Franco-American Gravies, Au Jus (1/4 cup)	10	1	0	2	0	310
Beef (1/4 cup)	30	2	1	4	0	300
Brown w/Onions (1/4 cup)	25	1	0	4	0	340
Creamy Mushroom (1/4 cup)	20	1	0	4	0	310
Mushroom (1/4 cup)	20	1	0	3	0	300
Turkey (1/4 cup)	25	1	0	3	0	290
Heinz Home Style Gravies, Blue Ribbon Country (1/4 cup)	25	1	0	4	1	210
Classic Chicken (1/4 cup)	30	1	0	3	0	340
Roasted Turkey (1/4 cup)	25	1	0	3	0	360
Savory Brown (1/4 cup)	25	1	0	3	0	300
Pepperidge Farm Gravies, Cream of Chicken (1/4 cup)	30	1	1	3	0	280
Golden Chicken w/Pieces of Chicken (1/4 cup)	25	1	0	3	0	270
Hearty Beef w/Pieces of Beef (1/4 cup)	25	1	0	4	0	360

	Calories	Fat g	Saturated Fat g	Carbohydrate g	Fiber g	Sodium mg
Pepperidge Farm Gravies *(continued)*						
Mushroom & Wine w/Mushrooms (¼ cup)	30	1	1	4	0	280
Roasted Onion & Garlic (¼ cup)	30	2	1	4	0	350
Seasoned Turkey w/Pieces of Turkey (¼ cup)	30	1	0	4	0	330
Stroganoff w/Sliced Mushrooms (¼ cup)	30	1	1	4	0	240
Pillsbury Gravy Mixes, Brown or Homestyle, prep w/water (¼ cup)	10	0	0	3	0	270
Chicken Style, prep w/water & skim milk (¼ cup)	20	0	0	4	0	260
Pioneer No-Fat Country Gravy Mix, prep w/water (¼ cup)	24	0	0	6	1	320
Weight Watchers Gravy Mixes, Brown w/Mushrooms, prep w/water (¼ cup)	10	0	0	2	NA	270
Brown w/Onions, prep w/water (¼ cup)	10	0	0	2	NA	310
Brown, prep w/water (¼ cup)	10	0	0	2	NA	360
Chicken, prep w/water (¼ cup)	10	0	0	2	NA	410
MARINARA, PASTA, AND SPAGHETTI SAUCES						
Campbell's Spaghetti Sauces, Extra Garlic & Onion (½ cup)	60	1	0	12	2	370
Flavored w/Ground Beef (½ cup)	90	3	1	14	3	540
Homestyle (½ cup)	70	0	0	15	2	410
Italian Style (½ cup)	50	0	0	11	2	410
Marinara (½ cup)	70	0	0	15	2	410
Mushroom & Garlic (½ cup)	80	2	1	14	3	570
Mushroom (½ cup)	60	1	0	11	2	390
Traditional (½ cup)	100	2	0	18	3	590
Del Monte Spaghetti Sauces, Traditional (½ cup)	80	1	0	15	<1	470
w/Garlic & Onions (½ cup)	70	1	0	15	<1	440
w/Green Peppers & Mushrooms (½ cup)	70	1	0	13	<1	320
w/Mushrooms (½ cup)	80	2	0	15	<1	520
Di Giorno Light Varieties Chunky Tomato w/Basil (½ cup)	70	0	0	16	2	290
Plum Tomato & Mushroom Sauce (½ cup)	70	0	0	15	2	310

	Calories	Fat g	Saturated Fat g	Carbohydrate g	Fiber g	Sodium mg
Healthy Choice Pasta Sauce, Extra Chunky, Mushrooms (1/2 cup)	50	1	0	10	2	390
Italian Style Vegetables (1/2 cup)	50	1	0	11	2	390
Super Chunky Pasta Sauce, Mushrooms & Sweet Peppers (1/2 cup)	50	1	0	11	2	390
Traditional (1/2 cup)	50	1	0	10	2	390
Hunt's Spaghetti Sauces, Chunky (4 oz)	50	<1	0	12	2	470
Homestyle Spaghetti Sauces, Plain (4 oz)	60	2	0	10	2	530
w/Meat (4 oz)	60	2	0	9	2	570
w/Mushrooms (4 oz)	50	1	0	10	2	530
Traditional (4 oz)	70	2	0	12	2	530
w/Meat or w/Mushrooms (4 oz)	70	2	0	12	2	560-570
Muir Glen Organic Fat Free Pasta Sauces, Garlic & Onion (1/2 cup)	60	0	0	13	4	300
Italian Herb (1/2 cup)	60	0	0	13	4	300
Tomato Basil (1/2 cup)	60	0	0	13	4	300
Organic Pasta Sauces, Low Fat Chunky Style (1/2 cup)	80	2	0	13	3	300
Mushrooms & Green Peppers (1/2 cup)	70	2	0	10	4	300
Newman's Own Sauces, Sockarooni, Spaghetti or Spaghetti w/Mushrooms (1/2 cup)	60	2	0	9	3	700
Prego Spaghetti Sauces, Extra Chunky, Garden Combination (1/2 cup)	90	1	1	16	3	480
Zesty Oregano (1/2 cup)	140	3	1	25	3	580
Three Cheese (1/2 cup)	100	2	1	20	3	480
Tomato & Basil (1/2 cup)	110	3	1	19	3	420
Pritikin Spaghetti Sauces, Chunky Garden Style (1/2 cup)	50	1	0	12	2	30
Marinara (1/2 cup)	60	0	0	13	2	260
Original (1/2 cup)	60	0	0	13	2	30
Ragú Fino Italian Pasta Sauces, Garden Medley, Sliced Mushroom or Zesty Tomato (1/2 cup)	90	3	0	14	2	580
Garlic & Basil or Tomato & Herb (1/2 cup)	90	3	0	15	2	580
Parmesan (1/2 cup)	100	3	1	15	2	580

	Calories	Fat g	Saturated Fat g	Carbohydrate g	Fiber g	Sodium mg
Ragú *(continued)*						
Light Pasta Sauces, Chunky Mushroom or Tomato & Herb (1/2 cup)	50	0	0	10	2	410
Garden Harvest (1/2 cup)	50	0	0	11	2	410
No Sugar Added (1/2 cup)	60	2	0	9	3	410
Pasta Sauce, Hearty Italian Tomato (1/2 cup)	120	3	1	19	3	580
Thick & Hearty Pasta Sauces, Mushroom or Tomato & Herb (1/2 cup)	120	3	1	19	3	580
Weight Watchers Spaghetti Sauces, w/Meat (1/2 cup)	60	1	0	10	4	430
w/Mushrooms (1/2 cup)	60	0	0	11	4	420
ORIENTAL SAUCES						
Betty Crocker Recipe Sauces, Pepper Steak (1/2 cup)	50	2	1	8	0	600
Sweet & Sour (1/2 cup)	160	0	0	40	0	350
Chelten House Sweet & Pungent Duck Sauce (2 tbsp)	50	0	0	12	0	140
Chun King Sweet & Sour Sauce (1/4 cup)	80	0	0	19	NA	25
Contadina Sweet 'N Sour Sauce (2 tbsp)	40	1	0	8	0	110
House of Tsang Sweet & Sour Concentrate (1 tsp)	10	0	0	3	0	15
Bangkok Padang (1 tbsp)	45	3	1	4	0	240
Hoisin (1 tsp)	15	0	0	3	0	105
Saigon Sizzle (1 tbsp)	40	1	0	8	0	350
Spicy Brown Bean (1 tsp)	15	0	0	3	0	125
Ka-me Sauces, Black Bean (1 tbsp)	10	0	0	2	1	550
Duck (2 tbsp)	80	0	0	20	0	480
Fish (1 tbsp)	10	0	0	1	0	1,300
Hoisin (2 tbsp)	45	0	0	10	1	620
Hot Chili w/Garlic (1 tbsp)	15	0	0	4	1	115
Lemon (1 tbsp)	45	0	0	11	0	125
Mandarin Orange or Plum (2 tbsp)	80	0	0	21	0	420-430
Oyster Flavored (1 tbsp)	10	0	0	3	0	460
Sweet & Sour w/Ginger (2 tbsp)	50	0	0	13	0	270
Szechuan (1 tbsp)	20	1	0	2	2	410
Tamari (1 tbsp)	10	1	0	1	0	930

Oriental Sauces (continued)	Calories	Fat g	Saturated Fat g	Carbohydrate g	Fiber g	Sodium mg
Tempura (2 tbsp)	15	0	0	3	0	1,790
Kraft Sweet 'n Sour Sauce (2 tbsp)	80	1	0	19	0	180
Sauceworks Sweet 'n Sour Sauce (2 tbsp)	60	0	0	14	0	125
La Choy Sauces, Sweet & Sour (1 tbsp)	25	<1	0	7	<1	40
Sweet & Sour Duck (1 tbsp)	25	<1	0	7	<1	40
Woody's Sweet 'n Sour Sauce (2 tbsp)	70	0	0	17	<1	610
PIZZA SAUCES						
Contadina Pizza Squeeze (1/4 cup)	35	2	0	6	1	350
Pizza Sauces, Flavored w/Pepperoni (1/4 cup)	40	2	1	6	1	420
Plain (1/4 cup)	35	2	0	6	1	350
w/Italian Cheeses (1/4 cup)	40	2	0	6	1	420
Prego Pizza Sauces, Traditional (1/4 cup)	40	2	0	6	2	230
w/Pepperoni Chunks (1/4 cup)	70	3	1	7	1	330
Progresso Pizza Sauce (1/4 cup)	35	1	0	5	1	140
Ragú Pizza Quick Sauces, Chunky Mushroom or Garlic & Basil (1/4 cup)	40	2	0	6	1	340
Chunky Tomato (1/4 cup)	40	2	0	7	1	300
Flavored w/Pepperoni (1/4 cup)	60	2	1	5	1	420
Traditional (1/4 cup)	40	2	0	5	1	340
Pizza Sauce 100% Natural (1/4 cup)	30	1	0	4	1	270
STIR-FRY SAUCES						
House of Tsang Stir Fry Sauces, Classic (1 tbsp)	25	1	0	4	0	570
Sweet & Sour (1 tbsp)	35	0	0	8	0	50
Szechuan Spicy (1 tbsp)	20	1	0	4	0	490
Ka-me Stir-Fry Sauce (1 tbsp)	10	0	0	1	0	570
TARTAR SAUCES						
Best Foods Reduced Fat Tartar Sauce (2 tbsp)	60	5	1	6	0	340
Hellmann's Reduced Fat Tartar Sauce (2 tbsp)	60	5	1	6	0	340
Kraft Nonfat Tartar Sauce (2 tbsp)	25	0	0	5	<1	210
TERIYAKI SAUCES						
Chun King Teriyaki Sauces, Lite (1 tbsp)	15	0	0	3	NA	470
Regular (1 tbsp)	15	0	0	3	NA	700

	Calories	Fat g	Saturated Fat g	Carbohydrate g	Fiber g	Sodium mg
House of Tsang Korean Teriyaki (1 tbsp)	30	1	0	6	0	430
Ka-me Teriyaki Sauce & Marinade (1 tbsp)	10	0	0	2	0	480
TOMATO SAUCES						
America's Choice Fresh Tomato Sauce (¼ cup)	20	0	0	4	1	300
Contadina Tomato Sauces, Italian or Thick & Zesty (¼ cup)	15	0	0	4	1	320-330
Del Monte Tomato Sauce, No Salt Added (¼ cup)	20	0	0	4	0	20
Hunt's Tomato Sauces, Herb Flavored (4 oz)	70	2	1	12	2	470
Italian (4 oz)	60	2	1	10	2	460
Meatloaf Fixin's (2 oz)	20	<1	0	5	<1	580
Special (4 oz)	35	<1	0	8	2	280
w/Bits (4 oz)	30	<1	0	7	2	620
w/Garlic (4 oz)	70	2	0	10	2	480
w/Mushrooms (4 oz)	25	<1	0	6	2	710
w/Onions (4 oz)	40	<1	0	9	2	650
Muir Glen Organic Tomato Sauce (¼ cup)	20	0	0	5	1	190
Old El Paso Sauces, Tomatoes & Green Chilies (¼ cup)	10	0	0	2	0	310
Tomatoes & Jalapenos (¼ cup)	15	0	0	3	1	290

SNACK FOODS

Foods included in this section of the Guide are low in fat and saturated fat *as purchased* or when *prepared as indicated in the Guide.* One serving of these products does not exceed the cutoff points of 3 grams of fat and 1 gram of saturated fat. Other foods that are good as snacks include choices from the dairy, fruit, vegetable, bread, cracker, and cereal sections of the Guide.

Chips

	Calories	Fat g	Saturated Fat g	Carbohydrate g	Fiber g	Sodium mg
CHIPS						
Higher-Fat						
Potato Chips, salted (14 chips = 1 oz)	154	10	1	16	1	180
Corn Chips, salted (17 chips = 1 oz)	164	11	2	15	1	170
Lower-Fat						
Amazing Taste Premium Baked Tortilla Chips, Yellow Corn (1 oz = about 14 chips)	110	0	0	25	<1	75
Baked Tostitos, Cool Ranch (11 chips)	120	3	1	21	1	170
Plain (13 chips)	110	1	0	24	2	140
Unsalted (13 chips)	110	1	0	24	2	0
Bugles, BBQ or Original Flavor (1½ cups)	130	3	1	24	<1	380-390
Burns & Ricker Fat Free Bagel Crisps (5 pieces)	100	0	0	22	1	280
Childers Fat Free Potato Chips, Barbecue, Lightly Salted, Onion & Chive or Salt & Vinegar (1 oz = about 30 chips)	100	0	0	22	0	120
Salt Free (1 oz = about 30 chips)	100	0	0	22	0	0

	Calories	Fat g	Saturated Fat g	Carbohydrate g	Fiber g	Sodium mg
Childers (continued)						
Fat Free Tortilla Chips, White Corn (1 oz = about 14 chips)	100	0	0	22	1	80
Guiltless Gourmet Baked Tortilla Chips, Chili & Lime Flavored (about 22 chips)	110	1	0	21	3	200
Nacho Flavored (about 22 chips)	110	1	0	22	1	200
Original Style (about 22 chips)	110	1	0	24	4	160
Original Style, No Salt (about 22 chips)	110	1	0	24	4	26
White Corn (about 22 chips)	110	1	0	24	2	140
Health Valley Fat-Free Cheese Puffs, Green Onion, Original Cheese or Zesty Chili (1 1/2 cups)	110	0	0	23	2	260
Louise's Fat-Free Potato Chips, Maui Onion or Original (1 oz = about 30 chips)	110	0	0	23	2	180
Mesquite Barbecue (1 oz = about 30 chips)	110	0	0	24	2	180
Vinegar & Salt (1 oz = about 30 chips)	100	0	0	23	2	300
Pacific Grain Products No Fries Snacks, BBQ Potato (1 oz = about 22 pieces)	120	2	0	23	1	140
Cheese Puff (1 oz = about 35 puffs)	120	2	0	23	1	190
Potato (1 oz = about 23 pieces)	120	2	0	23	1	200
Ranch-O's (1 oz = about 20 pieces)	120	2	0	23	1	180
Pop Secret Pop Chips, Butter Flavor (1 oz = 31 chips)	120	3	1	21	1	380
Original (1 oz = 31 chips)	120	3	1	21	1	380
Right Snax 98% Fat Free Spud Bakes Potato Snacks, Cheddar Cheese (1 oz = 25 crisps)	100	1	1	22	1	105
Mesquite Barbecue (1 oz = 25 crisps)	110	1	0	25	1	75
Original (1 oz = 25 chips)	110	1	1	22	1	200
Sour Cream & Onion (1 oz = 25 crisps)	100	1	0	21	2	110
Rubschlager Cocktail Chips, Caraway Rye (9 chips)	100	1	0	20	3	240
Chili Corn (9 chips)	110	1	0	20	2	240
Garlic (9 chips)	100	1	0	20	1	240
Pizza (9 chips)	100	1	0	20	2	240
Smart Temptations Baked Tortilla Chips, No Salt (12 chips)	120	1	0	25	2	0
Original (11 chips)	120	1	0	25	2	110

Chips (continued)	Calories	Fat g	Saturated Fat g	Carbohydrate g	Fiber g	Sodium mg
The Fat Free Gourmet Baked Tortilla Chips, Nacho Flavored or Salsa Flavored (1 oz = about 15 chips)	95	1	0	22	1	224
Natural Flavor (1 oz = about 15 chips)	92	1	0	22	1	189
Jalapeno & Cheese Flavored (1 oz = ¾ cup)	100	0	0	23	1	115
Potato Corns, Nacho Flavored (1 oz = about ¾ cup)	90	0	0	20	2	21
Ultra Slim-Fast Lite N' Tasty Cheese Curls (1 oz = 26 curls)	120	3	1	22	2	190
Weight Watchers Smart Snackers, Barbecue Flavored Curls (.5 oz)	60	2	0	11	1	110
DIPS						
Higher-Fat						
Seasoned Sour Cream Dip (2 tbsp)	54	5	3	1	0	210
Guacamole Dip (2 tbsp)	47	4	1	3	1	137
Lower-Fat						
Borden Fat Free Sour Cream Dips, French Onion (2 tbsp)	25	0	0	4	0	170
Ranch or Vegetable Ranch (2 tbsp)	25	0	0	4	0	150-160
Salsa, Hot or Mild (2 tbsp)	25	0	0	4	0	130
Chi-Chi's Fiesta Dips, Bean (2 tbsp)	35	2	1	4	1	140
Cheese (2 tbsp)	40	3	1	3	0	270
Doritos Dips, Cheese N' Salsa (2 tbsp)	20	2	1	5	<1	650
Salsa, Medium or Mild (2 tbsp)	15	0	0	3	1	200-220
Frito-Lay Bean Dips, Hot (2 tbsp)	35	1	0	5	2	220
Jalapeno (2 tbsp)	40	1	1	6	0	140
Cheese Dips, Jalapeno & Cheddar (2 tbsp)	50	3	1	3	0	280
Mild Cheddar (2 tbsp)	50	3	1	4	0	240
Guiltless Gourmet Dips, BBQ Black Bean (2 tbsp)	35	0	0	7	1	120
BBQ Pinto Bean (2 tbsp)	35	0	0	7	2	120
Black Bean (2 tbsp)	30	0	0	5	1	100
Nacho (2 tbsp)	25	0	0	5	0	150
Pinto Bean (2 tbsp)	30	0	0	6	2	130
Salsa (2 tbsp)	10	0	0	2	0	150

	Calories	Fat g	Saturated Fat g	Carbohydrate g	Fiber g	Sodium mg
Land O'Lakes No-Fat Dip, French Onion (2 tbsp)	30	0	0	5	0	320
Salsa (2 tbsp)	25	0	0	5	0	290
Ranch (2 tbsp)	30	0	0	6	0	180
Old El Paso Dips, Cheese 'n Salsa, Medium or Mild (2 tbsp)	25	3	1	3	0	300
Chunky Salsa, Medium or Mild (2 tbsp)	15	0	0	3	1	230
Jalapeno (2 tbsp)	30	1	0	4	2	125
Smart Temptations Dips, Garbanzo Bean, Mild or Spicy (2 tbsp)	20	0	0	4	2	130-140
Mild Black Bean or Spicy Pinto Bean (2 tbsp)	20	0	0	4	1	140-150
Mild Pinto Bean (2 tbsp)	20	0	0	4	1	130
Spicy Black Bean (2 tbsp)	20	0	0	4	2	160
The Fat Free Gourmet Bean Dips, Black (1 oz)	30	<1	0	5	NA	150
Pinto (1 oz)	20	<1	0	6	NA	160
Tostitos Picante Dips, Hot or Medium (2 tbsp)	15	0	0	3	1	250-260
Mild (2 tbsp)	15	0	0	2	1	140
FRUIT SNACKS						
Betty Crocker Assorted Fruit Snacks, Berry Bears (1 pouch)	90	1	0	21	0	30
Bugs Bunny & Friends, Rollerblade, Shark Bites or Tazmanian Devil (1 pouch)	90	1	0	21	0	25
Fruit Snacks, Berry Bears or Fruit Punch (1 pouch)	90	1	0	21	0	30
X-MEN Fun Snacks (1 pouch)	90	1	0	21	0	25
Gushers, Cherry (1 pouch)	90	1	0	21	0	90
Sour Berry (1 pouch)	90	1	0	20	0	45
Sour Cherry, Sour Grape, Sour Strawberry or Strawberry (1 pouch)	90	1	0	21	0	35
General Mills Fruit Roll-Ups, Cherry (2 rolls)	110	2	0	24	<1	80
Crazy Colors (2 rolls)	110	1	0	24	<1	80
Grape (2 rolls)	110	2	0	24	<1	105
Hot Colors (2 rolls)	110	1	0	24	<1	75
Raspberry or Strawberry (2 rolls)	110	1	0	24	<1	100

Fruit Snacks (continued)	Calories	Fat g	Saturated Fat g	Carbohydrate g	Fiber g	Sodium mg
Secret Pictures (2 rolls)	110	1	0	24	<1	90
Fruit-By-The-Foot, Cherry, Grape, Strawberry or Wild Fire (1 roll)	80	2	0	17	<1	40
Sun Belt Fruit Snacks Fruit Jammers (1 pkt)	100	1	1	23	0	20
Sunkist Fruit Rolls, Apple or Raspberry (1 roll)	70	0	0	17	1	20
Apricot or Cherry (1 roll)	70	0	0	17	2	15
Fruit Punch or Strawberry (1 roll)	70	0	0	17	2	20-25
Grape (1 roll)	80	0	0	17	2	35
Weight Watchers Smart Snackers, Apple Chips (.75 oz)	70	0	0	18	3	125
Smart Snackers Fruit Snacks, Apple, Cinnamon, Peach or Strawberry (.5 oz)	50	0	0	13	2	125

GRANOLA AND BREAKFAST BARS

Higher-Fat

	Calories	Fat g	Saturated Fat g	Carbohydrate g	Fiber g	Sodium mg
Chocolate-Coated Peanut Butter Granola Bar (1.4 oz)	204	13	5	22	1	41

Lower-Fat

	Calories	Fat g	Saturated Fat g	Carbohydrate g	Fiber g	Sodium mg
Fi-Bar Berry Best Low Fat, Cranberry Vanilla or Strawberry Vanilla (1 bar)	130	3	1	27	3	70-85
Raspberry Vanilla (1 bar)	130	3	1	27	3	50
One Gram Low Fat, Apple Cinnamon, Blueberry or Cranberry Apple (1 bar)	90	1	0	22	2	65
Health Valley Fat-Free Breakfast Bars, Apple, Apricot, Blueberry, Cherry, Strawberry or Strawberry-Apple (1 bar)	110	0	0	26	3	25
Cappuccino (1 bar)	110	0	0	26	3	30
Chocolate (1 bar)	110	0	0	26	4	30
Fat-Free Fruit Bar, Apple (1 bar)	140	0	0	35	3	0
Apricot (1 bar)	140	0	0	35	4	5
Date (1 bar)	140	0	0	34	3	5
Raisin (1 bar)	140	0	0	35	3	5
Fat-Free Granola Bar, Chocolate Chip (1 bar)	140	0	0	35	3	5

	Calories	Fat g	Saturated Fat g	Carbohydrate g	Fiber g	Sodium mg
Health Valley *(continued)*						
Fat-Free Granola Fruit Bars, Blueberry Apple, Date Almond, Raisin, Raspberry or Strawberry (1 bar)	140	0	0	35	3	5
Fruit & Fitness Bar (1 bar)	110	0	0	25	2	25
Kellogg's Cereal Bars, Rice Krispies Treats Squares (1 bar)	90	2	0	18	0	75
Low Fat Crunchy Granola Bars, Almond & Brown Sugar, Apple Spice or Cinnamon Raisin (1 bar)	80	2	0	16	1	60
Nutri-Grain Cereal Bars, Apple Cinnamon, Blueberry, Peach, Raspberry or Strawberry (1 bar)	140	3	1	27	1	60
Nature Valley Lowfat Bite-Sized Granola Bars, Oats & Honey (1 pouch)	120	2	0	24	1	135
Variety Pack (1 pouch)	120	2	0	24	1	110
Lowfat Chewy Granola Bars, Oatmeal Raisin or Variety Pack (1 bar)	110	2	0	21	1	65-70
Lowfat Crunchy Granola Bar, Cinnamon (1 pouch)	140	2	0	29	1	190
Quaker Lowfat Chewy Granola Bars, Apple Berry or Chocolate Chunk (1 bar)	110	2	1	22	NA	95-110
SnackWell's Cereal Bars, Apple Cinnamon or Strawberry (1 bar)	120	0	0	29	1	100-105
Blueberry (1 bar)	120	0	0	28	1	105
POPCORNS						
Higher-Fat						
Popcorn, Microwave, regular (2 3/4 cups = 1 oz)	137	6	1	20	4	182
Lower-Fat						
Most Brands, Popcorn prep w/o fat or salt (3 1/2 cups popped)	107	1	0	22	4	1
Estee Caramel Popcorn, No Sugar Added (1 cup)	120	2	0	26	1	90
Greenfield Healthy Foods Low Fat Caramel Popcorn (2/3 cup)	120	2	0	23	2	70

Popcorns (continued)	Calories	Fat g	Saturated Fat g	Carbohydrate g	Fiber g	Sodium mg
Health Valley Fat Free Caramel Corn Puffs Apple Cinnamon or Original (1 serving)	110	0	0	24	2	60
Jolly Time American's Best Pop Corn, White or Yellow (5 cups air popped)	100	1	0	24	6	0
White or Yellow (5 cups air popped)	100	1	0	24	6	0
Lance Fat Free Popcorn Delight (1 bar)	100	0	0	24	0	70
Louise's Fat-Free Caramel Popcorn (1 oz = about 7/8 cup)	100	0	0	24	1	80
Newman's Own Popcorn (3 tbsps unpopped)	110	2	0	27	7	0
Light Microwave Popcorn, Butter Flavored or Natural (3.5 cups popped)	110	3	1	20	3	90
Orville Redenbacher's Gourmet Hot Air Popping Corn (3 cups popped)	40	<1	0	10	3	0
Gourmet Light Butter Flavored or Light Natural Flavored Microwaved Popping Corn (3 cups popped)	70	3	1	8	3	110-115
Pop Secret Popcorn By Request, Butter Flavor or Natural Flavor (3 tbsp unpopped = 6 cups popped)	130	3	1	25	3	370
Ultra Slim-Fast Lite N' Tasty Popcorn, Caramel (1 oz)	120	2	0	25	2	80
Weight Watchers Smart Snackers Popcorn, Butter Toffee (.9 oz)	110	3	1	21	1	90
Caramel (.9 oz)	100	1	0	22	1	45
Microwave (1 oz)	90	1	0	22	7	0
PRETZELS						
Higher-Fat						
Chocolate-Covered Pretzels (3 = 1.2 oz)	138	4	2	24	1	415
Lower-Fat						
Most Brands, Pretzels (1 oz)	114	1	0	24	1	514
California Pretzels (1 oz)	110	2	0	22	1	350
Delicious Pretzels, Party (23 pieces)	120	1	0	23	1	400
Sticks (52 pieces)	120	0	0	24	1	560
Twists (10 pieces)	130	1	0	25	1	520
Estee, Reduced Sodium Pretzel Nuggets (30 nuggets)	120	2	0	24	1	180
Harry's Sourdough Pretzels (1 oz)	102	0	0	23	NA	548

	Calories	Fat g	Saturated Fat g	Carbohydrate g	Fiber g	Sodium mg
Keebler Fat Free Knots (7 pretzels)	120	0	0	26	1	400
Keystone Pretzels, Dutch (3 pretzels)	90	1	1	18	<1	210
Juniors, No Salt (22 pretzels)	90	0	0	17	<1	0
No Fat Sticks (50 sticks)	80	0	0	16	<1	440
Oat Bran (3 pretzels)	80	0	0	16	<1	110
Oat Bran, No Salt (3 pretzels)	70	0	0	15	<1	5
Lance Pretzels (9 pretzels)	140	1	0	28	<1	470
Mike-sell's Pretzels, Dutch (3 pretzels)	130	2	0	22	<1	600
Mini Twist (21 pretzels)	110	2	0	22	<1	710
Sticks (33 sticks)	110	1	0	22	<1	670
Thins (9 pretzels)	120	2	0	22	<1	600
Nabisco Mister Salty Fat Free Pretzels, Sticks (47 sticks)	110	0	0	23	1	370
Twists (9 twists)	110	0	0	23	1	380
Mister Salty Pretzels, Dutch (2 pretzels)	120	1	0	25	1	580
Mini (22 pretzels)	110	1	0	22	1	440
Pepperidge Farm Pretzel Goldfish (45 pieces)	120	3	1	22	<1	430
Pretzel Snack Sticks (9 sticks)	130	3	0	23	<1	440
Rold Gold Original Pretzel Chips (10 chips)	110	1	0	23	1	370
Rold Gold Pretzels, Bavarian (3 pretzels)	110	2	1	21	1	440
Fat Free Pretzels, Sticks (48 pretzels)	110	0	0	23	1	530
Thins (Less Sodium) (10 pretzels)	110	0	0	23	1	340
Tiny Twist (18 pretzels)	100	0	0	23	1	420
Hard Sour Dough (1 pretzel)	90	2	0	17	1	200
Rods (3 pretzels)	110	2	1	22	1	370
Sticks (48 pretzels)	110	1	0	23	1	430
Thin Twist (10 pretzels)	110	1	0	22	1	510
Tiny Twist (18 pretzels)	110	1	0	22	1	420
Tom Sturgis Old Fashioned Pretzels, Cheese (1 oz = about 5 pretzels)	120	2	1	23	2	500
The Fat Free Gourmet Pretzels, Sourdough (1 oz)	120	1	0	26	0	560
Sourdough, Unsalted (1 oz)	114	1	0	23	<1	60
Ultra Slim-Fast Lite N' Tasty Pretzel Twists (1 oz = 16 pretzels)	110	2	0	22	3	420

Pretzels (continued)	Calories	Fat g	Saturated Fat g	Carbohydrate g	Fiber g	Sodium mg
Weight Watchers Smart Snackers, Oat Bran Pretzel Nuggets (1.5 oz)	170	3	0	33	3	250

OTHER SNACKS

	Calories	Fat g	Saturated Fat g	Carbohydrate g	Fiber g	Sodium mg
Burns & Ricker Fat Free Party Mix (¾ cup)	120	0	0	23	1	210

SOUPS

The foods included in this section of the Guide are low in fat and saturated fat *as purchased* or when *prepared as indicated in the Guide*. One serving of these foods does not exceed the cutoff points of 3 grams of fat and 1 gram of saturated fat. Some cream soups are not listed in the Guide because the package directions include the addition of whole milk. However, these soups may not exceed the cutoff points when water, skim milk, or ½% or 1% low-fat milk is substituted for whole milk.

Bean Soups	Calories	Fat g	Saturated Fat g	Carbohydrate g	Fiber g	Sodium mg
BEAN SOUPS						
Aunt Patsy's Pantry Soup, Many Bean, prep w/onions, canned tomatoes & tomato sauce (1 cup)	200	1	0	39	7	.816
Buckeye Beans & Herbs Soup, Veggie Bean, prep w/onions, canned tomatoes & tomato sauce (1 cup)	200	1	0	39	7	816
Campbell's Soups, Black Bean, condensed, prep w/water (1 cup)	120	2	1	19	5	1,030
Chunky, Old Fashioned Bean 'N Ham, ready-to-serve (1 cup)	190	2	1	29	9	880
Old Fashioned Bean 'N Ham, ready-to-serve (11 oz can)	240	3	1	37	11	1,130
Home Cookin' Soups, Bean & Ham, ready-to-serve (1 cup)	180	2	1	33	9	720
Bean & Ham, ready-to-serve (10 ¾ oz can)	230	2	1	41	11	890
Health Valley Soups, Black Bean (1 cup)	110	0	0	28	10	290
No Salt (1 cup)	110	0	0	28	10	45

	Calories	Fat g	Saturated Fat g	Carbohydrate g	Fiber g	Sodium mg
Fat-Free Soup, Black Bean Vegetable (1 cup)	110	0	0	24	12	280
Five Bean Vegetable (1 cup)	140	0	0	32	13	250
Healthy Choice Soup, Bean & Ham (1 cup)	180	3	1	34	10	460
N.K. Hurst 15 Bean Soups, Beef (3 tbsp dry)	160	1	0	27	1	360
Cajun (3 tbsp dry)	160	1	0	27	1	140
Chicken (3 tbsp dry)	160	1	0	27	1	380
Chili (3 tbsp dry)	160	1	0	27	1	240
Ham (3 tbsp dry)	160	1	0	26	1	90
Nile Spice Soups, Black Bean (1.9 oz dry pkg)	190	2	0	34	2	570
Red Beans & Rice (1.8 oz dry pkg)	190	2	0	36	3	560
Old El Paso Soup, Black Bean w/Bacon (1 cup)	160	2	1	26	7	960
Progresso Soups, Bean & Ham (1 cup)	160	2	1	25	8	870
Hearty Black Bean (1 cup)	170	2	0	30	10	730
BEEF SOUPS						
Campbell's Soups, Beef Noodle, condensed, prep w/water (1 cup)	70	3	1	8	1	920
Beefy Mushroom, condensed, prep w/water (1 cup)	70	3	1	6	1	1,000
Chunky, Beef Pasta, ready-to-serve (1 cup)	150	3	1	18	2	970
Beef Pepper, ready-to-serve (1 cup)	140	3	1	18	3	830
Healthy Choice Soups, Beef & Potato (1 cup)	120	2	1	18	3	440
Chili Beef (1 cup)	190	1	0	33	18	490
Lipton Soups, Recipe Secrets, Beefy Mushroom (2 tbsp dry)	35	0	0	7	0	650
BROTHS AND CONSOMMÉS						
Campbell's Soups, Chicken Broth, condensed, prep w/water (1 cup)	30	2	1	2	0	770
Chicken Broth, Low Sodium, ready-to-serve (1 cup)	25	2	1	1	<1	60
Ready-to-serve (1 cup)	15	1	0	0	0	820
Consommé Beef Soup, condensed, prep w/water (1 cup)	25	0	0	2	0	820

	Calories	Fat g	Saturated Fat g	Carbohydrate g	Fiber g	Sodium mg
Campbell's (continued)						
Double Rich Double Strength Beef Broth, condensed, prep w/water (1 cup)	15	0	0	1	0	900
Healthy Request, Chicken Broth, ready-to-serve (1 cup)	20	0	0	1	0	480
College Inn Broth, Beef (1 cup)	20	0	0	0	0	1,140
Lower Sodium (1 cup)	20	0	0	0	0	620
Chicken, Lower Sodium (1 cup)	25	2	1	0	0	640
Health Valley Broth, Chicken (1 cup)	35	0	0	0	0	250
No Salt (1 cup)	35	0	0	0	0	75
Fat-Free Broth, Beef (1 cup)	20	0	0	0	0	160
No Salt (1 cup)	20	0	0	0	0	70
Chicken (1 cup)	30	0	0	0	0	170
Herb-Ox Bouillon Cubes, Beef (1 cube)	10	0	0	1	0	700
Chicken (1 cube)	10	0	0	1	0	1,040
Vegetable (1 cube)	10	0	0	1	0	1,000
Instant Bouillon Powder, Beef (1 tsp dry)	10	0	0	1	0	750
Chicken (1 tsp dry)	10	0	0	1	0	1,040
Instant Broth & Seasoning Packet, Beef (1 pkt)	10	0	0	1	0	900
Low Sodium (1 pkt)	15	0	0	2	0	5
Chicken (1 pkt)	10	0	0	1	0	760
Low Sodium (1 pkt)	15	0	0	1	0	20
Lipton Soups, Recipe Secrets, Italian Herb (1 tbsp dry)	40	0	0	8	1	520
Savory Herb w/Garlic (1 tbsp dry)	30	1	0	6	0	460
Recipe Soup Mix, Golden Herb w/Lemon (2 tbsp dry)	35	1	0	7	0	510
Pepperidge Farm Consommé Madrilene (2/3 cup)	50	1	0	6	0	910
Pritikin Broth, Chicken (1 cup)	15	0	0	1	0	290
Vegetable (1 cup)	10	0	0	2	0	290
Swanson Broth, Chicken (1 cup)	20	1	0	1	0	860
Clear Beef (1 cup)	20	1	1	1	0	820
Clear Chicken (1 cup)	30	2	1	1	0	1,000
Natural Goodness Clear Chicken (1 cup)	15	0	0	1	0	560
Vegetable (1 cup)	20	1	0	3	0	1,000

Broths and Consommés (continued)	Calories	Fat g	Saturated Fat g	Carbohydrate g	Fiber g	Sodium mg
Weight Watchers Instant Broth Mix, Beef (.16 oz dry)	10	0	0	0	0	820
Chicken (.16 oz dry)	10	0	0	1	0	900
CHICKEN SOUPS						
Campbell's Soups, Chicken & Stars, condensed, prep w/water (1 cup)	70	2	1	9	1	1,010
Chicken Alphabet w/Vegetables, condensed, prep w/water (1 cup)	80	2	1	11	1	880
Chicken Gumbo, condensed, prep w/water (1 cup)	60	2	1	9	1	990
Chicken Noodle O's, condensed, prep w/water (1 cup)	80	3	1	10	1	980
Chicken Noodle, condensed, prep w/water (1 cup)	70	3	1	9	1	950
Ready-to-serve (7¼ oz can)	60	2	1	8	1	870
Chicken Won Ton, condensed, prep w/water (1 cup)	45	1	0	5	1	940
Chicken w/Rice, condensed, prep w/water (1 cup)	70	3	1	9	0	830
Ready-to-serve (7¼ oz can)	50	2	1	5	0	780
Chicken w/Wild Rice, condensed, prep w/water (1 cup)	70	2	1	9	1	900
Healthy Request, Chicken Corn Chowder, ready-to-serve (1 cup)	140	3	1	22	2	480
Chicken Noodle, condensed, prep w/water (1 cup)	70	3	1	8	1	480
Chicken w/Rice, condensed, prep w/water (1 cup)	70	3	1	9	<1	480
Cream of Chicken, condensed, prep w/water (1 cup)	80	3	1	11	0	480
Hearty Chicken Rice, ready-to-serve (1 cup)	120	3	1	17	0	480
Home Cookin', Chicken Rice, ready-to-serve (1 cup)	115	3	1	15	2	770
Microwave Soups, Chicken Rice, ready-to-serve (10½ oz container)	120	3	1	20	2	1,130
Quality Soup Mix, Chicken Noodle w/White Meat (3 tbsp dry)	90	2	1	15	0	650
Healthy Choice Soups, Chicken Corn Chowder (1 cup)	150	3	1	27	7	430

	Calories	Fat g	Saturated Fat g	Carbohydrate g	Fiber g	Sodium mg
Healthy Choice *(continued)*						
Chicken Noodle (1 cup)	130	2	1	21	2	460
Hearty Chicken (1 cup)	140	3	1	20	3	480
Lipton Soups, Cup-A-Soup, Chicken Noodle, prep w/water (6 fl oz)	50	1	1	8	0	570
Cream of Chicken, prep w/ water (6 fl oz)	70	3	1	11	0	650
Hearty Chicken Noodle, prep w/water (6 fl oz)	60	1	1	10	0	540
Soup Mix, Chicken Noodle Hearty Soup, prep w/water (1 cup)	80	1	1	14	<1	660
Chicken Noodle Soup w/Chicken, prep w/water (8 fl oz)	80	3	1	12	0	650
Lunch Bucket Soups, Chicken Fiesta (7 1/2 oz container)	160	2	1	30	5	530
Chicken Noodle (7 1/4 oz container)	80	2	1	13	0	830
Old El Paso Soup, Chicken w/Rice (1 cup)	90	3	1	10	0	680
Pritikin Soups, Chicken & Rice (1 cup)	80	1	0	13	2	250
Chicken Pasta (1 cup)	100	1	0	18	1	290
Progresso Soups, Chicken & Wild Rice (1 cup)	100	2	1	15	2	820
Chicken Barley (1 cup)	110	3	1	14	3	720
Chicken Noodle (1 cup)	80	2	1	8	1	730
Chicken Rice & Vegetable (1 cup)	110	3	1	12	<1	750
Healthy Classics, Chicken Noodle (1 cup)	80	2	1	10	1	480
Chicken Rice w/Vegetables (1 cup)	90	2	0	12	1	450
Hearty Chicken & Rotini (1 cup)	90	2	1	8	0	860
Hearty Penne Pasta in Chicken Broth (1 cup)	70	1	0	11	0	930
Tortellini in Chicken Broth (1 cup)	80	2	1	10	2	750
Weight Watchers Soups, Chicken Noodle (10.5 oz can)	80	1	0	11	7	950
Chicken Noodle (7.5 oz tub)	80	1	0	13	0	450

CLAM CHOWDERS

Higher-Fat

	Calories	Fat g	Saturated Fat g	Carbohydrate g	Fiber g	Sodium mg
New England Clam Chowder, condensed, prep w/whole milk (1 cup)	161	7	3	16	1	980

	Calories	Fat g	Saturated Fat g	Carbohydrate g	Fiber g	Sodium mg
Lower-Fat						
**Campbell's Soups, Manhattan Style Clam Chowder, condensed, prep w/water (1 cup)	70	2	1	12	2	910
New England Clam Chowder Seashore Soup, condensed, prep w/water (1 cup)	90	3	1	13	1	970
Progresso Soups, Healthy Classics, New England Clam Chowder (1 cup)	120	2	1	20	1	530
Manhattan Clam Chowder (1 cup)	110	2	0	11	3	710
Weight Watchers New England Clam Chowder (7.5 oz)	90	0	0	16	2	330
LENTIL SOUPS						
Aunt Patsy's Pantry Red Lentil Soup, prep w/onions & tomatoes (1 cup)	220	1	0	42	6	792
Campbell's Home Cookin' Soups, Hearty Lentil, ready-to-serve (1 cup)	150	2	1	26	5	860
Ready-to-serve (10¾ oz can)	190	3	0	33	6	1,070
Health Valley Fat-Free Soups, Lentil & Carrot (1 cup)	90	0	0	25	14	220
Organic Soups, Lentil (1 cup)	90	0	0	20	9	240
No Salt (1 cup)	90	0	0	20	9	40
Pritikin Soup, Lentil (1 cup)	130	1	0	24	8	280
Progresso Soups, Healthy Classics, Lentil (1 cup)	130	2	0	20	6	440
Lentil & Shells (1 cup)	130	2	0	22	4	840
Lentil (1 cup)	140	2	0	22	7	750
Lentil (10.5 oz)	170	3	0	27	8	930
Ultra Slim-Fast Low Fat Lunch Soup, Lentil (15 oz can)	230	3	1	40	3	990
MINESTRONE SOUPS						
Campbell's Soups, Healthy Request, Hearty Minestrone, ready-to-serve (1 cup)	120	2	1	24	3	480
Minestrone, condensed, prep w/water (1 cup)	90	1	1	17	2	480
Home Cookin, Minestrone, ready-to-serve (1 cup)	120	2	1	19	3	990
Minestrone, condensed, prep w/water (1 cup)	100	2	1	16	4	960

	Calories	Fat g	Saturated Fat g	Carbohydrate g	Fiber g	Sodium mg
Health Valley Fat-Free Soup, Minestrone (1 cup)	80	0	0	21	11	210
Organic Soups, Minestrone (1 cup)	90	0	0	23	10	190
No Salt (1 cup)	90	0	0	23	10	115
Healthy Choice Soup, Minestrone (1 cup)	110	2	1	21	3	470
Pritikin Minestrone Soup (1 cup)	90	1	0	19	3	290
Progresso Soups, Healthy Classics, Minestrone (1 cup)	120	3	0	20	1	510
Hearty Minestrone w/Shells (1 cup)	120	2	0	20	4	700
Minestrone (1 cup)	130	3	1	19	5	850
Ultra Slim-Fast Low Fat Lunch Soup, Minestrone (15 oz can)	240	3	1	45	8	890
MUSHROOM SOUPS						
Higher-Fat						
Cream of Mushroom Soup, prep w/whole milk (1 cup)	204	14	5	15	0	1,076
Lower-Fat						
Campbell's Soups, Golden Mushroom, condensed, prep w/water (1 cup)	80	3	1	10	1	930
Healthy Request Cream of Mushroom, condensed, prep w/water (1 cup)	70	3	1	9	1	480
Health Valley Organic Soups, Mushroom Barley (1 cup)	60	0	0	15	8	220
No Salt (1 cup)	60	0	0	15	8	95
Lipton Cup-A-Soup, Creamy Mushroom, prep w/water (6 fl oz)	60	3	1	9	<1	610
Weight Watchers Soup, Cream of Mushroom (10.5 oz can)	70	1	0	15	1	1,260
NOODLE SOUPS						
Higher-Fat						
Ramen Noodle Soup (1 cup)	188	7	2	27	1	978
Lower-Fat						
Campbell's Soups, Cup-A-Soup, Ring Noodle, prep w/water (6 fl oz)	50	<1	0	9	<1	560
Curly Noodle w/Chicken Broth, condensed, prep w/water (1 cup)	80	3	1	12	1	840
Double Noodle in Chicken Broth, condensed, prep w/water (1 cup)	100	3	1	15	2	810

	Calories	Fat g	Saturated Fat g	Carbohydrate g	Fiber g	Sodium mg
Lowfat Ramen Noodle (1/2 block)	150	1	0	31	1	780
Quality Soup Mix, Noodle Soup w/Real Chicken Broth (3 tbsp dry)	100	2	1	18	1	790
Teddy Bear Pasta Shapes, condensed, prep w/water (1 cup)	80	2	1	12	2	840
Lipton Soup Mixes, Giggle Noodle w/Real Chicken Broth, prep w/water (8 fl oz)	80	2	1	11	0	730
Harvest Noodle, prep w/water (8 fl oz)	70	1	0	12	1	650
Hearty Noodle w/Vegetables or Ring-O-Noodle w/Real Chicken Broth, prep w/water (8 fl oz)	70	2	1	11	0	710
Noodle Soup w/Real Chicken Broth, prep w/water (8 fl oz)	60	2	1	9	0	710
ONION SOUPS						
Campbell's Soups, French Onion made w/Beef Stock, condensed, prep w/water (1 cup)	70	3	0	10	1	980
Quality Soup N' Recipe Mixes, Onion (1 tbsp dry)	25	0	0	5	0	660
Onion w/Chicken Broth (2 tbsp dry)	50	1	0	10	1	680
Lipton Recipe Secrets, Beefy Onion (1 tbsp dry)	25	1	0	5	0	610
Golden Onion (2 tbsp dry)	60	2	0	10	0	650
Onion Mushroom (2 tbsp dry)	35	1	0	6	0	620
Onion Recipe (1 tbsp dry)	20	0	0	4	0	610
Pepperidge Farm Soup, French Onion made w/Beef Stock (2/3 cup)	50	1	1	7	1	1,080
PEA SOUPS						
Aunt Patsy's Pantry, Plentiful Pea Soup, prep w/onions (1 cup)	210	1	0	39	5	768
Campbell's Soups, Chunky, Split Pea N' Ham, ready-to-serve (1 cup)	190	3	1	27	3	1,120
Healthy Request Soup, Split Pea w/Ham, ready-to-serve (1 cup)	170	3	1	27	6	480
Home Cookin' Soups, Split Pea w/Ham, ready-to-serve (1 cup)	170	2	1	30	6	880
Split Pea w/Ham, ready-to-serve (10 3/4 oz can)	210	2	1	37	8	1,100

	Calories	Fat g	Saturated Fat g	Carbohydrate g	Fiber g	Sodium mg
Campbell's *(continued)*						
Green Pea, condensed, prep w/water (1 cup)	180	3	1	29	5	890
Health Valley Fat-Free Soup, Split Pea & Carrot (1 cup)	110	0	0	17	4	230
Organic Soups, Split Pea (1 cup)	110	0	0	23	8	160
No Salt (1 cup)	110	0	0	23	8	115
Healthy Choice Soup, Split Pea & Ham (1 cup)	160	2	1	26	5	470
Pritikin Soup, Split Pea (1 cup)	140	1	0	29	10	290
Progresso Soups, Green Split Pea (1 cup)	170	3	1	25	5	870
Healthy Classics Soup, Split Pea (1 cup)	180	3	1	30	5	420
Real Fresh Soups, Split Pea (1 cup)	130	0	0	24	<1	740
Split Pea w/Bacon (1 cup)	140	1	0	22	<1	760
Ultra Slim-Fast Low Fat Lunch Soup, Split Pea (15 oz can)	230	3	1	42	8	1,270
TOMATO SOUPS						
Campbell's Soups, Healthy Request Soup, Tomato, condensed, prep w/water (1 cup)	90	2	1	18	1	460
Homestyle Cream of Tomato, condensed, prep w/water (1 cup)	110	3	1	21	1	860
Italian Tomato w/Basil & Oregano, condensed, prep w/water (1 cup)	100	1	0	23	2	820
Old Fashioned Tomato Rice, condensed, prep w/water (1 cup)	120	2	1	23	1	790
Tomato, condensed, prep w/water (1 cup)	100	2	0	18	2	730
Ready-to-serve (7¼ oz can)	110	2	1	21	2	790
Health Valley Organic Soups, Tomato (1 cup)	90	0	0	22	4	250
No Salt (1 cup)	90	0	0	22	4	25
Healthy Choice Soup, Tomato Garden (1 cup)	110	2	1	19	3	430
Lipton Cup-A-Soup, Tomato, prep w/water (6 fl oz)	90	2	1	19	1	490
Progresso Soups, Hearty Tomato & Rotini (1 cup)	90	1	0	16	3	820
Tomato (1 cup)	90	2	0	15	4	990

	Calories	Fat g	Saturated Fat g	Carbohydrate g	Fiber g	Sodium mg
TURKEY SOUPS						
Campbell's Soups, Healthy Request, Turkey Vegetable w/Wild Rice, ready-to-serve (1 cup)	120	3	1	17	2	480
Turkey Noodle, condensed, prep w/water (1 cup)	80	3	1	10	1	970
Turkey Vegetable, condensed, prep w/water (1 cup)	80	3	1	11	2	840
Healthy Choice Soup, Turkey w/White & Wild Rice (1 cup)	110	3	1	18	3	410
VEGETABLE SOUPS						
Higher-Fat						
Corn Chowder, prep w/whole milk (1 cup)	269	15	5	27	3	678
Lower-Fat						
Campbell's Soups, Beef w/Vegetables & Barley, condensed, prep w/water (1 cup)	80	2	1	11	2	920
Chicken Vegetable, condensed, prep w/water (1 cup)	80	2	1	12	2	940
Chunky Vegetable, ready-to-serve (1 cup)	130	3	1	22	4	870
Healthy Request, Cream of Broccoli, condensed, prep w/water (1 cup)	70	2	1	9	1	480
Cream of Celery, condensed, prep w/water (1 cup)	70	2	1	11	1	480
Hearty Chicken Vegetable, ready-to-serve (1 cup)	120	3	1	17	2	480
Hearty Vegetable Beef, ready-to-serve (1 cup)	140	3	1	20	3	480
Hearty Vegetable, condensed, prep w/water (1 cup)	90	1	1	16	2	480
Ready-to-serve (1 cup)	100	1	0	20	2	470
Southwest Style Vegetable, ready-to-serve (1 cup)	150	2	1	28	5	480
Tomato Vegetable, ready-to-serve (1 cup)	120	2	1	22	3	480
Vegetable Beef, condensed, prep w/water (1 cup)	80	2	1	11	2	480
Vegetable, condensed, prep w/water (1 cup)	90	2	1	15	2	480

	Calories	Fat g	Saturated Fat g	Carbohydrate g	Fiber g	Sodium mg
Campbell *(continued)*						
Hearty Vegetable w/Pasta, condensed, prep w/water (1 cup)	90	1	0	18	2	830
Home Cookin', Country Vegetable, ready-to-serve (1 cup)	110	1	0	19	2	760
Country Vegetable, ready-to-serve (10 ³/₄ oz can)	130	2	0	26	2	940
Southwestern Vegetable, ready-to-serve (1 cup)	130	3	1	24	4	750
Vegetable Beef, ready-to-serve (1 cup)	120	2	1	18	3	1,010
Homestyle Vegetable, condensed, prep w/water (1 cup)	70	2	1	10	2	970
Microwave Soups, Vegetable Beef, ready-to-serve (7 ³/₄ oz container)	90	2	1	13	2	780
Vegetable, ready-to-serve (7 ³/₄ oz container)	100	2	1	17	2	850
Old Fashioned Vegetable, condensed, prep w/water (1 cup)	70	3	1	10	2	950
Quality Soup N' Recipe Mix, Vegetable (2 tbsp dry)	35	0	0	7	0	650
Vegetable Beef, condensed, prep w/water (1 cup)	80	2	1	10	2	810
Vegetable, Low Sodium, ready-to-serve (7 ¹/₄ oz can)	90	2	1	14	2	30
Condensed, prep w/water (1 cup)	90	1	0	17	2	750
Ready-to-serve (7 ¹/₄ oz can)	70	2	1	12	1	730
Vegetarian Vegetable, condensed, prep w/water (1 cup)	70	1	0	14	2	770
Health Valley Soups, Fat-Free Soups, Carotene Vegetable Power (1 cup)	70	0	0	17	6	240
Country Corn & Vegetable (1 cup)	70	0	0	17	7	135
Garden Vegetable (1 cup)	80	0	0	17	4	250
Italian Plus Carotene (1 cup)	80	0	0	19	6	240
Tomato Vegetable (1 cup)	80	0	0	17	5	240
Vegetable Barley (1 cup)	90	0	0	19	4	210
Organic Soups, Potato Leek (1 cup)	70	0	0	15	3	230
No Salt (1 cup)	70	0	0	15	3	35
Vegetable (1 cup)	80	0	0	18	6	230
No Salt (1 cup)	80	0	0	18	6	80

	Calories	Fat g	Saturated Fat g	Carbohydrate g	Fiber g	Sodium mg
Super Broccoli Carotene (1 cup)	70	0	0	16	7	240
Healthy Choice Soups, Vegetable Beef (1 cup)	170	2	1	32	8	430
Country Vegetable (1 cup)	100	1	1	22	6	420
Garden Vegetable (1 cup)	110	1	1	22	6	450
Hormel Micro Cup, Beef Vegetable (1 cup)	90	1	0	14	2	740
Lipton Soups, Cup-A-Soup, Chicken Vegetable, prep w/water (6 fl oz)	50	1	1	9	<1	510
Hearty Harvest Vegetable, prep w/water (6 fl oz)	90	2	1	17	2	450
Spring Vegetable, prep w/water (6 fl oz)	50	1	1	9	<1	470
Recipe Secrets, Vegetable (3 tbsp dry)	30	0	0	7	1	580
Lunch Bucket Country Vegetable (7 1/4 oz container)	60	1	0	14	3	750
Nile Spice Soup, Chicken Flavored Vegetable (1.1 oz pkg)	120	2	1	20	1	600
Old El Paso Soups, Chicken Vegetable (1 cup)	110	3	1	13	0	620
Garden Vegetable (1 cup)	110	3	1	17	0	710
Pepperidge Farm Soup, Gazpacho (2/3 cup)	70	2	0	12	2	1,050
Pritikin Soups, Hearty Vegetable (1 cup)	90	1	0	20	3	290
Vegetarian Vegetable (1 cup)	100	0	0	23	3	290
Progresso Soups, Broccoli & Shells (1 cup)	70	1	0	14	3	720
Chicken, Vegetables & Penne Pasta (1 cup)	100	3	1	11	3	780
Escarole in Chicken Broth (1 cup)	25	1	0	2	0	980
Healthy Classics, Beef Vegetable (1 cup)	150	2	1	25	6	410
Cream of Broccoli (1 cup)	90	3	1	13	2	580
Garlic & Pasta (1 cup)	100	2	0	18	3	450
Tomato Garden Vegetable (1 cup)	100	1	0	19	4	480
Vegetable (1 cup)	80	2	0	13	1	470
Hearty Vegetable w/Rotini (1 cup)	110	1	0	20	3	720
Homestyle Chicken & Vegetable (1 cup)	100	3	1	10	1	680
Vegetable (1 cup)	90	2	1	15	3	850
Ultra Slim-Fast Low Fat Lunch Soup, Vegetable Bean (15 oz can)	240	3	1	42	8	990
Weight Watchers Soup, Vegetable Beef (7.5 oz)	80	1	0	13	0	450

Other Soups	Calories	Fat g	Saturated Fat g	Carbohydrate g	Fiber g	Sodium mg
OTHER SOUPS						
Higher-Fat						
Cheese Soup, condensed, prep w/whole milk (1 cup)	230	15	9	16	0	1,020
Lower-Fat						
Pepperidge Farm Crab Soup (²/₃ cup)	80	2	1	9	2	1,150

SWEETS AND TOPPINGS

Many products in this section of the Guide, such as jelly, syrup, and low-fat candy, are made primarily of sugar. Candy that contains chocolate, nuts, peanut butter, and/or caramel is high in fat. When sweets are eaten, it should be in addition to well-balanced meals and not as a replacement for foods needed for good health. One serving of the foods included in this section of the Guide provides a maximum of 3 grams of fat and 1 gram of saturated fat.

Candies	Calories	Fat g	Saturated Fat g	Carbohydrate g	Fiber g	Sodium mg
CANDIES						
Higher-Fat						
Chocolate-Coated Caramels (7, each ¾"diam)	183	8	5	27	0	65
Chocolate-Coated Coconut Candy Bars (2 snack size)	185	10	7	22	3	49
Chocolate-Coated Nougat w/Peanuts & Caramel (2.1 oz regular size bar)	271	13	7	36	2	130
Milk Chocolate Bar w/Almonds (1.5 oz bar)	216	14	7	22	3	30
Peanut Roll (1.4 oz)	204	13	2	19	2	112
Candy-Coated Chocolate Pieces (3 tbsp)	186	9	5	27	1	40
Chocolate-Coated Peanut Butter Cups (5 miniature)	192	12	6	19	2	113
Lower-Fat						
Most Brands, Candy Corn (40 pieces)	142	0	0	37	0	125
Gumdrops (1.4 oz)	153	0	0	39	0	17
Hard Candy (1.4 oz)	148	0	0	39	0	15
Marshmallows (6 regular)	137	0	0	35	0	20
Mints, uncoated (1.4 oz)	142	0	0	37	0	16

	Calories	Fat g	Saturated Fat g	Carbohydrate g	Fiber g	Sodium mg
Amazin' Fruit Gummy Bears (17 pieces)	130	0	0	31	0	45
Brach's Butterscotch Disks (3 pieces)	70	0	0	17	0	95
Candy Corn (26 pieces)	140	0	0	36	0	80
Cinnamon Imperials (52 pieces)	60	0	0	15	0	0
Dessert Mint (37 pieces)	160	0	0	40	0	30
Jelly Beans (14 pieces)	140	0	0	36	0	0
Kentucky Mints (17 pieces)	150	1	0	37	0	0
Lemon Drops (4 pieces)	70	0	0	16	0	5
Orange Slices (2 pieces)	130	0	0	32	0	20
Red Twists (5 pieces)	160	1	0	35	1	10
Sour Balls (3 pieces)	70	0	0	17	0	10
Sparkies (3 pieces)	70	0	0	17	0	30
Star Brites Peppermint Starlight Mints (3 pieces)	60	0	0	15	0	10
Estee Sugar Free Candies, Gum Drops (23 pieces)	140	0	0	36	0	0
Tropical Fruit Hard Candy (5 candies)	60	0	0	16	0	0
Jelly Belly 38 Flavor Assortment, Blueberry, Chocolate Fudge, Chocolate Pudding, Coconut, Jalapeno, Licorice, Strawberry Cheese Cake, Strawberry Daiquiri, Tangerine, Toasted Marshmallow, Top Banana or Tutti Fruitti (2 tbsp)	150	0	0	37	0	10
A&W Cream Soda, Butterscotch or Pineapple (2 tbsp)	150	0	0	37	0	20
A&W Root Beer, Champagne Punch, Green Apple, Ice Blue Mint, Mai Tai, Peach, Polynesian Punch, Raspberry or Sizzling Cinnamon (2 tbsp)	150	0	0	37	0	0
Black Forest Cake, Juicy Pear, Lemon or Pink Grapefruit (2 tbsp)	150	0	0	36	0	10
Bubble Gum (2 tbsp)	150	0	0	38	0	5
Buttered Popcorn, Lemon Lime, Orange Sherbet or Totally Mint (2 tbsp)	150	0	0	37	0	15
Cantaloupe, Grape Jelly, Pina Colada, Sassy Sours, Very Cherry or Wildberry (2 tbsp)	150	0	0	37	0	5
Cinnamon or Orange (2 tbsp)	150	0	0	37	0	25
Cotton Candy (2 tbsp)	150	0	0	37	0	30

	Calories	Fat g	Saturated Fat g	Carbohydrate g	Fiber g	Sodium mg
Island Punch or Peanut Butter (2 tbsp)	150	0	0	36	0	20
Watermelon (2 tbsp)	150	0	0	38	0	25
Kraft Butter Mints or Party Mints (7 pieces)	60	0	0	14	0	25
Caramels (5 pieces)	170	3	1	32	0	110
Nibs Bits, Cherry (22 pieces)	140	1	0	31	0	85
Licorice (22 pieces)	140	1	0	31	0	220
Panda All Natural Licorice, Bar (1 bar)	110	0	0	25	0	65
Chews (15 pieces)	135	0	0	31	0	80
All Natural Raspberry, Bar (1 bar)	115	0	0	26	0	65
Chews (15 pieces)	145	0	0	33	0	80
Pearson Coffee Nips (2 pieces)	60	2	1	12	0	45
Skittles Bite Size Candies, Original or Tart-N-Tangy (2.2 oz bag)	250	3	1	55	0	10
Tropical or Wild Berry (2.2 oz)	250	3	1	56	0	10
Starburst Fruit Chews, California, Original, Strawberry or Tropical Fruits (8 pieces)	160	3	1	33	0	20
Twizzlers Bites, Cherry (18 pieces)	140	1	0	31	0	120
Licorice (18 pieces)	130	1	0	31	0	210
Pull 'N' Peel, Cherry (1 pkg)	130	1	0	29	1	105
Strings, Strawberry (3 pieces)	150	0	0	35	0	100
Twists, Cherry (3 pieces)	120	1	0	27	0	105
Chocolate (5 pieces)	140	1	1	31	0	160
Licorice (3 pieces)	130	1	0	31	0	210
Strawberry (3 pieces)	130	1	0	31	0	100
Willy Wonka "New" Tart'N Tinys, Nerds or Sweet & Sour Hearts (1 tbsp)	60	0	0	14	0	0
Dinasour Eggs (10 pieces)	60	0	0	15	0	0
Egg Breakers or Gobstoppers (6 pieces)	60	0	0	15	0	0
Freckled Eggs (9 pieces)	50	0	0	13	0	0
Fruit Runts (15 pieces)	60	0	0	14	0	0
Goliath-Secret Centers (1 piece)	40	0	0	10	0	0
Heart Breakers (8 pieces)	60	0	0	15	NA	0
Merry Mix (11 pieces)	60	0	0	14	NA	0
Runts Mini Hearts (17 pieces)	60	0	0	14	NA	0
Wacky Wafer Bunnys (14 pieces)	60	0	0	15	NA	0

	Calories	Fat g	Saturated Fat g	Carbohydrate g	Fiber g	Sodium mg
HONEY						
Most Brands, Honey (1 tbsp)	64	0	0	18	0	1
Sue Bee Honey (1 tbsp)	60	0	0	17	0	0
JAMS, JELLIES, AND PRESERVES						
Most Brands, Fruit Spreads, Jams, Preserves or Marmalade (1 tbsp)	48	0	0	13	0	8
Jellies (1 tbsp)	45	0	0	12	0	7
America's Choice Jelly, Pure Apple or Pure Grape (1 tbsp)	60	0	0	14	0	10
Marmalade, Pure Orange (1 tbsp)	50	0	0	13	0	10
Pure Preserves, Apricot, Peach, Pineapple or Strawberry (1 tbsp)	50	0	0	13	0	10
Grape or Raspberry (1 tbsp)	60	0	0	14	0	10
Estee Low Calorie Fruit Spread, Apple Spice, Grape or Strawberry (1 tbsp)	10	0	0	2	0	20
Apricot (1 tbsp)	5	0	0	1	0	20
Gedney Minnesota State Fair Preserves, Apricot, Double Berry or Red Raspberry (1 tbsp)	50	0	0	12	NA	0
Strawberry (1 tbsp)	45	0	0	12	NA	0
Kraft Jams, Grape or Red Plum (1 tbsp)	60	0	0	14	0	10
Strawberry (1 tbsp)	50	0	0	13	0	10
Jellies, Apple or Strawberry (1 tbsp)	60	0	0	14	0	10
Apple-Strawberry, Blackberry, Grape, Guava or Red Currant (1 tbsp)	50	0	0	13	0	10
Marmalade, Orange (1 tbsp)	50	0	0	14	0	10
Preserves, Apricot, Red Raspberry or Strawberry (1 tbsp)	50	0	0	13	0	10
Blackberry (1 tbsp)	50	0	0	13	<1	10
Peach or Pineapple (1 tbsp)	50	0	0	14	<1	10
Reduced Calorie Fruit Spread, Grape or Strawberry (1 tbsp)	20	0	0	5	0	20
Smucker's Apple Butter, Autumn Harvest, Cider, Natural or Simply Fruit (1 tbsp)	36	0	0	9	NA	0
Extra Fruit Spread (1 tbsp)	45	0	0	9	0	0
Jellies (1 tbsp)	60	0	0	14	0	0

Jams, Jellies, and Preserves (continued)	Calories	Fat g	Saturated Fat g	Carbohydrate g	Fiber g	Sodium mg
Orange Marmalade, Preserves or Jams (1 tbsp)	50	0	0	13	0	0
Light Fruit Spreads or Slenderella Reduced Calorie Fruit Spread (1 tbsp)	21	0	0	6	NA	0
Low Sugar Spreads (1 tbsp)	25	0	0	6	0	0
Peach Butter (1 tbsp)	45	0	0	12	0	0
Pumpkin Butter, Autumn Harvest (1 tbsp)	36	0	0	9	NA	42
Simply Fruit Spreads (1 tbsp)	48	0	0	12	NA	0
Weight Watchers Fruit Spreads, Grape, Raspberry or Strawberry (1 tbsp)	24	0	0	6	0	0

MARSHMALLOWS

	Calories	Fat g	Saturated Fat g	Carbohydrate g	Fiber g	Sodium mg
Kraft Marshmallow Creme (2 tbsp)	100	0	0	27	0	30
Marshmallows, Funmallows (4 pieces)	110	0	0	26	0	20
Funmallows Miniature (1/2 cup)	100	0	0	25	0	20
Jet-Puffed (5 pieces)	110	0	0	25	0	30
Miniature (1/2 cup)	100	0	0	25	0	30
Teddy Bear Cocoa-Flavored (1/2 cup)	100	0	0	23	0	25

MOLASSES AND SYRUPS

	Calories	Fat g	Saturated Fat g	Carbohydrate g	Fiber g	Sodium mg
Most Brands, Molasses, Blackstrap (1 tbsp)	48	0	0	12	0	11
Light (1 tbsp)	55	0	0	14	0	8
Medium (1 tbsp)	55	0	0	14	0	8
Most Brands, Syrup, Maple, Pure (1/4 cup)	206	0	0	53	0	7
Pancake (1/4 cup)	221	0	0	60	0	95
America's Choice Syrups, Artificial Butter Flavor (1/4 cup)	220	0	0	54	0	60
Lite Reduced Calorie (1/4 cup)	100	0	0	26	0	115
Pancake & Waffle w/2% Real Maple Syrup (1/4 cup)	210	0	0	53	0	30
Strawberry (1/4 cup)	110	0	0	28	0	5
Aunt Jemima Syrups, Butter Rich (1/4 cup)	210	0	0	52	0	170
Butterlite (1/4 cup)	100	0	0	26	0	150
Lite (1/4 cup)	100	0	0	27	0	160
Pancake & Waffle (1/4 cup)	210	0	0	53	0	120
Brer Rabbit Molasses, Dark (1 tbsp)	50	0	0	14	0	10
Light (1 tbsp)	60	0	0	15	0	10
Syrup, Dark (1/4 cup)	240	0	0	61	0	5
Light (1/4 cup)	240	0	0	62	0	0

Molasses and Syrups (continued)	Calories	Fat g	Saturated Fat g	Carbohydrate g	Fiber g	Sodium mg
Estee Lite Syrup, Blueberry (¼ cup)	80	0	0	20	0	70
Maple (¼ cup)	80	0	0	20	0	125
Golden Griddle Syrup, Pancake (4 tbsp)	220	0	0	57	0	55
Hershey's Syrup, Chocolate (2 tbsp)	100	0	0	24	0	25
Strawberry (2 tbsp)	110	0	0	28	0	5
Hungry Jack Microwave Syrups, Butter Maple or Regular (¼ cup)	210	0	0	52	0	90
Butter Maple Lite or Lite (¼ cup)	100	0	0	24	<1	180
Karo Syrup, Dark or Light Corn (2 tbsp)	120	0	0	30	0	35-45
Pancake (4 tbsp)	240	0	0	60	0	130
Log Cabin Country Kitchen Syrup, Butter Flavored (¼ cup)	200	0	0	53	0	200
Lite Reduced Calorie (¼ cup)	100	0	0	26	0	160
Regular (¼ cup)	200	0	0	53	0	110
Lite Reduced Calorie Syrup (¼ cup)	100	0	0	26	0	180
Regular (¼ cup)	200	0	0	52	0	60
Mrs. Richardson's Syrup, Lite (¼ cup)	100	0	0	26	0	160
Smucker's Syrups, Fruit (2 tbsp)	100	0	0	26	NA	0
Sunrise Syrup, All Natural Syrup (¼ cup)	210	0	0	53	0	90
Vermont Maid Syrup, Lite (¼ cup)	100	0	0	26	<1	140
Regular (¼ cup)	210	0	0	53	0	25
Weight Watchers Syrup, Reduced Calorie (¼ cup)	110	0	0	27	0	150
SWEETENERS						
Most Brands, Sugar, Brown, packed (1 tsp)	17	0	0	4	0	2
Powdered Confectioners' (1 tsp)	10	0	0	2	0	0
White (1 tsp)	16	0	0	4	0	0
Most Brands, Sugar Substitutes, Aspartame (1 pkt)	4	0	0	1	0	0
Saccharin (1 pkt)	4	0	0	1	0	2
Sweet 'N Low Sugar Substitutes, Brown or White	0	0	0	0	0	0
Sweet Magic Calorie Free Sugar Substitute (1 pkt)	0	0	0	0	0	60
Sweet One Sugar Substitute (1 pkt)	0	0	0	0	1	0
Weight Watchers Sweetener Sugar Substitute (1 pkt)	4	0	0	1	0	30

	Calories	Fat g	Saturated Fat g	Carbohydrate g	Fiber g	Sodium mg
TOPPINGS						
Hershey's Fudge Toppings, Butterscotch Caramel (2 tbsp)	130	2	1	28	0	170
Chocolate Caramel (2 tbsp)	120	2	1	26	0	210
Double Chocolate (2 tbsp)	120	2	1	24	<1	75
Kraft Toppings, Artificially Flavored Butterscotch (2 tbsp)	130	2	1	28	0	150
Caramel (2 tbsp)	120	0	0	28	0	90
Chocolate Flavored (2 tbsp)	110	0	0	26	1	30
Pineapple (2 tbsp)	110	0	0	28	0	15
Strawberry (2 tbsp)	110	0	0	29	0	15
Smucker's Light Topping, Hot Fudge (2 tbsp)	90	0	0	23	2	92
Special Recipe Topping, Butterscotch Caramel (2 tbsp)	130	1	1	30	<1	70
Dark Chocolate Flavored (2 tbsp)	130	1	(1)	31	NA	45
Sundae Syrups, Caramel Flavored, Chocolate Flavored or Butterscotch (2 tbsp)	110	0	0	27	0	70
Strawberry (2 tbsp)	90	0	0	26	0	0
Toppings, Butterscotch Flavored (2 tbsp)	130	0	0	31	<1	110
Caramel Flavored (2 tbsp)	130	0	0	31	<1	110
Chocolate Flavored Syrup (2 tbsp)	130	0	0	27	0	35
Chocolate Fudge (2 tbsp)	130	2	1	28	1	60
Hot Caramel (2 tbsp)	120	3	1	29	0	60
Marshmallow (2 tbsp)	120	0	0	29	NA	0
Peanut Butter-Caramel (2 tbsp)	150	2	(0)	29	NA	120
Pecans in Syrup Topping (2 tbsp)	130	1	(0)	28	NA	0
Walnuts in Syrup Topping (2 tbsp)	130	1	(0)	27	NA	0
Pineapple (2 tbsp)	130	0	0	32	NA	0
Strawberry (2 tbsp)	100	0	0	26	0	0
Swiss Milk Chocolate Fudge (2 tbsp)	140	1	(0)	31	NA	70

VEGETABLES

Vegetables contain little or no fat or saturated fat unless an ingredient containing fat is added in preparation. Frying vegetables or seasoning them with fat adds approximately 2 grams of fat per ½ cup; frying potatoes in deep fat or dipping vegetables in batter (breading) and frying them adds approximately 4 grams of fat per ½-cup serving. Butter, bacon, bacon fat, salt pork, cream sauce, and cheese are high in fat and saturated fat and should not be added to vegetables. One serving of the products included in this section of the Guide does not exceed the cutoff points of 3 grams of fat and 1 gram of saturated fat. Fresh, frozen, canned, and dehydrated vegetables are listed separately in the Guide since they are found in different sections of the supermarket. Most of the fresh vegetables and many of the processed foods are listed as "most brands." Avocado and olives (which, technically, are fruits) are listed in the Fats section beginning on page 141.

The sodium values given for fresh vegetables are for foods that have not been salted. Although most plain frozen vegetables are unsalted, combination vegetables and vegetable mixes may be seasoned with salt. Many canned vegetables are high in sodium because of the salt and other sodium-containing compounds added in processing.

Canned Vegetables	Calories	Fat g	Saturated Fat g	Carbohydrate g	Fiber g	Sodium mg
CANNED VEGETABLES						
ARTICHOKES, CANNED						
Progresso Artichoke Hearts (2 pieces)	35	0	0	6	1	240
ASPARAGUS, CANNED						
Asparagus, drained (½ cup spears)	23	1	0	3	3	472
No Salt Added, drained (½ cup)	34	1	0	6	2	5

Canned Vegetables (continued)

	Calories	Fat g	Saturated Fat g	Carbohydrate g	Fiber g	Sodium mg
BAMBOO SHOOTS, CANNED						
Bamboo Shoots, drained (1/2 cup sliced)	12	0	0	2	1	5
BEANS, CANNED						
Most Brands, Baked Beans w/Pork & Tomato Sauce (1/2 cup)	124	1	1	25	5	557
Broadbeans (1/2 cup)	121	1	0	22	6	202
Garbanzo (1/2 cup)	134	2	0	22	4	199
Kidney (1/2 cup)	114	1	0	20	7	438
Lima, drained (1/2 cup)	108	0	0	20	7	225
No Salt Added, drained (1/2 cup)	108	0	0	20	7	2
Pinto (1/2 cup)	118	0	0	22	6	206
Allens Mexican Chili Beans (1/2 cup)	120	1	0	22	8	300
Refried Beans (1/2 cup)	150	3	1	24	11	360
Seasoned Black Beans (1/2 cup)	120	2	1	20	7	410
B&M Baked Beans, 99% Fat Free (1/2 cup)	160	1	0	31	7	220
Barbecue (1/2 cup)	170	2	1	32	6	360
Brick Oven (1/2 cup)	180	2	1	32	7	390
Extra Hearty (1/2 cup)	190	2	1	36	8	450
Red Kidney (1/2 cup)	170	2	1	32	6	440
Yellow Eye (1/2 cup)	170	2	1	28	7	460
w/Honey (1/2 cup)	170	2	0	30	8	450
Brown Beauty Beans, Mexican Chili (1/2 cup)	120	1	0	22	8	300
Mexican w/Jalapenos (1/2 cup)	120	1	0	21	7	370
Bush's Beans, Baked (1/2 cup)	150	1	0	29	7	550
w/Onions (1/2 cup)	150	2	1	26	6	500
Chili Hot (1/2 cup)	120	1	1	20	6	480
Garbanzo (1/2 cup)	130	2	1	22	9	500
Great Northern w/Pork (1/2 cup)	110	2	1	17	6	460
Pintos, Cowboy (1/2 cup)	120	1	1	20	6	360
w/Bacon & Jalapeno (1/2 cup)	110	2	1	17	6	550
w/Bacon (1/2 cup)	110	1	1	18	6	540
w/Pork (1/2 cup)	120	3	1	17	6	530
Pork & Beans, Deluxe (1/2 cup)	160	2	1	28	8	480
Fanci Pak (1/2 cup)	160	2	1	28	7	350
Regular (1/2 cup)	120	2	1	22	6	550
Vegetarian (1/2 cup)	140	1	0	24	6	550

	Calories	Fat g	Saturated Fat g	Carbohydrate g	Fiber g	Sodium mg
Campbell's Baked Beans, Brown Sugar & Bacon Flavored (¹/2 cup)	170	3	1	29	7	490
Tangy Barbecue Flavor (¹/2 cup)	170	3	1	29	6	460
Chili Beans in a Zesty Sauce (¹/2 cup)	130	3	1	21	6	490
Homestyle Beans (¹/2 cup)	150	2	1	27	7	490
Old Fashioned Beans (¹/2 cup)	180	3	1	32	6	460
Old Fashioned Barbecue Beans (¹/2 cup)	170	3	1	29	6	460
Pork & Beans in Tomato Sauce (¹/2 cup)	130	2	1	24	6	420
Vegetarian Beans in Tomato Sauce (¹/2 cup)	130	2	1	24	6	460
Chi-Chi's Ranchero Beans (¹/2 cup)	100	1	0	18	3	540
Del Monte Country Three-Bean Salad (¹/2 cup)	100	0	0	23	1	510
Friend's Baked Beans, Original (¹/2 cup)	170	1	0	32	7	390
Red Kidney (¹/2 cup)	160	1	0	32	6	510
Green Giant Three Bean Salad (¹/2 cup)	70	0	0	16	3	470
Heartland Iron Kettle Baked Beans (¹/2 cup)	150	1	0	29	5	500
Hunt's Chili Beans (4 oz)	100	<1	0	18	6	490
Pork & Beans (4 oz)	135	1	0	26	8	430
Joan of Arc Three Bean Salad (¹/2 cup)	70	0	0	16	3	470
Las Palmas, No Fat Refried Beans (¹/2 cup)	110	0	0	19	6	470
Refried Beans (¹/2 cup)	110	2	1	17	5	500
Old El Paso Beans, Black (¹/2 cup)	100	1	0	17	7	400
Garbanzo (¹/2 cup)	120	3	0	20	7	280
Mexe (¹/2 cup)	110	1	0	19	7	630
Pinto (¹/2 cup)	110	1	0	19	7	420
Refried (¹/2 cup)	110	2	1	17	5	500
Black (¹/2 cup)	120	2	0	18	6	340
Fat Free (¹/2 cup)	110	0	0	20	6	480
Vegetarian (¹/2 cup)	100	1	0	16	6	490
w/Green Chilies (¹/2 cup)	110	1	0	19	6	720
Ortega Refried Beans (¹/2 cup)	140	3	1	23	5	580
Progresso Black Beans (¹/2 cup)	100	1	1	17	7	400
Cannellini Beans (¹/2 cup)	100	1	0	18	5	270
Chick Peas (¹/2 cup)	120	3	0	20	7	280
Fava Beans (¹/2 cup)	110	1	0	20	5	250
Pinto Beans (¹/2 cup)	110	1	0	18	7	250

	Calories	Fat g	Saturated Fat g	Carbohydrate g	Fiber g	Sodium mg
Red Kidney Beans (¹/₂ cup)	110	1	0	20	8	280
Trappey's Baby Green Lima Beans w/Bacon (¹/₂ cup)	120	1	1	22	6	330
Baby White Lima Beans w/Bacon (¹/₂ cup)	130	2	1	21	6	350
Great Northern Beans w/Sausage (¹/₂ cup)	100	1	1	18	7	460
Jalapinto Pinto Beans w/Bacon (¹/₂ cup)	120	1	1	22	8	540
Large White Butterbeans w/Sausage (¹/₂ cup)	110	1	0	21	6	300
Light Red Kidney Beans w/Jalapeno (¹/₂ cup)	110	1	0	19	6	420
Mexi-Beans w/Jalapenos (¹/₂ cup)	130	2	1	22	8	460
Navy Beans w/Bacon or Navy Beans w/Bacon & Jalapeno (¹/₂ cup)	110	2	1	17	7	420
New Orleans Style Light Red Kidney Beans w/Bacon (¹/₂ cup)	110	1	1	20	6	410
Pinto Beans w/Bacon (¹/₂ cup)	120	1	1	20	7	270
Pork & Beans (¹/₂ cup)	110	1	1	21	7	710
Red Kidney Beans w/Chili Gravy (¹/₂ cup)	110	1	0	20	7	510
Seasoned Black Beans (¹/₂ cup)	120	2	1	20	7	410
Van Camp's Baked Beans, Fat Free (¹/₂ cup)	130	0	0	28	5	430
Premium (¹/₂ cup)	140	1	0	29	5	520
Brown Sugar Beans (¹/₂ cup)	170	3	1	31	6	410
Butterbeans (¹/₂ cup)	110	1	0	22	7	430
Mexican Style Chili Beans (¹/₂ cup)	110	2	1	21	8	430
Vegetarian Beans in Tomato Sauce (¹/₂ cup)	110	1	0	23	5	400
Wagon Master Pork & Beans (¹/₂ cup)	110	1	1	21	7	710
BEAN SPROUTS, CANNED						
Chun King Bean Sprouts (3 oz)	5	0	0	<1	NA	15
BEETS, CANNED						
Beets, drained (¹/₂ cup sliced)	26	0	0	6	2	116
Harvard (¹/₂ cup)	62	0	0	15	2	119
No Salt Added, drained (¹/₂ cup sliced)	37	0	0	8	2	65
Pickled, undrained (¹/₂ cup sliced)	90	0	0	22	2	199

	Calories	Fat g	Saturated Fat g	Carbohydrate g	Fiber g	Sodium mg
CARROTS, CANNED						
Carrots, drained (¹/₂ cup slices)	17	0	0	4	1	176
No Salt Added, drained (¹/₂ cup slices)	33	0	0	6	2	48
CORN, CANNED						
Most Brands, Cream Style (¹/₂ cup)	104	1	0	24	2	413
Whole Kernel, drained (¹/₂ cup)	66	1	0	15	2	265
No Salt Added, drained (¹/₂ cup)	66	0	0	17	3	4
Del Monte Cream Style Corn, Golden, 50% Less Salt (¹/₂ cup)	90	1	0	20	2	180
No Salt Added (¹/₂ cup)	90	1	0	20	2	10
White (¹/₂ cup)	100	0	0	21	2	360
Whole Kernel Corn, 50% Less Salt (¹/₂ cup)	60	1	0	11	3	130
Golden, No Salt Added (¹/₂ cup)	60	1	0	11	3	10
White (¹/₂ cup)	80	0	0	17	2	360
Green Giant Mexicorn (¹/₃ cup)	60	0	0	14	2	430
Ka-me Baby Corn, Stir-Fry (pre-cut) Corn (¹/₂ cup)	20	0	0	3	2	10
GINGER ROOT, CANNED						
Ka-me Ginger Root, slices (20 pieces)	0	0	0	1	0	70
GREEN BEANS, CANNED						
Most Brands, Green Beans or Snap Beans, drained (¹/₂ cup)	14	0	0	3	2	171
No Salt Added, drained (¹/₂ cup)	18	0	0	4	2	9
Bush's Green Beans, w/Ham Flavor & Potatoes (¹/₂ cup)	40	0	0	7	3	560
w/Ham Flavor (¹/₂ cup)	35	0	0	6	2	500
Del Monte Green Beans, 50% Less Salt (¹/₂ cup)	20	0	0	4	2	180
Italian (¹/₂ cup)	30	0	0	6	3	360
No Salt Added (¹/₂ cup)	20	0	0	4	2	10
Seasoned (¹/₂ cup)	20	0	0	4	2	360
GREEN CHILIES, CANNED						
Most Brands, Hot Chili Peppers, drained (1 pepper)	10	0	0	2	0	472
Chi-Chi's Green Chilies, diced (2 tbsp)	10	0	0	1	0	5
Whole (³/₄ pepper)	10	0	0	1	0	5

	Calories	Fat g	Saturated Fat g	Carbohydrate g	Fiber g	Sodium mg
Old El Paso Green Chilies, chopped (2 tbsp)	5	0	0	1	1	110
Whole (1 chili)	10	0	0	2	1	230
Ortega Green Chilies, diced (2 tbsp)	10	0	0	2	0	20
Whole (1 pepper)	15	0	0	3	<1	30
Jalapeño Peppers, diced (2 tbsp)	10	0	0	3	0	25
Whole (2 peppers)	10	0	0	3	0	25
Pancho Villa Green Chiles, diced (2 tbsp)	5	0	0	1	1	110
HOMINY, CANNED						
Most Brands, Hominy (1/2 cup)	58	1	0	11	2	168
Bush's Hominy, Golden w/Peppers (1/2 cup)	70	1	0	14	3	570
White w/Peppers (1/2 cup)	80	1	0	16	4	500
MIXED VEGETABLES, CANNED						
Most Brands, Mixed Vegetables, drained (1/2 cup)	36	0	0	7	2	182
Peas & Carrots (1/2 cup)	36	0	0	7	2	182
No Salt Added (1/2 cup)	38	0	0	8	3	54
Allens Okra, Tomatoes & Corn (1/2 cup)	30	0	0	6	4	280
Chun King Chow Mein Vegetables (3 oz)	10	0	0	<1	NA	15
Del Monte Mixed Vegetables w/Corn (1/2 cup)	40	0	0	8	2	360
Saucy Fiesta Vegetables (1/2 cup)	80	0	0	17	1	480
Savory Italian Medley (1/2 cup)	60	0	0	14	1	510
Sweet & Sour Oriental Vegetables (1/2 cup)	70	0	0	17	<1	370
Sweet & Tangy Garden Medley (1/2 cup)	130	1	0	27	2	520
Green Giant Garden Medley Vegetables (1/2 cup)	40	0	0	15	3	360
Mixed Vegetables (1/2 cup)	60	0	0	19	4	460
House of Tsang Vegetables & Sauce, Cantonese Classic (1/2 cup)	70	1	0	13	1	930
Hong Kong Sweet & Sour (1/2 cup)	160	0	0	40	0	580
Szechuan Hot & Spicy (1/2 cup)	70	1	0	14	1	1,090
Tokyo Teriyaki (1/2 cup)	100	0	0	22	0	1,240
Ka-me Stir-Fry Vegetables (1/2 cup)	20	0	0	4	2	10
La Choy Vegetables, Chop Suey (1/2 cup)	10	<1	0	2	<1	320
Fancy Mix (1/2 cup)	12	<1	0	2	1	30
Trappey Okra, Tomatoes & Corn (1/2 cup)	30	0	0	6	4	280

Canned Vegetables (continued)	Calories	Fat g	Saturated Fat g	Carbohydrate g	Fiber g	Sodium mg
MUSHROOMS, CANNED						
Most Brands, Mushrooms (1/2 cup pieces)	19	0	0	4	2	332
BinB Mushrooms, Pieces & Stems, Sliced or Whole (1 can = 3 oz)	30	0	0	4	2	460
w/Garlic, sliced (1 can = 3 oz)	35	1	0	4	1	410
Ka-me Mushrooms Stir-Fry or Straw, whole, peeled (1/2 cup)	20	0	0	3	2	380
OKRA, CANNED						
Trappey Creole Okra Gumbo (1/2 cup)	35	1	0	6	3	290
PEAS, BLACKEYE, CANNED						
Bush's Blackeye Peas, w/Bacon & Jalapeno (1/2 cup)	120	3	1	16	5	660
w/Bacon (1/2 cup)	110	1	1	18	5	630
w/Snap Beans (1/2 cup)	110	1	0	17	5	550
Trappey Blackeye Peas, w/Bacon & Jalapeno (1/2 cup)	110	2	1	19	5	470
w/Bacon (1/2 cup)	120	2	1	19	5	350
PEAS, COWBOY, CANNED						
Bush's Cowboy Peas (1/2 cup)	120	1	0	19	5	500
PEAS, CROWDER, CANNED						
Bush's Crowder Peas (1/2 cup)	110	1	0	18	5	500
PEAS, FIELD, CANNED						
Trappey Field Peas, w/Bacon (1/2 cup)	90	1	1	15	5	380
w/Snaps & Bacon (1/2 cup)	110	1	1	19	4	380
PEAS, GREEN, CANNED						
Most Brands, Green Peas, drained (1/2 cup)	59	0	0	11	3	186
No Salt Added, drained (1/2 cup)	66	0	0	12	5	74
Del Monte Peas, 50% Less Salt (1/2 cup)	60	0	0	11	4	180
No Salt Added (1/2 cup)	60	0	0	11	4	10
PEPPERS, CANNED						
Progresso Roasted Peppers (1/2 cup)	10	0	0	1	0	60
POTATOES, CANNED						
Potatoes, drained (1/2 cup)	54	0	0	12	2	234
PUMPKIN, CANNED						
Libby's Solid Pack Pumpkin (1/2 cup)	60	1	0	15	4	5

	Calories	Fat g	Saturated Fat g	Carbohydrate g	Fiber g	Sodium mg
SAUERKRAUT, CANNED						
Most Brands, Sauerkraut (1/2 cup)	22	0	0	5	4	780
Bush's Bavarian Kraut (1/2 cup)	60	1	0	14	3	470
Claussen Sauerkraut (1/4 cup)	5	0	0	1	1	210
SPINACH, CANNED						
Most Brands, Spinach, drained (1/2 cup)	25	1	0	4	3	210
No Salt Added, drained (1/2 cup)	30	0	0	6	2	92
Del Monte Spinach, 50% Less Salt (1/2 cup)	30	0	0	4	2	180
No Salt Added (1/2 cup)	30	0	0	4	2	85
SWEET POTATOES AND YAMS, CANNED						
Most Brands, Sweet Potatoes in syrup, mashed (1/2 cup)	138	0	0	32	2	50
Drained (1/2 cup)	106	0	0	25	1	38
Royal Prince Sweet Potatoes, Candied (1/2 cup)	210	1	0	50	2	30
Orange-Pineapple (1/2 cup)	210	1	0	43	3	30
TOMATO PASTE						
Most Brands, Tomato Paste (2 tbsp)	28	0	0	6	1	259
No Salt Added (2 tbsp)	28	0	0	6	1	21
Contadina Tomato Paste, Italian (2 tbsp)	40	1	0	7	1	320
Hunt's Tomato Paste, Italian Style or w/Garlic (2 oz)	50	<1	0	11	2	430-440
TOMATO PUREE						
Most Brands, Tomato Puree (1/2 cup)	49	0	0	12	2	499
Muir Glen Organic Tomato Puree (1/4 cup)	20	0	0	5	1	20
TOMATOES, CANNED						
Most Brands, Tomatoes (1/2 cup)	24	0	0	5	1	196
Low Sodium (1/2 cup)	24	0	0	5	1	16
America's Choice Tomatoes, Crushed in Puree w/Basil (1/4 cup)	25	0	0	5	1	170
Italian Diced (1/2 cup)	50	2	0	7	1	270
Italian Stewed (1/2 cup)	35	0	0	8	1	270
Italian Style or Mexican Style, Stewed (1/2 cup)	35	0	0	7	2	270

	Calories	Fat g	Saturated Fat g	Carbohydrate g	Fiber g	Sodium mg
Chi-Chi's Diced Tomatoes & Green Chilies (¼ cup)	20	0	0	4	0	340
Contadina Tomatoes, Italian Style Pear Tomatoes or Recipe Ready Tomatoes (½ cup)	25	0	0	4	1	200-220
Pasta Ready Tomatoes (½ cup)	50	2	0	7	1	550
Primavera (½ cup)	50	2	1	8	1	600
w/Crushed Red Pepper (½ cup)	60	3	1	8	1	690
w/Mushrooms (½ cup)	50	2	1	9	1	640
w/Olives (½ cup)	60	3	1	8	1	640
Stewed Tomatoes, Italian Style (½ cup)	40	0	0	8	1	260
Mexican Style (½ cup)	40	0	0	9	1	220
Del Monte Tomatoes, Salsa Style Chunky (½ cup)	35	0	0	8	2	560
Wedges (½ cup)	35	0	0	9	2	380
Stewed, Cajun Style (½ cup)	35	0	0	9	2	460
Chunky Chili Style (½ cup)	30	0	0	6	2	600
Chunky Pasta Style (½ cup)	45	0	0	11	2	560
Italian Style (½ cup)	30	0	0	8	2	420
Mexican Style (½ cup)	35	0	0	9	2	400
No Salt Added (½ cup)	35	0	0	9	2	50
Pizza Style (½ cup)	35	0	0	9	2	670
Green Giant Stewed Tomatoes, Classic Recipe (½ cup)	35	0	0	15	2	360
Italian Recipe (½ cup)	30	0	0	15	2	360
Mexican Recipe (½ cup)	35	0	0	17	2	400
Hunt's Tomatoes, Angela Mia Crushed (4 oz)	35	<1	0	7	<1	260
Italian Flavored Tomatoes, Crushed (4 oz)	40	<1	0	9	<1	460
Stewed (4 oz)	40	<1	0	9	<1	370
Whole (4 oz)	25	<1	0	6	<1	420
Italian Style Pear Shaped (4 oz)	20	<1	0	5	<1	320
Muir Glen Organic Tomatoes, Crushed w/Basil (¼ cup)	25	0	0	4	1	85
Diced or Stewed (½ cup)	25	0	0	4	1	190
Ground Peeled (¼ cup)	10	0	0	2	1	100
Whole Peeled (½ cup)	30	0	0	5	1	260

	Calories	Fat g	Saturated Fat g	Carbohydrate g	Fiber g	Sodium mg
Canned Vegetables (continued)						
Progresso Peeled Tomatoes, Imported w/Basil (1/2 cup)	25	0	0	4	1	200
w/Basil (1/2 cup)	25	0	0	4	1	220
WATERCHESTNUTS, CANNED						
Waterchestnuts, drained (1/2 cup)	34	0	0	9	2	10
ZUCCHINI, CANNED						
Most Brands, Zucchini, Italian-Style, undrained (1/2 cup)	18	0	0	4	1	443
Del Monte Zucchini, In Tomato Sauce (1/2 cup)	30	0	0	7	1	490
Zesty Italian (1/2 cup)	40	0	0	9	0	520
Progresso Italian Style Zucchini (1/2 cup)	40	2	0	7	2	400
DRIED VEGETABLES						
BEANS, DRIED						
Most Brands, cooked w/o fat or salt, Kidney (1/2 cup cooked)	112	0	0	20	7	2
Lentils (1/2 cup cooked)	115	0	0	20	5	2
Lima (1/2 cup cooked)	90	0	0	17	5	48
Navy (1/2 cup cooked)	129	1	0	24	6	1
Pinto (1/2 cup cooked)	117	0	0	22	6	2
White (1/2 cup cooked)	122	0	0	22	5	5
N.K. Hurst Pinto Beans w/Spanish Seasoning (3 tbsp dry)	120	1	0	22	6	350
TOMATOES, SUN-DRIED						
Sun-Dried Tomatoes, dry pack (1 tbsp)	9	0	0	2	0	71
FRESH VEGETABLES (COOKED VEGETABLES PREP W/O FAT OR SALT)						
Alfalfa Sprouts, raw (1 cup)	10	0	0	1	1	2
Artichokes, cooked (1 medium)	60	0	0	13	4	114
Asparagus, cooked (1/2 cup)	25	0	0	4	2	4
Beans, Green or Snap, cooked (1/2 cup)	16	0	0	4	2	8
Beets, slices, cooked (1/2 cup)	37	0	0	8	2	65
Broccoli, chopped, cooked (1/2 cup)	26	0	0	4	3	22
Chopped, raw (1/2 cup)	12	0	0	2	1	12
Spears, cooked (1 spear)	10	0	0	2	1	8

Fresh Vegetables (continued)	Calories	Fat g	Saturated Fat g	Carbohydrate g	Fiber g	Sodium mg
Brussels Sprouts, cooked (1/2 cup)	33	0	0	6	4	18
Cabbage, Chinese, cooked (1/2 cup)	10	0	0	2	1	29
Raw (1/2 cup)	5	0	0	1	0	23
Cabbage, Red, cooked (1/2 cup)	16	0	0	3	2	6
Raw (1/2 cup shredded)	9	0	0	2	1	6
Cabbage, cooked (1/2 cup)	16	0	0	3	2	6
Raw (1/2 cup shredded)	9	0	0	2	1	6
Carrots, cooked (1/2 cup slices)	35	0	0	8	2	51
Raw (7 1/2" x 1" diam)	31	0	0	7	2	25
Cauliflower, cooked (1/2 cup)	17	0	0	3	1	16
Raw (1/2 cup)	13	0	0	3	1	15
Celery, cooked (1/2 cup diced)	13	0	0	3	2	68
Raw (1 stalk = 7 1/2" x 1")	6	0	0	1	1	35
Chayote, cooked (1/2 cup)	19	0	0	4	3	1
Corn, cooked (1/2 cup)	66	0	0	17	3	4
Cucumbers, raw (1/2 cup slices)	7	0	0	1	0	1
Eggplant, cooked (1/2 cup cubes)	13	0	0	3	1	1
Endive, raw (1/2 cup chopped)	2	0	0	0	0	3
Garlic, raw (1 clove)	4	0	0	1	0	1
Ginger Root, raw (5 slices)	8	0	0	2	0	1
Greens, Beet, cooked (1/2 cup)	14	0	0	3	2	174
Dandelion, cooked (1/2 cup)	14	0	0	3	1	8
Mustard, cooked (1/2 cup)	14	0	0	3	2	20
Turnip, cooked (1/2 cup)	14	0	0	3	2	21
Jicama or Yambean, raw (1 cup slices)	53	0	0	11	2	8
Kale, cooked (1/2 cup chopped)	18	0	0	4	1	10
Raw (1/2 cup chopped)	10	0	0	2	1	6
Kohlrabi, cooked (1/2 cup slices)	24	0	0	6	2	17
Leeks, cooked (1/4 cup)	7	0	0	2	1	1
Raw (1/4 cup)	7	0	0	2	1	4
Lettuce, Iceberg (1/4 head)	9	0	0	1	1	6
Mushrooms, cooked (1/2 cup chopped)	21	0	0	4	2	2
Raw (1 whole)	4	0	0	1	0	1
Raw (1/2 cup)	12	0	0	2	1	2
Okra, cooked (1/2 cup slices)	30	0	0	7	4	2
Onion, Green (scallion) (1 med)	5	0	0	1	0	2

Fresh Vegetables (continued)	Calories	Fat g	Saturated Fat g	Carbohydrate g	Fiber g	Sodium mg
Onions, cooked (1/2 cup chopped)	46	0	0	11	2	3
Raw (1/2 cup chopped)	30	0	0	7	2	2
Parsley (1/2 cup chopped)	5	0	0	1	1	8
Parsnips, cooked (1/2 cup slices)	63	0	0	15	3	8
Peas, Cowpeas, cooked (1/2 cup)	99	1	0	18	8	3
Green, cooked (1/2 cup)	62	0	0	11	4	70
Peppers, Bell, Green or Red, raw (1/2 cup chopped)	14	0	0	3	1	1
Peppers, Hot Chili, raw (1)	18	0	0	4	1	3
Potato w/Skin, baked (1 med)	133	0	0	31	2	10
Boiled (1/2 cup chopped)	68	0	0	16	1	5
Pumpkin, cooked (1/2 cup)	42	0	0	10	1	6
Radicchio, raw (1/2 cup shredded)	5	0	0	1	0	4
Radishes, raw, 1" diam (10)	1	0	0	0	0	1
Rutabagas, cooked (1/2 cup pieces)	33	0	0	7	1	17
Shallots, raw (1 tbsp)	3	0	0	1	0	2
Snow Peas, cooked (1/2 cup)	34	0	0	6	1	3
Raw (1/2 cup)	29	0	0	5	1	3
Spinach, cooked (1/2 cup)	25	0	0	5	2	77
Raw (1/2 cup)	6	0	0	1	1	22
Squash, Summer, cooked (1/2 cup slices)	18	0	0	4	1	1
Raw (1/2 cup slices)	9	0	0	2	1	2
Squash, Winter, cooked (1/2 cup cubes)	40	1	0	9	3	1
Sweet Potatoes, baked (1/2 cup chopped)	91	0	0	21	2	9
Baked (1/2 cup mashed)	131	0	0	31	3	13
Taro, cooked (1/2 cup slices)	74	0	0	17	1	4
Tomatillos (1)	11	0	0	2	0	0
Tomatoes, cooked (1/2 cup)	32	1	0	7	2	13
Fresh (1 tomato = 2 3/5" diam)	26	0	0	6	1	11
Turnips, cooked (1/2 cup pieces)	14	0	0	4	2	39
Watercress (1/2 cup chopped)	2	0	0	0	0	7
Zucchini, boiled (1/2 cup slices)	14	0	0	4	1	3

FROZEN VEGETABLES

ASPARAGUS, FROZEN

	Calories	Fat g	Saturated Fat g	Carbohydrate g	Fiber g	Sodium mg
Asparagus, cooked w/o fat or salt (4 spears)	17	0	0	3	1	2

	Calories	Fat g	Saturated Fat g	Carbohydrate g	Fiber g	Sodium mg
BROCCOLI, FROZEN						
Higher-Fat						
Broccoli w/Cheese Sauce (1/2 cup)	120	8	4	7	2	412
Lower-Fat						
Most Brands, Broccoli, cooked w/o fat or salt (1/2 cup)	26	0	0	5	3	22
Green Giant Broccoli, in Cheese Flavored Sauce (2/3 cup)	70	3	1	9	2	520
Spears in Butter Sauce (4 oz)	50	2	1	7	2	330
BRUSSELS SPROUTS, FROZEN						
Most Brands, Brussels Sprouts, cooked w/o fat or salt (1/2 cup)	33	0	0	6	4	18
CARROTS, FROZEN						
Carrots, cooked w/o fat or salt (1/2 cup slices)	33	0	0	8	2	48
CAULIFLOWER, FROZEN						
Most Brands, Cauliflower, cooked w/o fat or salt (1/2 cup)	17	0	0	3	1	16
Green Giant Cauliflower in Cheese Flavored Sauce (1/2 cup)	60	3	1	8	2	510
CORN, FROZEN						
Most Brands, Corn, cooked w/o fat or salt (1/2 cup)	66	0	0	17	3	4
Ore-Ida Cob Corn (1 ear)	180	3	0	33	4	5
Mini-Gold (1 ear)	90	1	0	16	2	0
GREEN BEANS, FROZEN						
Most Brands, Green or Snap Beans, cooked w/o fat or salt (1/2 cup)	18	0	0	4	2	9
GREENS, FROZEN						
Turnip Greens, cooked w/o fat or salt (1/2 cup)	16	0	0	4	3	24
MIXED VEGETABLES, FROZEN						
Most Brands, Peas & Carrots, cooked w/o fat or salt (1/2 cup)	38	0	0	8	3	54
Peas & Onions, cooked w/o fat or salt (1/2 cup)	43	0	0	0	3	40

	Calories	Fat g	Saturated Fat g	Carbohydrate g	Fiber g	Sodium mg
Green Giant American Mixtures						
Vegetables, California Style (¾ cup)	25	0	0	5	2	15
Heartland Style (1 cup)	30	0	0	6	3	35
Manhattan Style (1 cup)	25	0	0	4	2	15
New England Style (⅔ cup)	70	2	0	13	3	70
San Francisco Style (¾ cup)	30	0	0	6	2	20
Santa Fe (¾ cup)	60	0	0	13	2	10
Seattle Style (¾ cup)	25	0	0	5	2	15
Western Style (¾ cup)	50	2	0	9	2	10
Create A Meal! Vegetables (vegetables only),						
Lo Mein Stir Fry (2⅓ cups)	160	1	0	32	5	1,070
Sweet & Sour Stir Fry (1¾ cups)	130	0	0	29	5	390
Teriyaki Stir Fry (1¾ cups)	100	0	0	19	4	870
International Mixtures Vegetables,						
Japanese Style Teriyaki (4 oz)	50	0	0	9	2	400
Oriental Style Rice (8 oz)	180	1	0	0	4	980
Mixed Vegetables in Butter Sauce (¾ cup)	70	2	1	11	3	240
Ore-Ida Stew Vegetables (⅔ cup)	50	0	0	11	<1	50
OKRA, FROZEN						
Okra, cooked w/o fat or salt (½ cup)	34	0	0	8	4	3
ONIONS, FROZEN						
Ore-Ida Onions, chopped (¾ cup)	25	0	0	6	1	20
PEAS, GREEN, FROZEN						
Most Brands, Peas, cooked w/o fat or salt (½ cup)	62	0	0	11	4	70
POTATOES, FROZEN						
Higher-Fat						
French-Fried Potatoes, deep-fried & salted (17 med)	217	14	2	22	2	113
Lower-Fat						
Ore-Ida Country Style, Dinner Fries, baked (about 8 fries)	110	3	1	19	1	20
Hash Browns, baked (1 cup)	60	0	0	13	1	10
Potato Wedges w/Skin, baked (about 9 fries)	110	3	1	19	2	15
Potatoes O'Brien, baked (¾ cup)	60	0	0	13	2	15

	Calories	Fat g	Saturated Fat g	Carbohydrate g	Fiber g	Sodium mg
Ore-Ida *(continued)*						
Shredded Hash Browns, baked (1 patty)	70	0	0	15	1	25
Southern Style Hash Browns, baked (¾ cup)	70	0	0	17	2	25
SNOW PEAS, FROZEN						
Snow Peas, cooked w/o fat or salt (½ cup)	34	0	0	6	1	3
SPINACH, FROZEN						
Most Brands, Spinach, cooked w/o fat or salt (½ cup)	27	0	0	5	2	82
Green Giant Cut Leaf Spinach in Butter Sauce (½ cup)	40	2	1	5	2	280
SUCCOTASH, FROZEN						
Succotash, cooked w/o fat or salt (½ cup)	76	0	0	15	4	42
SWEET POTATOES, FROZEN						
Higher-Fat						
Candied Sweet Potatoes, prep w/margarine & salt (1 med)	251	6	1	48	3	278
Lower-Fat						
Most Brands, Sweet Potatoes, cooked w/o fat or salt (½ cup chopped)	91	0	0	21	2	9
Mrs. Paul's Candied Sweet Potatoes (5 oz)	330	1	1	80	3	130
Candied Sweet Potatoes 'N Apples (1 cup)	270	0	0	66	3	90

APPENDIX

RECIPE SUBSTITUTIONS TO LOWER
FAT AND/OR DIETARY CHOLESTEROL*

Instead of Using	Try Substituting
Bacon	Canadian bacon or lean ham
Baking chocolate (1 square)	Cocoa powder (3 tablespoons) plus tub margarine (1 tablespoon) or oil (1 teaspoon)
Butter	Tub margarine
Cheese, regular	Low-fat or reduced-fat cheese (3 to 5 grams or less fat per ounce)
Cottage cheese, regular	Fat-free or low-fat cottage cheese
Coconut	Coconut extract (texture of finished product will be different)
Cream — whipping cream or half and half	Canned evaporated skim milk (can be whipped)
Cream cheese	Reduced-fat or fat-free cream cheese
Eggs, whole	Egg whites (2 equal 1 whole egg) or egg substitute
Fudge sauce	Chocolate syrup
Ground beef or hamburger meat	Extra lean ground beef or turkey (10% or less fat)
Margarine, tub	Reduced amount of tub margarine or equal amount of a reduced-fat margarine or spread may be suitable for some recipes
Milk, evaporated	Canned evaporated skim milk
Milk, whole or 2%	Skim, 1/2%, or 1% low-fat milk or canned evaporated skim milk
Nuts	Reduce amount in recipe by 1/2 to 1/3
Oil	Can reduce amount by 1/4 to 1/3 in many recipes; may substitute equal amount of applesauce in some quick-bread or muffin recipes
Shortening or lard (1/2 cup)	Tub margarine (1/2 cup) or oil (1/3 cup)
Sour cream	Low-fat or fat-free sour cream or plain, fat-free yogurt
Tuna, oil-pack	Tuna, water pack

*From *The New Living Heart Diet,* by DeBakey, M.E., Gotto, A.M., Scott, L.W., et al., Simon & Schuster, New York, 1996.

RECIPE SUBSTITUTIONS TO LOWER SODIUM

Regular Product	Amount	Use Product Labeled	Sodium Reduced Approximately mg*
Baking powder	1 teaspoon	Low-sodium baking powder (3 teaspoons)	485
Beans, pinto, canned	1 cup	Cooked from dry without salt	410
Broth or meat stock, salted, beef or chicken	1 cup	Low-sodium bouillon Beef Chicken	580 720
Buttermilk	1 cup	Skim, $1/2$%, or 1% low-fat milk (1 cup minus 1 tablespoon) plus lemon juice or vinegar (1 tablespoon)	130
Cheese, American processed	1 ounce	Low-sodium Low-fat and low-sodium	230 320
Cheese, cheddar	1 ounce	Low-sodium Low-fat and low-sodium	60 90
Cottage cheese	$1/2$ cup	No salt added Dry curd	435 450
Garlic salt	$1/4$ teaspoon	Garlic powder	240
Tomatoes, canned	1 cup	No salt added	360
Tomato juice	1 cup	Salt-free	850
Tomato paste	$1/2$ cup	No salt added	950
Tomato sauce	$1/2$ cup	No salt added	705
Tuna, canned in water	2 ounces	Unsalted Low-sodium	165 75
Vegetables, canned	1 cup	No salt added	225–520

mg = milligrams.
* Values rounded to nearest 5.
† Refers only to "low sodium" broth or bouillon; "light in salt" or other reduced-sodium broth or bouillon is higher in sodium.
From *The New Living Heart Diet,* by DeBakey, M.E., Gotto, A.M., Scott, L.W., et al., Simon & Schuster, New York, 1996.

SUPPLEMENTING MEAL-TYPE PRODUCTS

Meal-type products may start out low in calories and fat, but the calorie and fat content of the finished meal depends on all of the foods in it. Here are some examples of quick-to-prepare foods that can be served with meal-type products that are low in calories and fat. Menus for three sample meals at different calorie levels are on the following page. The calories listed for the foods shown below are estimates only, and will vary somewhat with your individual choices.

Suggested foods to supplement meal-type products	Serving Size	Approximate Calories
Tossed green salad	2 cups	30
Salad dressing, fat-free	2 tablespoons	10
Vegetable, cooked (ex. spinach, broccoli, green beans, summer squash)	1 cup	60
Bread, regular	1 slice	80
Diet	2 slices	80
Roll, hard type	1 average	80
Fresh fruit	1 average piece	60
Skim milk	1 cup	90
Frozen yogurt, low-fat or nonfat	1/2 cup	110
Tub margarine, regular	1 teaspoon	35
Diet	2 teaspoons	35

The following sample menus for adults are based on three calorie levels — 1,200, 1,500, and 2,200. Each one includes a lunch or dinner meal. The goal for dividing calories among the meals is about 20% for breakfast, 40% for lunch, and 40% for dinner. This division of calories does not include snacks.

1,200 Calorie Eating Plan
Example of Lunch or Dinner Providing 500 Calories

Foods	Serving Size	Approximate Calories
Frozen dinner	1	300
Tossed green salad	2 cups	30
Salad dressing, fat-free	2 tablespoons	10
Broccoli, steamed	1 cup	60
Bread, diet	1 slice	40
Tub margarine, diet	1 teaspoon	18
Fresh fruit	1 average piece	60
Total for the meal		518

1,500 Calorie Eating Plan
Example of Lunch or Dinner Providing 600 Calories

Foods	Serving Size	Approximate Calories
Frozen dinner	1	300
Tossed green salad	2 cups	30
Salad dressing, fat-free	2 tablespoons	10
Summer squash, steamed	1/2 cup	30
Bread, diet	1 slice	40
Tub margarine, diet	2 teaspoons	35
Skim milk	1 cup	90
Fresh fruit	1 average piece	60
Total for the meal		595

2,200 Calorie Eating Plan
Example of Lunch or Dinner Providing 900 Calories

Foods	Serving Size	Approximate Calories
Frozen dinner	1	300
Tossed green salad	2 cups	30
Salad dressing, fat-free	2 tablespoons	10
Green beans, cooked	1 cup	60
Hard rolls	2 average	160
Tub margarine, regular	3 teaspoons	105
Skim milk	1 cup	90
Fresh fruit	1 average piece	60
Frozen yogurt, low-fat	1/2 cup	110
Total for the meal		925

DO YOU FIND EATING OUT A CHALLENGE?

The average adult eats away from home approximately four times each week, or about 198 meals per year. Fortunately, today most restaurants offer at least a few lower-fat selections. The authors of this guide have written a book designed to help you choose heart-healthy foods when eating away from home. In addition to listing the calories, fat, saturated fat, and cholesterol for more than 1,600 foods served in American and ethnic restaurants and in fast food establishments, *The Living Heart Guide to Eating Out* also provides 160 helpful tips on choosing foods lower in fat and sodium. Here are a few of the tips for choosing lower-fat restaurant foods.

- Order your food "à la carte" instead of ordering a complete meal, which may contain more food than you wish to eat.
- Don't hesitate to tell your serving person how you want your food prepared.
- Avoid fried foods.
- Ask for reasonable substitutions, such as a baked potato or a salad for the French fries that may come with a meal.
- Top your baked potato with green onions, salsa, lemon juice, hot peppers, mustard, or a small amount of margarine or low-fat ranch or French dressing instead of butter, sour cream, or bacon bits.
- Select lower-fat sandwiches of lean roast beef, lean ham, sliced turkey or chicken, or grilled chicken, rather than hamburgers or sandwiches containing a creamy filling, such as tuna, chicken, ham, or egg salad.
- Choose lower-fat breads, such as sliced bread, hard rolls, plain dinner rolls, and sandwich buns, rather than higher-fat biscuits, cornbread, and croissants.

An order form for *The Living Heart Guide to Eating Out* is on page 286, the last page of this book.

PRODUCT NAME TRADEMARKS

The following is a list of trademarks of products appearing in this book. Some manufacturers specified whether a product name was a trademark (indicated by ™) or a registered trademark (indicated by ®). Other manufacturers listed their trademarked names without specifying the type of trademark; these products are listed below without an accompanying symbol.

Allen® Canning Company: Allens®, Royal Prince®, TRAPPEY'S®

American Pop Corn Company: Jolly Time®

Beatrice Cheese, Inc.: HEALTHY CHOICE®

Best Foods/CPC International: Arnold®, Arnold Bakery®, Bakery Light™, Best Foods®, Bran'nola®, Brick Oven®, Brownberry®, Golden Griddle®, Hellmann's®, Karo®, Mazola®, Mueller's®, No Stick™, Sahara®, Super Shapes®, Thomas'®

Bremner Biscuit Company: BREMNER®

Buckeye Beans & Herbs: BUCKEYE BEANS & HERBS®

Cabot Creamery: CABOT®

Campbell Soup Company: Beach Haven, Campbell's, Campbell's Simmer Chef, Campbell's Kitchen, Chunky, Double Noodle, Franco-American, Garfield, Healthy Request, Healthy Treasures, Home Cookin', Marie's, Mrs. Paul's, Natural Goodness, Open Pit, Prego, Prego Extra Chunky, SpaghettiO's, Swanson, Tomato Del Mar, V8, V8 Picante

Chelten House Products Inc.: Chelten House, Dockside, Medford Farms

Citrus World, Inc.: FLORIDA'S NATURAL®

Coca-Cola Foods: Minute Maid®, FIVE ALIVE®, Hi-C®

Coca-Cola USA: Coca-Cola®, Coca-Cola Classic®, Coke®, Fanta®, Fresca®, Mello Yello®, Minute Maid®, Mr. Pibb®, PowerAde™, Tab®

ConAgra Frozen Foods: HEALTHY CHOICE®

Eden Foods, Inc.: EDENBLEND®, EDENRICE®, EDENSOY®

Frito-Lay, Inc.: COOL RANCH®, DORITOS®, FRITO-LAY®, ROLD GOLD®, TOSTITOS®

Frozfruit Corporation: FROZFRUIT®

Gerber Cheese Co., Inc.: SWISS KNIGHT®

Gisé Inc.: GISÉ®

Golden Jersey Products, Inc.: Golden Jersey

Guiltless Gourmet, Inc.: GUILTLESS GOURMET®

Hansen Beverage Company: HANSEN'S® Natural

Health Valley Foods: Health Valley®

Hershey Foods Corporation: DELMONICO® Pasta, HERSHEY®, NIBS®, P&R® Pasta, SAN GIORGIO® Pasta, SKINNER® Pasta, SPECIAL DARK®, TWIZZLERS®

Hormel Foods Corporation: BANGKOK PADANG™, CHI-CHI'S®, CHI-CHI'S™, HERB-OX®, HONG KONG™, HORMEL®, HORMEL™, HOUSE OF TSANG™, KOREAN™, MANDARIN™, NOT-SO-SLOPPY-JOE®, SAIGON SIZZLE™

Hunt-Wesson, Inc.: LA CHOY®

International Trading Company: Hafnia®

Keebler Company: Cinnamon Crisp®, Club®, Elfin Delights®, Graham Selects®, Keebler®, Toasteds®, Town House®, Zesta®

Kellogg Company: Kellogg's®, All-Bran®, Apple Cinnamon Rice Krispies™, Apple Cinnamon Squares®, Apple Jacks®, Apple Raisin Crisp®, Blueberry Squares™, Bran Buds®, Cocoa Krispies®, Common Sense®, Complete® Bran Flakes, Corn Pops®, Crispix®, Double Dip Crunch®, Eggo®, Froot Loops®, Frosted Krispies®, Frosted Mini-Wheats®, Fruitful Bran®, Fruity Marshmallow Krispies®, Healthy Choice™ from Kellogg's, Just Right®, Kellogg's Corn Flakes®, Kellogg's Frosted Bran®, Kellogg's Frosted Flakes®, Kenmei® Rice Bran, Müeslix®, Nut & Honey Crunch®, Nut & Honey Crunch O's®, Nutri-Grain®, Product 19®, Raisin Squares®, Rice Krispies®, Rice Krispies Treats® Cereal, Rice Krispies Treats™ Squares, Smacks®, Special K®, Strawberry Squares®

Kraft General Foods USA: ALPHA-BITS, BRAN'NOLA, BREAKSTONE'S, BREAK-STONE'S FREE, BREYERS, CAPRI SUN, CATALINA, CHEEZ WHIZ LIGHT, CHIFFON, COOL WHIP, COUNTRY TIME, COUNTRY KITCHEN, COUNTRY KITCHEN LITE, CRANBERRY BREEZE, CRYSTAL LIGHT, DI GIORNO, DI GIORNO LIGHT VARIETIES, DREAM WHIP, D-ZERTA, ENTENMANN'S, FROSTED WHEAT BITES, FRUIT WHEATS, FRUIT & FIBRE, FUNMALLOWS, GENERAL FOODS INTERNATIONAL COFFEE, GOLDEN CRISP, GOOD SEA-SONS, GRAPE-NUTS, GREAT BLUEDINI, HARVEST MOON, HONEY BUNCH-ES OF OATS, HONEYCOMB, INCREDIBERRY, JELL-O, JELL-O AMERICANA, JELL-O Brand FREE, JELL-O 1-2-3, KAHLUA CAFE, KNUDSEN, KNUDSEN CAL 70, KNUDSEN FREE, KNUDSEN LIGHT, KOOL-AID, KOOL-AID BURSTS, KRAFT, KRAFT 100%, KRAFT DELICIOUSLY RIGHT, KRAFT FREE, KRAFT HANDI-SNACKS, KRAFT HEALTHY FAVORITES, KRAFT LIGHT, KRAFT THICK'N SPICY, KRAFT TOUCH OF BUTTER, KRAFT-JET-PUFFED, LIGHT N' LIVELY, LIGHT N' LIVELY FREE, LIGHT N' LIVELY FREE 70 CALORIES, LIGHT N' LIVELY FREE 50 CALORIES, LOG CABIN, LOG CABIN LITE, MAUI PUNCH, MINUTE, MIRACLE WHIP, MIRACLE WHIP FREE, MIRACLE WHIP LIGHT, MOUNTAIN COOLER, MR. FREEZE, NABISCO, OVEN FRY, PACIFIC COOLER, PARKAY, PEBBLES, PHILADELPHIA BRAND FREE, PINK SWIMMINGO, POST,

POST TOASTIES, POSTUM, PURPLESAURUS REX, ROCK-A-DILE RED, SAFARI PUNCH, SALSA, SAUCEWORKS, SEALTEST, SEALTEST FREE, SEALTEST LIGHT, SEVEN SEAS, SEVEN SEAS FREE, SEVEN SEAS VIVA, SHAKE'N BAKE, SHAKE'N BAKE PERFECT POTATOES, SHREDDED WHEAT'N BRAN, SPOON SIZE, STRAWBERRY COOLER, SURFER COOLER, TANG, TEAM, THE BUDGET GOURMET, TOMBSTONE, VELVEETA LIGHT, YO YOGI BERRY

Lady J, Inc.: LADY J™

Lance Inc.: CAPTAIN'S WAFERS, LANCE, SESAME TWINS, WHEATSWAFERS, WHEAT TWINS

Lawry's Foods, Inc.: Lawry's®

Lifeline Food Company, Inc.: Lifetime®, Healthy Farms®

M. A. Gedney Company: GEDNEY®, STATE FAIR™

Mama Tish's Italian Specialties, Inc.: Mama Tish's®, Original Italian Ices®

Mazzone Enterprises, Inc.: Mazzone's®

Miceli Dairy Products Company: Miceli's®

"Mike-sells" Potato Chip Co: Mike-sell's®

Muir Glen Organic Tomato Products: MUIR GLEN®

Natural Nectar Corporation: FI-BAR®

Ocean Spray Cranberries, Inc.: CITRUS REFRESHERS™ Juice Drinks, CRANAPPLE®, CRAN-BLUEBERRY®, CRAN-CHERRY™, CRAN-GRAPE®, CRANICOT®, CRAN-RASPBERRY®, CRAN-STRAWBERRY™, CRANTASTIC® Fruit Punch, ISLAND GUAVA™, LIGHTSTYLE®, MANGO-MANGO™, MAUNA LA'I®, OCEAN SPRAY®, PARADISE PASSION™

Pepperidge Farm, Incorporated: Pepperidge Farm

Pet Incorporated: B&M, DOWNYFLAKE, FRIEND'S, HEARTLAND, LAS PALMAS, OLD EL PASO, PANCHO VILLA, PET, PROGRESSO, SEGO, VAN DE KAMP'S

Riviana Foods Inc.: Carolina, Mahatma, Success, Water Maid

Rubschlager Baking Corporation: RUBSCHLAGER®

Rymer Foods Inc.: MENU MAKER®

The Willy Wonka Candy Factory: DINASOUR EGGS®, Everlasting GOBSTOPPER®, FRECKLED EGGS®, Fruit RUNTS®, Heart Breakers®, NERDS®, Sweet N Sour Hearts®, TART n TINYS®, WACKY WAFER Bunnys®

U.S. Mills, Inc.: Apple Stroodles, Aztec, Banana-O's, Barley Plus, Erewhon, Galaxy Grahams

Yarnell's Ice Cream: GUILT FREE®, Yarnell's®

YZ Enterprises, Inc.: ALMONDINA®

Michael E. DeBakey, M.D., is a preeminent, internationally acclaimed medical educator and worldwide medical statesman. As a medical student, he devised a pump that became an essential component of the heart–lung machine, which made open-heart surgery possible. Among the first to complete successful heart transplantation in the United States, he has pioneered innumerable new diagnostic and successful therapeutic procedures for heart disease, including the first successful resection and graft replacement of an aneurysm of the thoracic aorta, first successful coronary artery bypass, first successful carotid endarterectomy, and first successful use of an artificial left ventricular assist device. Currently, he is Chancellor of Baylor College of Medicine, Distinguished Service Professor of its Department of Surgery, Director of The DeBakey Heart Center and Senior Attending Surgeon at The Methodist Hospital.

Antonio M. Gotto, Jr., M.D., D.Phil., is one of the world's most important specialists in research on fats in the blood and their role in the development of coronary heart disease. He serves as Principal Investigator of the Baylor College of Medicine Specialized Center of Research in Arteriosclerosis of the National Institutes of Health. Currently, he serves as Distinguished Service Professor and Chairman of the Department of Medicine at Baylor College of Medicine and Chief of the Internal Medicine Service at The Methodist Hospital, both of Houston, Texas. He is a past president of the American Heart Association and is currently President of The International Atherosclerosis Society.

Lynne W. Scott, M.A., R.D., is Assistant Professor in the Department of Medicine and Director of the Diet Modification Clinic at Baylor College of Medicine and The Methodist Hospital. She serves as a member of the National Cholesterol Education Program Expert Panel on Blood Cholesterol Levels in Children and Adolescents. She is a registered dietitian and clinical researcher investigating the effect of dietary components on blood cholesterol. She has 50 publications in the area of nutrition and serves on several nutrition committees of the national American Heart Association.

John P. Foreyt, Ph.D., is a clinical psychologist and Director of The DeBakey Heart Center's Nutrition Research Clinic at Baylor College of Medicine and The Methodist Hospital. Currently, he is Professor in the Department of Medicine at Baylor College of Medicine. He has published 13 books and more than 150 articles in the areas of behavior modification, cardiovascular risk reduction, obesity, and eating disorders.

Mary Carole McMann, M.P.H., R.D., is a registered dietitian and a nutrition counselor in the Diet Modification Clinic at Baylor College of Medicine and The Methodist Hospital. She is a contributing author for four books in the Living Heart series and is Associate Editor of *Panic in the Pantry* (1992). She has written numerous magazine, newsletter, and newspaper articles on health-related subjects.

Suzanne M. Jaax, M.S., R.D., is a registered dietitian in the Diet Modification Clinic at Baylor College of Medicine and The Methodist Hospital. She is involved in research on cholesterol, including the nutrition component of a study investigating regression on coronary atherosclerosis. She is also involved in a study investigating the effect of very low fat diets on skin cancer. She is a contributing author for four books in the Living Heart series.

To order additional copies of any MasterMedia book, send a check for the price of the book plus $2.00 postage and handling for the first book, $1.00 for each additional book to:

MasterMedia Limited
17 East 89th Street
New York, NY 10128
(212) 260-5600
(800) 334-8232 please use MasterCard or VISA on 1-800 orders
(212) 546-7638 (fax)

AGING PARENTS AND YOU: A Complete Handbook to Help You Help Your Elders Maintain a Healthy, Productive and Independent Life, by Eugenia Anderson-Ellis, is a complete guide to providing care to aging relatives. It gives practical advice and resources to adults who are helping their elders lead productive and independent lives. Revised and updated. ($9.95 paper)

BALANCING ACTS! Juggling Love, Work, Family, and Recreation, by Susan Schiffer Stautberg and Marcia L. Worthing, provides strategies to achieve a balanced life by reordering priorities and setting realistic goals. ($12.95 paper)

BEYOND SUCCESS: How Volunteer Service Can Help You Begin Making a Life Instead of Just a Living, by John F. Raynolds III and Eleanor Raynolds, C.B.E., is a unique how-to book targeted at business and professional people considering volunteer work, senior citizens who wish to fill leisure time meaningfully, and students trying out various career options. The book is filled with interviews with celebrities, CEOs, and average citizens who talk about the benefits of service work. ($19.95 cloth)

BOUNCING BACK: How to Turn Business Crises Into Success, by Harvey Reese. Based on interviews with entrepreneurs from coast to coast, this fascinating book contains cautionary tales that unfold with gripping suspense. Reese has discovered a formula for success that should be "must reading" for every new or budding entrepreneur. ($18.95 hardbound)

BREATHING SPACE: Living and Working at a Comfortable Pace in a Sped-Up Society, by Jeff Davidson, helps readers to handle information and activity overload and gain greater control over their lives. ($10.95 paper)

CITIES OF OPPORTUNITY: Finding the Best Place to Work, Live and Prosper in the 1990's and Beyond, by Dr. John Tepper Marlin, explores the job and living options for the next decade and into the next century. This consumer guide and handbook, written by one of the world's experts on cities, selects and features forty-six American cities and metropolitan areas. ($13.95 paper, $24.95 cloth)

THE CONFIDENCE FACTOR: How Self-Esteem Can Change Your Life, by Dr. Judith Briles, is based on a nationwide survey of six thousand men and women. Briles explores why women so often feel a lack of self-confidence and have a poor opinion of themselves. She offers step-by-step advice on becoming the person you want to be. ($9.95 paper, $18.95 cloth)

CRITICISM IN YOUR LIFE: How to Give It, How to Take It, How to Make It Work for You, by Dr. Deborah Bright, offers practical advice, in an upbeat, readable, and realistic fashion, for turning criticism into control. Charts and diagrams guide the reader into managing criticism from bosses, spouses, children, friends, neighbors, in-laws, and business relations. ($17.95 cloth)

DARE TO CHANGE YOUR JOB—AND YOUR LIFE, by Carole Kanchier, Ph.D., provides a look at career growth and development throughout the life cycle. ($9.95 paper)

THE DOLLARS AND SENSE OF DIVORCE, by Dr. Judith Briles, is the first book to combine practical tips on overcoming the legal hurdles by planning finances before, during, and after divorce. ($10.95 paper)

HERITAGE: The Making of an American Family, by Dr. Robert Pamplin, Jr., traces the phenomenal history of the Pamplin family from the Crusades to an eye-opening account of how they built one of the largest private fortunes in the United States. Heritage is an inspiring paradigm for achievement based on a strong belief in God and integrity. ($24.95, hardbound; $12.95 paperbound)

HOW TO GET WHAT YOU WANT FROM ALMOST ANYBODY, by T. Scott Gross, shows how to get great service, negotiate better prices, and always get what you pay for. ($9.95 paper)

LIFETIME EMPLOYABILITY: How to Become Indispensable, by Carole Hyatt, is both a guide through the mysteries of the business universe brought down to earth and a handbook to help you evaluate your attitudes, your skills, and your goals. Through expert advice and interviews of nearly 200 men and women whose lives have changed because their jobs or goals shifted, *Lifetime Employability* is designed to increase your staying power in today's down-sized economy. ($12.95 paper)

LEADING YOUR POSITIVELY OUTRAGEOUS SERVICE TEAM, by T. Scott Gross, provides a step-by-step formula for developing self-managing, excited service teams that put the customer first. T. Scott Gross tackles the question businesses everywhere are asking: "How do I get ordinary people to give world-class service?" A must-have for creating tomorrow's corporation today! ($12.95 paper)

THE LOYALTY FACTOR: Building Trust in Today's Workplace, by Carol Kinsey Goman, Ph.D., offers techniques for restoring commitment and loyalty in the workplace. ($9.95 paper)

MANAGING IT ALL: Time-Saving Ideas for Career, Family, Relationships, and Self, by Beverly Benz Treuille and Susan Schiffer Stautberg, is written for women who are juggling careers and families. Over two hundred career women (ranging from a TV anchorwoman to an investment banker) were interviewed. The book contains many humorous anecdotes on saving time and improving the quality of life for self and family. ($9.95 paper)

MANAGING YOUR CHILD'S DIABETES, by Robert Wood Johnson IV, Sale Johnson, Casey Johnson, and Susan Kleinman, brings help to families trying to understand diabetes and control its effects. ($10.95 paper)

MANN FOR ALL SEASONS: Wit and Wisdom from The Washington Post's *Judy Mann,* by Judy Mann, shows the columnist at her best as she writes about women, families, and the impact and politics of the women's revolution. ($9.95 paper, $19.95 cloth)

OUT THE ORGANIZATION: New Career Opportunities for the 1990's, by Robert and Madeleine Swain, is written for the millions of Americans whose jobs are no longer safe, whose companies are not loyal, and who face futures of uncertainty. it gives advice on finding a new job or starting your own business. ($12.95 paper)

POSITIVELY OUTRAGEOUS SERVICE: New and Easy Ways to Win Customers for Life, by T. Scott Gross, identifies what the consumers of the nineties really want and how businesses can develop effective marketing strategies to answer those needs. ($14.95 paper)

POSITIVELY OUTRAGEOUS SERVICE AND SHOWMANSHIP: Industrial Strength Fun Makes Sales Sizzle!!!!, by T. Scott Gross, reveals the secrets of adding personality to any product or service. ($12.95 paper)

THE PREGNANCY AND MOTHERHOOD DIARY: Planning the First Year of Your Second Career, by Susan Schiffer Stautberg, is the first and only undated appointment diary that shows how to manage pregnancy and career. ($12.95 spiralbound)

PRELUDE TO SURRENDER: The Pamplin Family and the Siege of Petersburg, by Dr. Robert Pamplin, Jr., offers an exciting and moving narrative, interspersed with facts, of the American Civil War and the ten-month siege and battles of Petersburg, Virginia, as seen through the eyes of Dr. Pamplin's ancestors, the Boisseau family. ($10.95 hardbound)

REAL LIFE 101: The Graduate's Guide to Survival, by Susan Kleinman, supplies welcome advice to those facing "real life" for the first time, focusing on work, money, health, and how to deal with freedom and responsibility. ($9.95 paper)

A SEAT AT THE TABLE: An Insider's Guide for America's New Women Leaders, by Patricia Harrison, provides practical and insightful advice for women who are interested in serving on a board of directors, playing a key role in politics and becoming a policy- or opinion-maker in public or private sectors. This is one book every woman needs to own. ($19.95 hardbound)

SIDE-BY-SIDE STRATEGIES: How Two-Career Couples Can Thrive in the Nineties, by Jane Hershey Cuozzo and S. Diane Graham, describes how two-career couples can learn the difference between competing with a spouse and becoming a supportive power partner. Published in hardcover as *Power Partners.* ($10.95 paper, $19.95 cloth)

STEP FORWARD: Sexual Harassment in the Workplace, What You Need to Know, by Susan L. Webb, presents the facts for identifying the tell-tale signs of sexual harassment on the job, and how to deal with it. ($9.95 paper)

TAKING CONTROL OF YOUR LIFE: The Secrets of Successful Enterprising Women, by Gail Blanke and Kathleen Walas, is based on the authors' professional experience with Avon Products' Women of Enterprise Awards, given each year to outstanding women entrepreneurs. The authors offer a specific plan to help women gain control over their lives, and include business tips and quizzes as well as beauty and lifestyle information. ($17.95 cloth)

TEAMBUILT: Making Teamwork Work, by Mark Sanborn, teaches business how to improve productivity, without increasing resources or expenses, by building teamwork among employers. ($19.95 cloth)

A TEEN'S GUIDE TO BUSINESS: The Secrets to a Successful Enterprise, by Linda Menzies, Oren S. Jenkins, and Rickell R. Fisher, provides solid information about starting your own business or working for one. ($7.95 paper)

TWENTYSOMETHING: Managing and Motivating Today's New Work Force, by Lawrence J. Bradford, Ph.D., and Claire Raines, M.A., examines the work orientation of the younger generation, offering managers in businesses of all kinds a practical guide to better understand and supervise their young employees. ($22.95 cloth)

WORK WITH ME: How to Make the Most of Office Support Staff, by Betsy Zazary, shows you how to find, train, and nurture the "perfect" assistant and how to best utilize your support staff professionals. ($9.95 paper)

YOUR HEALTHY BODY, YOUR HEALTHY LIFE: How to Take Control of Your Medical Destiny, by Donald B. Louria, M.D., provides precise advice and strategies that will help you to live a long and healthy life. Learn also about nutrition, exercise, vitamins, and medication, as well as how to control risk factors for major diseases. Revised and updated. ($12.95 paper)

ORDER FORM — BOOKS IN THE LIVING HEART SERIES

The Living Heart Guide to Eating Out is a guide to heart-healthy eating away from home. It includes 160 tips on selecting foods lower in fat and sodium in American and ethnic restaurants, as well as fast-food establishments. The book lists the amounts of calories, fat, saturated fat, and cholesterol in 1,630 restaurant foods. It is a convenient pocket size.

*The **New** Living Heart Diet* provides information on the role of diet in losing weight, preventing and treating high blood cholesterol and triglyceride, decreasing high blood pressure, and managing diabetes. The book also has chapters on vegetarian eating and vitamins and minerals. It includes 311 recipes, 72 menus, and nutrient analysis for 1,000 foods.

*The **New** Living Heart* uses easily understood terms to describe how the heart works, how it can fail, and what interventions are available for prevention and treatment of heart disorders. A number of cardiac tests are described, along with how to prepare for them and what to expect. Available October 1996.

Print Name _____

Address_____

_____

City_____State _____Zip _____

Please send the book(s) indicated below:

_____ copy(s) of *The Living Heart Brand Name Shopper's Guide,* Third Edition, at $14.95 each   = $ _____

_____ copy(s) of *The Living Heart Guide to Eating Out* at $9.95 each   = $ _____

_____ copy(s) of *The **New** Living Heart Diet* at $16.00 each   = $ _____

_____ copy(s) of *The **New** Living Heart* (Call for price)   = $ _____

Add $2.00 for postage and handling for the first book and $1.50 for each additional book $ _____

Total Enclosed $ _____

Make payment by check or money order payable to Diet Modification Clinic. (We cannot accept credit cards.)

Please return to:

Diet Modification Clinic   Phone (713) 798-4150
6565 Fannin, F770
Houston, TX 77030-2707